QUESTIONS AND UNCERTAINTIES
ABOUT PROSTATE CANCER

Questions and Uncertainties about Prostate Cancer

EDITED BY

W.B. Peeling
MA, MB, BChir, FRCS
Professor and Consultant Urological Surgeon
Royal Gwent Hospital, Newport, Gwent

FOREWORD BY
J.P. Blandy

Blackwell
Science

© 1996 by
Blackwell Science Ltd
Editorial Offices:
Osney Mead, Oxford OX2 0EL
25 John Street, London WC1N 2BL
23 Ainslie Place, Edinburgh EH3 6AJ
238 Main Street, Cambridge
  Massachusetts 02142, USA
54 University Street, Carlton
  Victoria 3053, Australia

Other Editorial Offices:
Arnette Blackwell SA
  1, rue de Lille, 75007 Paris
France

Blackwell Wissenschafts-Verlag GmbH
  Kurfürstendamm 57
  10707 Berlin, Germany

  Zehetnergasse 6
  A-1140 Wien
  Austria

First published 1996

Set by DP Photosetting, Aylesbury, Bucks
Printed and bound in Great Britain
by Hartnolls Ltd, Bodmin, Cornwall

DISTRIBUTORS

Marston Book Services Ltd
PO Box 87
Oxford OX2 0DT
(*Orders:* Tel: 01865 791155
          Fax: 01865 791927
          Telex: 837515)

North America
Blackwell Science, Inc.
238 Main Street
Cambridge, MA 02142
(*Orders:* Tel: 800 215-1000
          617 876-7000
          Fax: 617 492-5263)

Australia
Blackwell Science Pty Ltd
54 University Street
Carlton, Victoria 3053
(*Orders:* Tel: 03 9347 0300
          Fax: 03 9349 3016)

A catalogue record for this title
is available from the British Library

ISBN 0-86542-965-0

Library of Congress
Cataloging-in-Publication Data

Questions and uncertainties in prostate cancer/
  edited by W. B. Peeling.
      p. cm.
  Includes bibliographical references and
  index.
  ISBN 0-86542-965-0
  1. Prostate–Cancer.   I. Peeling, W. B.
RC280.P7Q47   1996
616.99′463–dc20   95-39904
                                       CIP

Contents

Contents

List of Contributors

Damien M. Bolton FRACS FRCS, *Senior Associate, University of Melbourne, Department of Surgery, St Vincent's Hospital, Fitzroy, Victoria 3065, Melbourne, Australia*

David G. Bostwick MD, *Consultant in Pathology and Professor of Pathology, Department of Pathology and Laboratory Medicine, Mayo Clinic and Mayo Medical School, Rochester, Minnesota 55905, USA*

Winsor G. Bowsher FRCS, *Consultant Urological Surgeon, Department of Urology, Glan Hafren NHS Trust, Royal Gwent Hospital, Cardiff Road, Newport, Gwent, NP9 2UB, UK*

Peter Boyle PhD, *Director, Division of Epidemiology and Biostatistics, European Institute of Oncology, via Ripamonti 435, 20141 Milan, Italy*

Michael K. Brawer MD, *Professor, Department of Urology, University of Washington and Chief, Section of Urology, Seattle VA Medical Center, Washington, USA*

Charles B. Brendler MD, *Professor and Chairman, Department of Surgery, Section of Urology, University of Chicago, MC 6038, South Maryland Avenue, Chicago, Illinois 60637, USA*

Ruth L. Byrne MBBS FRCS, *University Department of Surgery, Medical School, Framlington Place, Newcastle upon Tyne, NE2 4HH, UK*

Fernando Calais da Silva, *Consultant Urologist, Department of Urology, Hospital do Desterro, Avenue Elias Garcia, 81–60, Lisbon 1050, Portugal*

Michael P. Chetner MD MSc FRCS(C), *Chief, Division of Urology, Department of Surgery, University of Alberta, Caritas Hospitals, Edmonton, Alberta, Canada*

Richard Clements MA BM BCh FRCS FRCR, *Consultant Radiologist, Glan Hafren NHS Trust, Royal Gwent Hospital, Cardiff Road, Newport, Gwent, NP9 2UB, UK*

Louis Denis MD, *Department of Urology, Vrije Universiteit Brussel, AZ Middelheim, Antwerp, Belgium*

List of Contributors

Jonathan I. Epstein MD, *Department of Pathology, The Johns Hopkins Medical Institutions, Baltimore, Maryland 21287, USA*

Sophie D. Fosså MD, *Department of Medical Oncology and Radiotherapy, The Norwegian Radium Hospital, Montebello 0310, Oslo, Norway*

Peder H. Graverson MD, *Senior Registrar, Department of Urology, D-2112, Rigshospitalet, University of Copenhagen, Blegdamsvej 9, DK- 2100 Copenhagen Ø, Denmark*

Fouad K. Habib Phd DSc CChem FRSC, *Reader in Biochemistry, Department of Surgery/Urology, University of Edinburgh, Western General Hospital, Crewe Road South, Edinburgh, EH4 2XU, UK*

Maha Hussain MD FACP, *Assistant Professor, Division of Hematology/Oncology, Department of Medicine, Wayne State University, Detroit, Michigan, USA*

Peter Iversen MD, *Associate Professor of Urology, Department of Urology, D-2112 Rigshospitalet, University of Copenhagen, Blegdamsvej 9, DK-2100 Copenhagen Ø, Denmark*

David A. Levy MD, *Chief Resident Urologist, Department of Urology, Case Western Reserve University School of Medicine, University Hospitals of Cleveland, 2074 Abington Road, Cleveland, Ohio 44106, USA*

Patrick Maisonneuve ING, *Division of Epidemiology and Biostatistics, European Institute of Oncology, via Ripamonti 435, 20141 Milan, Italy*

Pavel Napalkov MD, *Division of Epidemiology and Biostatistics, European Institute of Oncology, via Ripamonti 435, 20141 Milan, Italy*

David E. Neal MS FRCS, *University Department of Surgery, Medical School, Framlington Place, Newcastle upon Tyne, NE2 4HH, UK*

Donald W.W. Newling, *Department of Urology, Free University Hospital (AZVU), De Boelelaan 1117, Post Bus 7057, 107 MB, Amsterdam, The Netherlands*

W. Brian Peeling, *Professor and Consultant Urological Surgeon, Glan Hafren NHS Trust, Royal Gwent Hospital, Cardiff Road, Newport, Gwent, NP9 2UB, UK*

Justin Peters FRACS, *Consultant Urological Surgeon, Department of Urology, St Vincent's Hospital, Fitzroy, Victoria 3065, Melbourne, Australia*

Martin I. Resnick MD, *Lester Persky Professor of Urology and Chairman, Department of Urology, Case Western Reserve University School of Medicine, University Hospitals of Cleveland, 2074 Abington Road, Cleveland, Ohio 44106, USA*

Carrie W. Rinker-Schaeffer PhD, *Department of Surgery, Section of Urology, University of Chicago, MC 6038 South Maryland Avenue, Chicago, Illinois 60637, USA*

Robert J. Shearer FRCS, *Consultant Urological Surgeon, Department of Urology, Royal Marsden Hospital, Fulham Road, London, SW3 6JJ, UK*

Philip H. Smith FRCS, *Department of Urology, St James' University Hospital, Beckett Street, Leeds, LS9 7TF, UK*

Gary D. Steinberg MD, *Department of Surgery, Section of Urology, University of Chicago, MC 6038 South Maryland Avenue, Chicago, Illinois 60637, USA*

Foreword

More than any other malignancy, cancer of the prostate is set about with questions and uncertainties – even basic matters such as definition, incidence and treatment turn out to bristle with controversy – to say nothing of the matter of screening. Alarmists point to the rising number of new cases found every year (in the West) but usually fail to add that even in these affluent countries, cancer of the prostate causes death in only three per thousand in each age cohort – or that this minute proportion has remained steady. Is the apparent increase in incidence real? Should it cause alarm: or is it perhaps an artifact due to the advent of prostatic-specific antigen and transrectal ultrasound?

What do we mean by prostate cancer? Do we mean the little foci of cancer present in the prostate of almost every grandfather? If they only kill 0.3% clearly some 99.7% of them must be harmless. True, they cannot all be. How can we detect the tiny fraction that is going to prove lethal? Is there a certain critical mass or a certain tumour pattern which will signify the threat of invasion and metastasis? May we at last trust more sophisticated indices of malignancy, e.g. a specific oncogene?

What of treatment? How can radical surgery be justified for so-called organ-confined cancer when tumour is so often present at the margin of the specimen, and when molecular biology suggests that cancer cells are already in the bloodstream? Perhaps they do not matter. Perhaps micrometastases do not signify either. What a muddle: if we cannot tell which cancer is going to be dangerous some believe we should treat them all, others consider we should treat none. What are the arguments for and against – and what treatment have we in mind?

Of all methods of treatment radical prostatectomy offers the classical clean answer so attractive to the surgeon – cut it out root and branch. Radical surgery can give results that match the expected survival rate. So also can watchful waiting: indeed there is evidence that doing nothing may actually improve the quality of life for the majority of patients. If we do not really know that treatment does good, should we recommend it? Can we justify a programme of screening in order to offer a treatment whose efficacy is unknown? Can we tell the patient he has cancer, but is better off having nothing done about it? For the patient as for the surgeon it is always far easier to choose a decisive operation than to refrain. Is it right? These questions are not easy: they are thoroughly discussed in these pages.

We have known for half a century that most cancers of the prostate depend on a regular supply of androgens, and that orchidectomy or hormone therapy can make metastases miraculously disappear. But even after all these years there remain questions unanswered: is total androgen blockade really any better than a single agent such as orchidectomy or luteinizing hormone releasing hormone agonist? Is there any advantage in treating metastases with either, if there are no symptoms? Need hormone therapy be given continuously, or is it perhaps even better to give it intermittently, as with antimicrobials?

The anxious patient in the consulting room expects and deserves advice based on sound knowledge of the pros and cons of each argument. Where there is uncertainty there is all the more need for the urologist to be master of the facts: these reviews tackle the issues head on, clearly point out the difficulties and dilemmas and deal in depth with both sides of each question. They do not, and cannot be expected to, provide easy answers to such difficult questions, but they should leave the urologist better informed and in a far better position to offer wise counsel.

John P. Blandy

Preface

Prostate cancer has yet to reveal many secrets. Consequently, urologists and others who treat men with this disease are faced with many questions and uncertainties about its behaviour and the best management for their patients. It is no surprise, therefore, that there is much debate and often considerable disagreement about many major points in the spectrum of this disease. In this book, which is not intended to be a textbook about prostate cancer, I have selected 20 such topics for discussion which reflect, in my view, the most important features about prostate cancer that need to be aired at the moment. Undoubtedly, not everyone will agree with the selection but I would expect few to disagree that, while it is recognized that prostate cancer is a major threat to public health, we do not understand its aetiology, there is limited information about its natural history, there is even less knowledge about the biology of metastatic disease, and at the moment there is no way of differentiating aggressive cancers from indolent tumours. With clinical issues, detection and assessment of prostate cancer needs more precision and there is debate about the best treatment not only for early disease but also for advanced prostate cancer. Some progress has been made in predicting clinical response although treatment of hormone-relapsed patients is still a matter of palliation till the inevitable end comes.

However, I make no apology for including two final chapters about the thorny problem of screening for prostate cancer, for this is probably the most burning issue to face urologists and health planners nowadays. Debate about this can often stir emotions of many otherwise mild-mannered people who will engage in hotly disputed dialogue that sometimes adheres to fact. There is also pressure for screening from members of the general public who are being informed, largely from media sources, that prostate cancer is now equal to lung cancer as a cause of male deaths from malignancy, so they want to know what urologists and others are doing about it.

As with most multi-author books, some overlap of material cannot be avoided, such as with prostate-specific antigen and transrectal ultrasound but these have usually interlocked to give useful views from several perspectives. Some of the authors are younger urologists or scientists on whom will fall the responsibility of following the trail for the next 15 to 20 years for that is the time scale involved with study of early prostate cancer which surely is the area of priority with this disease. I am, therefore, extremely grateful to all the authors who have contributed to this book for their time, knowledge and patience. Their contributions are witness to the vast efforts being made worldwide to understand the enigmas of prostate cancer and to refine methods of detection and treatment so that reduced morbidity and mortality from prostate cancer can be achieved as an ultimate goal.

Brian Peeling
Royal Gwent Hospital

Part 1
Biological and Scientific Aspects

1 / Prostate Cancer: The Threat to Health and Strategies for Control

P. Boyle, P. Maisonneuve and P. Napalkov

Introduction

Prostate cancer is an important public health problem with over a quarter of a million new cases diagnosed worldwide in the single year 1985 [1]. It was predicted that in the USA alone 38 000 men would die of prostate cancer in 1994 [2], while in the countries of the European Community (EC) it accounts for more than 35 000 deaths each year [3].

The incidence of the disease is increasing rapidly in most regions of the world [4] and will pass a half-a-million cases worldwide by the end of this century if the risk remains fixed at 1980 levels or could reach 700 000 or more if the observed trends in increase continue [5]. Whereas there are large increases in the incidence of prostate cancer apparent throughout the world, the mortality rate has remained constant in generations of men born since the early years of this century [6].

Prostate cancer exhibits large ethnic and international differences, being particularly common in Afro-Americans, among whom it is second rank after lung cancer. Different populations around the world experience different levels of prostate cancer with an international variation in incidence around two orders of magnitude [7]. However, when migration takes place groups of migrants tend to acquire the prostate cancer pattern of their new home [8]. Furthermore, groups within a community whose lifestyle habits differentiate themselves from other members of the same community generally have notably different prostate cancer rates, e.g. Seventh Day Adventists and Mormons [9].

For reasons such as these it is widely accepted that the risk of prostate cancer has environmental determinants, defining environment in its broadest sense to include a wide range of lifestyle factors including dietary, social and cultural practices. Although these are theoretically avoidable, for prostate cancer only a few avoidable causes have been clearly identified, although a large number of factors have been investigated. Within our current knowledge, only a small proportion of prostate cancer is avoidable.

Public health importance of prostate cancer: to the year 2000

In many countries of the world, prostate cancer is the second most common form of cancer in men [5]. It was estimated that there were 6 million cases of cancer diagnosed worldwide in 1980, of which 235 000 were cancer of the prostate, which may be compared with over half-a-million of each of stomach, lung, breast and large bowel and nearly 300 000 cancers of the oesophagus [10].

The incidence of prostate cancer is increasing steadily in many countries around the world. The highest increase in incidence rates is reported from the Afro-American population in the USA with an overall increase taking place in most western countries. Although the incidence of prostate cancer is remarkably lower in the developing world, the increase is also quite substantial [6].

In the 12 member states of the EC, it is estimated that in 1980 there were 85 000 new cases of prostate cancer, making this the second commonest form of cancer (after lung cancer) in men [3]. In the USA prostate cancer has overtaken lung cancer in terms of absolute incidence, although it remains second to lung cancer as a cause of cancer death. Most importantly, given that in several countries the increased number of children born after the Second World War will be in their mid 50s in the early part of the 20th century (at an age when cancer risk is becoming an important consideration) and coupled with the trends in increasing life expectancy (see Brody [11], for example), the consequences will be an increase in absolute terms in the number of cases of prostate cancer diagnosed [5]. In the absence of treatment improvements and with the prospects for prevention by modification of lifestyle remote within current knowledge, there will also be an increase in the number of deaths from prostate cancer worldwide. The situation would be further augmented by the presence of a temporal trend in risk which is widely reported from many countries and unlikely to be entirely artefact [5].

The numbers of cases of prostate cancer in the year 2000 and beyond are set to increase. For a disease which currently presents a near 10% lifetime risk in North Americans, the knowledge of risk factors is extremely limited and, consequently, the prospects for primary prevention are poor. The rise in the number of cases of prostate cancer requiring treatment will have important implications for the provision of treatment facilities, including the training and supply of specialists competent to treat these patients. If it stopped here it would merely reflect an economic challenge but, unfortunately, increased numbers of cases will bring with it increased numbers of deaths from the disease. The prospects for preventing the situation building up for the year

2000 are poor and work in hand today needs to progress to help limit the impact of the continuing expansion in absolute numbers of cases set to take place throughout the early decades of the next century. For this reason, prostate cancer is of great importance in public health, and a major effort is required to reduce the impact of these unavoidable increases.

Temporal trends in prostate cancer incidence and mortality

The entity *prostate cancer* is not easy to interpret. Prostate cancer is composed of three distinct components: (i) *clinical prostate cancer*, which are symptomatic cases in which a clinical diagnosis is possible; (ii) *occult prostate cancer*, where the primary lesion remains small or hidden but which produces clinically overt metastases; and (iii) *latent prostate cancer*, which is clinically unrecognizable through signs and symptoms and is generally an unexpected (or incidental) finding at transurethral resection of the prostate (TURP) for benign prostatic hyperplasia (BPH), or is screen-detected in asymptomatic patients. The rubric prostate cancer which is recorded at a cancer registry is a combination of each of these three entities.

Trends in incidence

Higher rates in black men than in white men, increases in overall trends in incidence and mortality rates and large geographical variations in occurrence are distinctive and recognized features of the descriptive epidemiology of prostate cancer [9].

The leading 23 rates of prostate cancer are reported from North America and the black population of Bermuda. The highest rates of prostate cancer have been recorded in the black population of the USA and are now over 100 per 100 000: the lowest incidence rates (Asia and northern Africa) are around 1, indicating a 100-fold difference in the incidence of prostate cancer worldwide (Table 1.1). In the USA incidence rates of prostate cancer are higher in Afro-Americans than in Caucasians. The relative risk for prostate cancer in Afro-Americans is generally reported to be around a factor of 1.7 when compared to Caucasians (Table 1.2).

In contrast to the distribution pattern of overt prostatic cancers, the frequency of the smaller non-invasive lesions denoted latent carcinoma does not appear to show much international variation [12]. This observation itself presents further difficulties in interpreting the international prostate cancer incidence pattern. The lifetime cumulative risk of prostate cancer (up until age 75) approaches 10% in some population groups at the present time, compared

Table 1.1 Highest and lowest recorded incidence rates of prostate cancer in the mid 1980s (prostate, male, ICD9 185).

Registry	Cases	Rate
USA, Atlanta: Black	832	102
USA, Bay Area: Black	944	95.6
USA, Detroit: Black	2210	94.2
USA, Alameda: Black	497	93.5
USA, Los Angeles: Black	1734	82.7
USA, Seattle	7712	82.4
USA, Utah	3019	77.9
USA, New Orleans: Black	582	72.9
USA, Connecticut: Black	296	65
Bermuda: Black	45	64
Kuwait: Kuwaitis	27	4.4
India: Ahmadabad	143	4.1
Thailand, Chiang Mai	59	4
Thailand, Khon Kaen	19	2.7
India, Madras	100	2.1
Algeria, Setif	21	2
China, Beijing	323	1.7
Gambia	6	1.2
China, Tianjin	84	1.2
China, Qidong	20	0.8

Data abstracted from *Cancer Incidence in Five Continents*, vol. VI, IARC, Lyon. The time period covered: around 1983–1988 [1].

Table 1.2 Prostate cancer incidence rates (IR: per 100 000) in blacks (Afro-Americans*) and whites (Caucasians†), and relative risk (RR) for prostate cancer in blacks when compared to whites (1983–1988).

Cancer registry	IR in blacks*	IR in whites†	RR
Bermuda	64.04	22.91	2.8
USA, Georgia, Atlanta	101.96	59.69	1.7
USA, California, Alameda County	93.47	55.24	1.7
USA, California, San Francisco Bay Area	95.6	57.8	1.7
USA, California, Los Angeles County	82.67	51.89	1.6
USA, Michigan, Detroit	94.15	61.63	1.5
USA, Connecticut	65	47.22	1.4
USA, Louisiana, New Orleans	72.85	53.94	1.4
USA, SEER	81.97	61.79	1.3

Data abstracted from *Cancer Incidence in Five Continents*, vol. VI, IARC, Lyon. The time period covered: around 1983–1988 [1].
* Afro-Americans for all the quoted registries, except Bermuda (where not specified).
† Caucasians for all the quoted regions, except Bermuda (where whites and other).
SEER, surveillance, epidemiology and end results.

to the 40% incidence of latent prostate carcinoma found in men over the age of 80 years [13, 14]. This makes prostate cancer a unique malignancy with a very high prevalence of histologically identified tumours and relatively low clinical manifestation. Adenocarcinoma of the prostate, whilst exhibiting the histological signs of malignancy, may never have been life-threatening nor cause any clinical symptom in the lifetime of the individual. Obviously any medical procedures or tests which can detect such prostate cancers will have the effect of increasing reported incidence in the absence of any real increase in underlying risk [15, 16]. TURP for BPH is normally accompanied by histological examination of all fragments removed and in 8–22% of all TURPs an incidental diagnosis of prostate cancer is made [14, 17]. Again, it is obvious that the increases in TURP rates since the 1970s will have led to corresponding increases in prostate cancer cases reported to the Cancer Registry: in fact, in Scotland, this phenomenon appears to account for all the increases seen in the reported incidence rate of prostate cancer between 1977 and 1988 [4].

Japanese migrants to the USA have experienced a marked increase in prostatic cancer, although the rates of the Japanese in the San Francisco Bay Area and in Los Angeles are still less than half of those of whites. Contrasts between US Chinese and those elsewhere are even greater. In Singapore, the risk in foreign-born Chinese was 70% of that in the Singapore-born from 1968 to 1982. Polish migrants to the USA also acquired higher mortality rates on migration [18], again emphasizing the influence of environmental factors on the risk of this form of cancer. Recent studies suggest that several weak oestrogenic components present in the predominantly vegetarian diet in Asian countries may play a protective role in the development of latent adenocarcinoma to clinical prostate cancer [19].

Prostate cancer incidence data are presently available from over 160 cancer registries throughout the world [1]. However, a few of them have long temporal series available covering uninterrupted time spans. Table 1.3 presents data covering over 25 years regarding prostate cancer incidence in selected cancer registries internationally. It is clear that there has been an increasing incidence of prostate cancer throughout the time period. Overall in Europe [20], the incidence is increasing in the Nordic countries and Switzerland at between 5 and 10% every 5 years. In Hungary (Szabolcs and Vas), Spain (Navarra) and Italy (Varese) the incidence rates are lower but the rate of increase observed is greater, being over 20% every 5 years. The rate of increase is slightly less in France (Bas-Rhin) and the UK. The exception to this general increase is the significant and steady decline in Warsaw City (Poland), which is interesting, but may reflect a local departure from the national pattern in Poland where mortality is still increasing [20]. Taken together, the data from

Chapter 1

Table 1.3 Evolution of prostate cancer incidence (selected cancer registries, 1960–1988).

Cancer registry	Volume 1	Volume 2	Volume 3	Volume 4	Volume 5	Volume 6
USA, Alameda: Black	*	65.26	75.02	100.2	87.85	93.47
USA, Alameda: White	*	38.03	40.38	44.46	49.56	55.24
USA, Connecticut	33.84	33.03	37.73	42.66	*	*
Canada, Manitoba	30.59	31.06	37.62	43.22	44.36	54.71
Norway	25.04	29.8	33.07	38.89	42.04	43.83
UK, Birmingham	17.3	18.39	17.7	18.57	18.9	24.97
India, Bombay	*	6.54	7.97	6.85	8.2	6.9
Japan, Miyagi	3.83	3.23	2.74	4.88	*	*

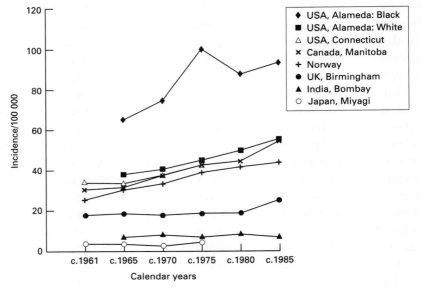

Data abstracted from *Cancer Incidence in Five Continents*, vols I–VI, IARC, Lyon.
The time periods covered are: volume 1 (around 1960–1963), volume 2 (around 1963–1966), volume 3 (around 1968–1972), volume 4 (around 1973–1977), volume 5 (around 1978–1982) and volume 6 (around 1983–1988) [1].
* No data available for this period.

southern Europe suggest that prostate cancer is increasing more rapidly than elsewhere in Europe at more than 25% every 5 years.

In North America, there have also been considerable increases in the age-standardized incidence rate of prostate cancer. In Connecticut, generally considered the gold standard of United States cancer registries, the incidence rate has increased from 33.8 per 100 000 person-years) to 47.2 over the 25-year period (Table 1.3). Large increases have taken place in other United

States registries and they are also apparent in Canada. Overall, the increases in North American populations are substantial being in the order of 15–25% every 5 years [20]. The incidence is generally rising more rapidly in Afro-American men than among Caucasian men [20]. Such are the underlying trends in the risk of prostate cancer that the lifetime risk of an Afro-American born around 1915 is 10% whereas the lifetime risk of an Afro-American born around 1940 appears to be closer to 15%.

Outside these developed countries with western cultures there have also been increases taking place. In Japan the overall incidence rate increased in Miyagi and Osaka prefectures and there were increases in Singapore also, although the rates remain less than one-tenth those found in the USA. There was no increase in non-Maoris in New Zealand and in the population of Bombay in India (Table 1.3). In Beijing (People's Republic of China) the incidence rate is low and unchanging and while the rates in Chinese in Hong Kong and Singapore are approximately four times higher, the increases are small – of the order of 6% every 5 years [20].

Interpretation of these increases in incidence is not entirely straightforward. As discussed earlier, the entity recorded at a cancer registry (prostate cancer) is the combination of three separate forms. Between registries, and within each registry as time advances, changes may take place in the incidence of prostate cancer recorded due to the influences of changes in either of the component entities. Thus, if there is a large increase in latent prostate cancer due to an increased rate of TURP or widespread use of prostate-specific antigen (PSA) test, this will influence the registration of prostate cancer and, hence, the overall incidence rate of prostate cancer recorded. Unfortunately, the data required to simplify the interpretation of such changes are not available from the registries.

Another way to assess the magnitude of the problem of prostate cancer is by considering the cumulative lifetime (up to age 75) risk. Based on 1985 incidence and mortality rates remaining unchanged throughout their lifetime, white men in the USA have an 8.7% lifetime risk of developing prostate cancer and Afro-American men a lifetime risk of 9.4%. With regard to mortality from prostate cancer, the lifetime risks among whites and Afro-Americans in the USA are currently 2.6% and 4.3% respectively.

Another feature of prostate cancer is the association between incidence (and mortality) rates and age, which is more striking than that for most other cancers. From an incidence rate of the order of 1–2 per 100 000 per annum in the 40s, the incidence rises dramatically to peak at 1200 per 100 000 in white men and 1600 per 100 000 in Afro-American men in their 80s.

This association with age has enormous consequences for the future.

Assuming that age-specific incidence rates remain fixed at 1980 levels, the number of cases of prostate cancer in men aged over 65 in the EC will rise through 80 000 in 1990 to 92 000 in the year 2000. This increase in numbers of cases will be seen in every one of the 12 member states, being most pronounced in France, Germany and Spain [5]. Since in these countries life expectancy is increasing – boys born now can expect to live to 80 years of age [11] – more and more men, living to older age, will result in increases in the absolute number of cases of prostate cancer diagnosed, even if the risk to an individual man remains fixed at 1980 levels. This increase is programmed to continue into the 21st century and to be exacerbated in many countries since those born in the post Second World War 'baby boomers' will be in their early 50s in the year 2000 and as they age will give rise to increasing numbers of cancers. This is the first group of men expected to go through life without the twin hazards of high infant mortality rates and a devastating war.

Looking around the world, the age-adjusted incidence of prostate cancer is increasing at an average annual rate of around 3% per annum. Some of this increase is undoubtedly associated with diagnostic artefact but the combined effect of this increase on incidence and the changing age structure of the population will be more pronounced for prostate cancer than for any other site in most populations of the world. Again, assuming that the age-specific rates throughout the world remain fixed at their 1980 levels, the numbers of prostate cancers diagnosed throughout the world will increase from 235 000 in 1980 to 352 000 in 2000 if ageing is the only contribution considered. If, however, the temporal trend of increases in age-specific rate continues, the result will be to increase the total burden to 492 000 new cases in the year 2000. It is clear that, even although the incidence rate may increase noticeably, the ageing population will be the strongest determinant of the international prostate cancer burden in coming years.

Trends in mortality

In view of the problems with latent carcinoma of the prostate varying between countries for a variety of reasons, compounded recently by the increasing use of TURP as a treatment for BPH, which is associated with a 16% yield of unexpected focal carcinoma upon microscopical inspection, and the increasing use of the PSA test for prostate cancer [21], examination of mortality data may give a clearer picture of changes in life-threatening prostate cancer through time, particularly since there has been little change in survival after treatment.

There are two interesting features to trends in mortality from prostate cancer. First, the overall age-adjusted mortality rate is higher than the truncated rates (calculated on ages 35–64) and, second, the overall age-adjusted mortality rate increases much faster than the truncated rates if both are increasing.

In an attempt to investigate the nature of any changes in risk pattern for prostate cancer and to quantify any effect found, all available data in the World Health Organization (WHO) mortality database were employed in an age–period cohort analysis of the changes in rates employing the method of DeCarli and La Vecchia [22]. In analysing and interpreting temporal changes in prostate cancer rates it is necessary to have mortality data available for a sufficiently long period of time and to be based upon large enough numbers of prostate cancer deaths to result in reasonably stable rates. Of more than 100 countries included in the WHO mortality database, 24 met the above criteria and have been included in the analysis of prostate cancer mortality rates [6].

For each country, data have been analysed for 10, 5-year age groups from 35–39 to 80–84 years and for between six and eight 5-year time periods. Correspondingly, there are between 15 (1880–1950) and 17 (1870–1950) birth cohorts. For the first and last time periods where data are not available for the whole of the 5-year period, rates have been based on years for which data are available. Results for time periods are expressed as relative risks, relative to the first available 5-year time period and for cohorts as risks relative to the birth cohort born during a period centred on 1915: this was chosen as the earliest cohort which had data available in all the time periods considered. Cohort effects have been calculated for birth cohorts until 1940, since estimates for later cohorts are based on, at most, two observations.

The findings from statistical modelling indicate a clear pattern. First of all, the relative risks found in birth cohorts (relative to the 1910 cohort) are small. There is a clear pattern of increasing risk in cohorts until those born around 1910. Subsequently in most countries the relative risk has either increased slowly or has remained fairly constant. In Scotland, England and Wales, Northern Ireland and the Irish Republic (Eire), there have been steady increases in risk among birth cohorts until those born approximately 1900 and subsequent birth cohorts have experienced very little change in risk. There have been small and steady increases in risk in the grouping of central and eastern European countries (Austria, Hungary, Czechoslovakia and (the former Federal Republic of) Germany), which seem to have stabilized among cohorts born since approximately 1930. Similarly, there have been small increases in risk experienced in Italy, Spain, Portugal, the Netherlands and Switzerland which have also stabilized since around 1930. The patterns observed in the Nordic countries seem to be a little different with more noticeable increases in risk taking place among recent birth cohorts. Despite a

11

10-fold increase in risk between cohorts born around 1870 and 1910 in Japan, there has been a much smaller increase taking place in subsequent birth cohorts. There have been very little changes throughout the entire period of observation in cohort-specific prostate cancer risks in the populations of Australia, New Zealand, Canada and the USA [23].

Discussion of trends in incidence and mortality from prostate cancer

Increases in the incidence of prostate cancer have been reported recently from several geographic areas with the largest increases – around 30% between 1980 and 1988 – noted among Caucasian men in the USA and southern Europe [24].

It is felt that increasing surgical intervention for BPH, widespread use of the PSA test and needle biopsies, leading to a fortuitous finding of latent carcinoma, could contribute to such observed increases in incidence [15, 16]. The type of cancer found in such circumstances, generally T1a–c, is not commonly lethal and in many instances does not interfere with the normal lifespan [25]. Small latent prostate cancers are considered to have a lower potential for malignant behaviour [26]. Both 5- and 10-year survival rates for state T1a–c prostatic adenocarcinomas reported in many studies are around 75–87% [27, 28] and average local and/or distant progression rates rarely reported more than 10% [29]. This may explain the differences observed in the temporal trends in incidence and mortality from prostate cancer.

The problem of increasing diagnosis and incidence would be of greater importance if it were leading to increases in the mortality rate from this condition. In the USA there is surprisingly little correlation between incidence and mortality rates for prostate cancer in the SEER cancer registry regions [30] and a slightly negative correlation ($r = -0.17$) among those European countries with both incidence and mortality data available [4]. Furthermore, the artificial increases in incidence would help to obscure the real trend in risk being experienced. Thus, in these circumstances, trends in mortality may be a better indicator of changing prostate cancer risk than incidence. It is clear from examination of these data that there is no great change taking place in the mortality rate from this disease: the cohort-relative risks are all small (less than 1.5) when compared with those observed for other sites such as oral cancer where 10-fold risks were observed [31]. There appears to be little independent contribution from the time period, indicating that artefactual changes brought about by systematic changes in death registration practices are not contributing to the changing mortality pattern [6]. Similar observations have previously been made in Australia and in England and Wales [32].

It is reassuring that the large increases reported in incidence of prostate cancer do not appear to be confirmed by changes in mortality data. In fact, given the lack of improvement in outcome among men with T2 disease and above, it would seem that the risk of a man developing this (frequently fatal) form of the disease has not been increasing in most countries whose data have been available for examination. The increasing incidence appears to relate to forms of prostate cancer which are not fatal and it appears that this could be related to increases in the relative and absolute frequency of T1a–c disease probably related to increasing prostatectomy for BPH, increasingly aggressive histopathological examination of resected specimens and increasing use of PSA testing. It is important to identify the contribution of each of these individually since they have important consequences for future practice. In particular, if PSA testing is finding a large number of non-fatal adenocarcinomas, it could be of significance for prostate cancer screening programmes which are currently an important, although very contentious, issue [33].

Analytical epidemiology of prostate cancer

Hormones, sexual activity and marital status

The prostate is a primarily androgen-dependent gland controlled essentially by levels of plasma testosterone, of which 90–95% of the daily production is synthesized and secreted by the testes. Within the prostate cell, testosterone is converted into the active androgen dihydrotestosterone (DHT), which is essential for the growth and development of the prostate gland. Labrie *et al.* [34] demonstrated that 60% of intraprostatic DHT in human prostate originated from testicular testosterone with 40% from the adrenals after transformation of inactive adrenal precursors into active androgens. The precise role of oestrogens in the prostate remains unknown, although it was suggested that they can synergistically promote biological effects of androgens [19]. Current research has indicated an important role of several growth factors which have been derived from the prostate in the pathogenesis of prostate cancer [35, 36]. However, despite major increases in knowledge of our understanding of the endocrine and biochemical processes that regulate prostatic growth and function [36], there is currently no consistent evidence of any primary endocrine disturbance that is necessarily implicated in the aetiology of prostate cancer.

Sexual activity, which may be a reflection or an indirect measure of hormonal status, has been related to the occurrence of prostate cancer [37, 38] with a general observation that prostate cancer cases seem to have a greater

13

sexual drive than controls of the same age but at the same time appear to be less sexually active. It has also been reported that prostate cancer cases experience puberty at an earlier age than controls and experience first sexual intercourse at a later age [37]. Although the studies have not been entirely consistent, prostate cancer mortality rates appear to be associated with marital status, being higher in divorced and widowed men than in married and, especially, single men [39]. Among married men, the risk of prostatic cancer may be higher in those men with children than among those without children [40].

Interpretation of these pieces of information is not at all straightforward. These variables can only be proxies of some other potential exposure factor and their meaning may well have changed with time. For example, *marital status* had a different meaning as a synonym for sexual activity 30 years ago than today due to changes in society and its attitudes. For a variety of reasons, including these, the available information regarding these variables is difficult to interpret in any aetiological sense, but the most plausible inference is general support for a hormonal influence in the pathogenesis of prostate cancer. A link with sexually transmitted diseases has been proposed as an alternative explanation but appears unlikely [9].

Diet and nutritional practices

Until the very recent past, the nutritional epidemiology of prostatic cancer could be characterized as comprising a series of studies which have produced tantalizing results but have suffered from limitations in their design and methodology. In recent times, the focus has fallen on four aspects of this association.

Total caloric intake, fat intake and intake of meat

Hypotheses relating prostatic cancer risk to a high-fat diet are attractive on theoretical grounds (through the possible influence of fat on hormone metabolism in men [41]) and arose initially from observations on the international distribution of prostatic cancer mortality [42]. Several correlation studies have reported a positive correlation between prostatic cancer occurrence, generally mortality, and national per capita fat disappearance statistics as well as strong correlations between prostate cancer mortality rates and those of other forms of cancer suspected as being associated with a high fat intake such as breast and ovarian cancer [9].

The US Health Professionals Follow-up Study was used to examine this association among 47855 men aged 40–75 at recruitment and initially free from cancer, and who had been followed up for 4 years. This is one of the first studies to include the (methodologically essential) adjustment for total caloric intake. In these men a total of 300 prostate cancers were diagnosed, including 127 advanced cases. Total fat consumption was directly related to the risk of advanced cancer: the risk, after adjustment for age and total energy intake, in the highest fifth of the intake range compared to the lowest fifth was 1.79 (95% confidence interval (CI) 1.04, 3.07) with the test for linear trend just falling short of the usually accepted level of statistical significance (being $P = 0.06$). The association observed was due mainly to saturated fat (relative risk (RR) = 1.63) but was not found with vegetable fat. Among the food groups considered, red meat represented the group with the strongest association with prostate cancer risk (RR) in the highest fifth being 2.64 (95% CI 1.21, 5.77); (P value for linear trend = 0.02). Fat from fish or dairy products was unrelated to risk apart from a positive association with butter. Saturated fat, monounsaturated fat and α-linoleic acid were associated with advanced prostate cancer, although only the association with α-linoleic acid remained after simultaneous adjustment for saturated fat, monounsaturated fat and linoleic acid [43].

Further positive associations (without adjustment for total caloric intake) have been reported for animal fat in a prospective study of US Seventh Day Adventists [44] and, more recently, a random population-based study in Hawaii [45]. It is interesting that the relative risk estimates in the Hawaiian and US health professionals studies are very similar despite the differences in methodology and study population.

Discrepancies in the effects reported between case-control and cohort studies may be attributed in part to the time at which exposure was classified: if dietary fat intake has its effect at a late stage in disease development then positive results would be anticipated in case-control studies and cohort studies with relatively short follow-up periods. In contrast, negative results should come from prospective studies with long follow-up periods, as has been observed for the Lutheran Brotherhood Cohort Study [46].

Studies have generally supported the hypothesis that prostate cancer risk is increased by a diet with an increasing content of fat [9]; of at least 13 case-control studies, 10 have shown some positive evidence but early cohort studies were less consistent. In total, there is evidence suggesting that the risk of prostate cancer is influenced by a diet which is high in calories, high in fat and high in meat [43], although the exact mechanism of carcinogenesis remains unknown. It is often suggested that fat exerts its effect through modification of the endogenous hormonal milieu [41]. Unfortunately there have been few studies of prostate cancer which have had a satisfactory dietary methodology and the putative associations cannot at the present time be considered causal.

Vitamin A, β-carotene and retinoids

It is difficult to escape the impression given from a number of studies that the risk of prostate cancer is increased by increasing reported intake of vitamin A, particularly retinol [9]. Recent results from an intervention trial in smokers leave the question of an association unresolved. Among 29 133 Finnish male smokers entered into a randomized trial of β-carotene versus placebo there were 138 cases of prostate cancer reported in the β-carotene group (a rate of 16.3 per 10 000) compared to 112 (13.2 per 10 000) in the placebo group [47]. The age-adjusted relative risk for β-carotene appears to be approximately 1.24 (the confidence interval cannot be calculated from the data presented). This finding is consistent with several previous observations that the risk of prostate cancer appears to be elevated among those men who received β-carotene but it is in a sense reassuring that if the excess is significant, then it is not very large in magnitude (around 25%). However, it is clear that this putative association deserves to be a continued priority for future research, particularly in light of the increasing tendency to undertake trials of carotenoids and retinoids in the prevention of malignant disease and that the general populations of many countries are already anticipating these findings and increasingly taking vitamins including these compounds.

Vitamin E

An interesting finding, although one which was completely unexpected, from this same study [47] was a striking negative association between risk of prostate cancer and intake of vitamin E. Among men randomized to α-tocopherol (50 mg daily) there were 99 incident cases of prostate cancer observed (rate 11.7 per 10 000) compared to 151 cases among those men receiving the placebo (17.8 per 10 000): the approximate age-adjusted relative risk was 0.66. This is the first evidence that vitamin E may be protective against prostate cancer; it is a post hoc inference and obviously requires confirmation before it can be acted upon and recommendations made to the general public. It is clearly identified, due to the magnitude of the effect, as a major priority in prostate cancer research at the present time.

Vitamin D

International correlation studies suggest that vitamin D could be closely linked to the risk of prostate cancer [48]. Such a potential association was examined in the cohort of members of the Kaiser Permanente Medical Care plan in

Oakland and San Francisco whose serum was collected between 1964 and 1971 [49]. A total of 90 cases of prostate cancer in Afro-American men and 91 cases in Caucasian men were identified from the cohort of 250 000 men sampled: controls were selected matched for age, race and day of serum storage. In these groups of cases and controls, levels of the major metabolites of vitamin D (25-hydroxyvitamin D (25-D_3) and 1,25 dihydroxyvitamin D (1,25-D)) were measured and examined in respect to prostate cancer risk. The mean serum level of 1,25-D was 1.81 pg/ml lower in cases than in matched controls: this difference was statistically significant ($P = 0.02$). The risk of prostate cancer decreased with higher levels of 1,25-D, especially in men with lower levels of 25-D_3. However, the mean levels of 25-D_3 were similar in cases of prostate cancer and in controls. In men aged 57 years or older, 1,25-D was found to be an important risk for palpable and anaplastic tumours but not for tumours found incidentally at the time of surgery to treat the symptoms of benign prostatic hyperplasia or well-differentiated tumours [49]. Thus, vitamin D may be specifically relevant to the promotional events and clinically important tumours which are of public health importance. It should be considered together with the other dietary factors listed above in the aetiology of prostate cancer.

Body mass index

Body mass index (BMI; weight/height^2, generally expressed as kg/m^2) is determined by a complex interaction of genetic factors, total caloric intake, basal metabolic rate and total exercise. In the American Cancer Society cohort, overweight males were shown to have a 30% increased risk of prostate cancer when compared to men within 10% of their ideal body weight [50]. A study from Northern Italy found a substantial dose–response gradient [51]. Setting the risk to be 1.0 in the lowest tertile of body mass index, the risk rose through 2.3 (95% CI 2.1, 4.8) to 4.4 (1.9, 9.9) in the highest group: the test for linear trend was highly significant ($P < 0.0001$). In view of this potential association, and the possible link to caloric intake, careful adjustment for BMI in the analysis of all nutritional data sets in prostate cancer epidemiology is essential [9].

Occupational factors

There have been a wide variety of occupations postulated as being involved in the aetiology of prostate cancer ranging through French polishers, engine drivers, rubber workers, coal miners and chemists [9].

In a current review of literature published since 1970, van der Gulden *et al.* [52] analysed the results of 56 incidence and mortality studies of association between prostate cancer and socioeconomic status (SES). The studies were grouped according to SES indicators used, including educational level, income, occupational position and combination of all three. Of 56 studies, 32 showed no significant relationship between various SES indicators and risk of prostate cancer. Eight of 26 demonstrated a positive association between educational level and prostate cancer (non-significant in two of them) and in three the association was negative (non-significant in one). Among 11 studies that used income as an indicator of the SES, four found a positive association and one negative. The risk of prostate cancer was associated with occupational position in six studies, although in two non-significantly. Of seven large studies that evaluated the combination of all three indicators (education, income and occupation), only one found a positive association between SES and risk of prostate cancer. In the remaining three studies, one of which showed a positive association, the SES indicator was unknown to the authors. According to the results of their own study that was based on 345 cases of both clinical and incidental prostate cancer and 1346 referents (patients with BPH), no significant relationship was found between various SES variables and prostate cancer, with the exception of a slight but non-significant risk for the men living in rural areas.

A general feature of the studies which have investigated these associations with occupation is the tendency for findings from one study not to be replicated in the following studies, which themselves identify a new set of occupations found to be associated with this disease.

However, the one association which emerges consistently from the great majority of studies in employment in agriculture, although not in a specific manner – although farmers appear to be at a higher risk of prostate cancer, the specific exposures which produce this increased risk have not yet been identified. A recent large study was conducted using the extensive record linkage system available in Canada employing census and cancer mortality and incidence databases [53]. Using farmers in Manitoba, Saskatchewan and Alberta, a total of 1148 prostate cancer deaths were discovered among over 2.2 million person-years of risk. The study explored the relationship between prostate cancer mortality and various farm practices as indicated on the 1971 Census of Agriculture, including exposure to chickens, cattle, pesticides and fuel. A weak but statistically significant association was found between the number of acres sprayed with herbicides in 1970 and subsequent prostate cancer mortality risk. When the authors restricted the analysis to farmers believed to be the subject of the least amount of misclassification, the risk associated with acres sprayed with herbicides increased (RR = 2.23 for 250 or more acres sprayed; 95% CI 1.30, 3.84; test for trend $P < 0.01$).

A study reported from the USA demonstrated that a substantial portion of the excess prostate cancer mortality among blacks from three south-eastern states with the highest mortality rates of prostate cancer may be associated with farming [54]. The authors examined death certificates from three south-eastern states of the USA and found 891 cases of adenocarcinoma of the prostate among black men in farm-related occupations compared to 228 similar cases in 21 other states. In contrast, the numbers of deaths from prostate cancer in blacks who were not engaged in farming were 3904 in three south-eastern states and 4536 in 21 other states. Using the estimates of risk, the prevalence of subjects who had farm-related occupations, along with directly measured rates of prostate cancer, the authors calculated the proportion of the mortality in the south-eastern and other states that might be attributed to farming. When cases attributable to farming were removed, the difference in mortality rates between two regions decreased by 37.8%.

Although not of themselves conclusive evidence, the results obtained from these studies highlight the importance of conducting further studies on this topic.

Cirrhosis and viral infections

There have been several studies which have found a decreased risk of prostate cancer in men with liver cirrhosis: if true, it could be due to the tendency for cirrhosis to cause relative hyperoestrogenism, due to increased oestrone, and increased conversion to oestrogen from androgenic hormones. Since oestrogens provide effective palliative treatment in patients with prostate cancer, it could be imagined that oestrogen would reduce the risk of developing prostate cancer. Although evidence to support this association is weak, it could be interesting to extend this to viral infections of the liver, such as hepatitis A, B and C. In this study, the opportunity exists to compare this factor in population at widely different levels of this exposure.

Genetic factors

Prostate cancer has been found to occur significantly more frequently in the male relatives of index cases than in controls [55]. Prostate cancer rates worldwide are high in black populations of North America, the Caribbean and Africa. This is all consistent with the existence of a genetic component to prostate cancer risk.

Among the common forms of cancer, prostate cancer has been shown to demonstrate among the strongest evidence for family aggregation [56]. A number of studies have shown that brothers of cases have overall a threefold increased risk of prostate cancer with an even higher risk being associated with earlier onset [57]. In rare cases, extended families show suggestions of inherited predisposition because the risk for disease can be seen over multiple generations. In general, these few families are suggestive of a dominantly inherited predisposition, with onset being diagnosed from age 60 years onwards.

In a study of familial prostate cancer from Sweden, investigators used the twin-population approach to evaluate the role of genetic factors in the development of this disease. The incidence of prostate cancer was studied among 4840 male twin pairs from the Swedish Twin and Cancer Registries. Of 458 prostate cancers that were identified during this study, 16 occurred in both monozygotic and 6 in both dizygotic twins. The authors demonstrated that the concordance rate for prostate cancer was more than four times higher in monozygotic than in dizygotic twins [58].

In an examination of three groups – (i) 422 first-degree female relatives of patients with bilateral breast cancer; (ii) 320 first-degree relatives of male patients with breast cancer; and (iii) 633 relatives of unselected female patients – observed numbers of breast cancers in relatives were compared with expected numbers based on population-based incidence estimates. A family history of prostate cancer increased the breast cancer risks in each of these groups compared with families without prostate cancer. The authors concluded that a family history of prostate cancer increased the risk of breast cancer in family members [59]. Interestingly, male carriers of BRCA1 are at increased risk of prostate cancer (increased risk of around three- to fivefold) [60]. This could suggest that a first step in a strategy for prostate cancer should be to examine the families for evidence of BRCA1 segregation.

Technical improvements over the last 10 years have meant that a molecular approach to studying family aggregation to cancer is feasible and valuable. Two areas of study have been particularly important. In the first, tumours are examined for changes in DNA over their normal cellular counterpart (these studies are termed loss of heterozygosity studies). While of the order of 15% of tumours show deletions of each region, some regions show a much higher frequency of change, sometimes of the order of 75% of tumours. In the second approach, families with multiple cases of specific cancers are samples looking for regions of DNA which are common to affected relatives. Such regions may indicate the location of a gene or genes which code for inherited predisposition. Both of these types of studies have yielded valuable insights into the process of carcinogenesis and on some occasions the genes implicated in the two types of studies have been shown to be identical; that is, the genes of relevance for inherited predisposition are also those involved in somatic mutations in common cancer.

The situations with prostate cancer is similar to that also observed for breast cancer and bowel cancer. For each site, relatives of cases have an increased risk of approximately threefold and in occasional families pedigrees are consistent with the inheritance of a highly penetrant but rare dominant gene. For breast cancer, BRCAl has been mapped to human chromosome 17q; this gene accounts for the majority of families with breast and ovarian cancer and about one-half of families with only breast cancer [61]. The genetics of colorectal cancer are continuing to become better understood [62].

Benign prostatic hyperplasia

Prostate cancer is frequently found in men with BPH. The frequency of incidental prostate cancer during TURP for BPH was reported to range from 13–22% [14]. Of course, both are common diseases in men and it is to be expected that even if the diseases occur independently of each other, then there will be men who are found with both diseases. The incidence of prostate cancer and BPH increases with age and both diseases are androgen-associated conditions. BPH arises exclusively in the transition zone; however this is the site of origin of about 10–20% of prostatic adenocarcinomas [13]. In addition, TURP leads to a detailed investigation of prostate tissue so that detection bias may increase the reported risk of current prostate cancer and screening bias reduce the risk of later prostate cancer.

The key question is whether, after allowing for these, the subsequent incidence of prostate cancer in men who have had a diagnosis of BPH is increased. The causal nature of this relationship between BPH and subsequent prostate cancer has been controversial for years.

The two most frequently quoted studies have produced contrasting findings. In one of these studies both retrospective and prospective approaches were used [63]. The results obtained from the prospective study demonstrate a relative risk of prostate cancer 3.7 times greater among BPH patients and indicate that prostatectomy produces a considerable reduction in subsequent prostate cancer risk. The retrospective study of patients with prostate cancer and controls admitted with BPH has shown a relative risk of 5.1 for the prostate cancer group. These findings are at variance with the results of a prospective study of BPH patients who had a subtotal prostatectomy and controls in which the prostate cancer risk of the BPH group was estimated to be 0.9 [64].

21

A large study has recently been reported from Rhode Island involving follow-up of a historical cohort of 4853 men who had either a transurethral resection or a prostatectomy who were identified in hospital discharge records and followed up for subsequent prostate cancer. Among those men who had a suprapubic prostatectomy, the risk of prostate cancer was found to be 1.01 (0.77, 1.31), compared to the rate expected from local cancer incidence statistics. Among men who had a TURP the risk was 1.18 (0.94, 1.47) [65]. Neither of these risks is statistically significant and the upper confidence boundaries are much smaller than the point estimates from the study of Armenian *et al.* [63].

A recent follow-up study from Sweden [66] suggested that neither BPH nor TURP increased the risk of developing clinical prostate cancer in patients who underwent transurethral resection of a clinically benign prostate gland. The clinical incidence of prostate cancer was reported as 0.30% in the TURP group and 0.25% in the control group. In a retrospective case-control study of 198 patients who had TURP and 203 age-matched controls, investigators did not observe any significant difference in the incidence of prostatic adeno-carcinoma. Contrary to other studies, all patients with stage T1 prostate cancer found by TURP were included in the comparison between two groups. The reported odds ratio for development of clinically evident prostate cancer was 0.8 (95% CI 0.2, 3.1), and for death from prostate cancer 1.3 (95% CI 0.24, 7.45). The authors concluded that neither TURP itself nor BPH increases the subsequent risk of clinical prostate cancer.

In contrast, Kearse *et al.* [29], in a long-term follow-up study of 269 patients who underwent TURP, found that a significant number (7.8%) subsequently developed clinical prostate cancer. Comparing these data with reports on disease progression in incidentally discovered prostate cancer, the authors suggested that the risk of progression and death from prostate cancer is similar in patients who underwent transrectal ultrasound (TRUS) for benign prostatic hyperplasia and for those who had incidentally discovered prostate cancer at TRUS. The authors suggested that this finding may be a result of both combination of increasing patient age and the common hormonal basis for the development of BPH and prostate cancer.

Although most of the studies failed to demonstrate any significant relationship between history of BPH and development of prostatic adenocarcinoma, some common features in the natural history of these diseases and the frequent incidental findings of prostate cancer in TRUP specimens may be considered as a sufficient reason for further studies [36].

Vasectomy

Several studies have suggested that vasectomy may predispose to prostate cancer: other equally good studies have found that it does not. All of these studies have limitations but, when taken together, the available evidence does not support such an association [67].

A recent case-control study from the USA involved a larger number of prostate cancer cases than any of the previous studies and was conducted in both black and white populations. The study was based on 965 cases of prostate cancer, of whom 471 were Afro-Americans and 494 were whites. Although the authors found some statistically non-significant increase in risk for prostate cancer among Afro-Americans who underwent vasectomy, the low prevalence of this procedure in Afro-Americans could not explain the significantly higher incidence of prostate cancer in Afro-American populations than in whites. Both in whites and in Afro-Americans, the increased risk for prostate cancer was only restricted to the group of men who had a vasectomy at less than age 35 [68].

Scrutiny of the available studies reveals that none of them satisfies more than four of eight basic methodological criteria and that all the studies are deficient in avoiding detection bias and obtaining accurate vasectomy histories. The attempted meta-analysis indicates that the evidence on this topic is conflicting [69].

At the present time, it seems unlikely, but not impossible, that there is a biological mechanism supporting a relationship between vasectomy and prostate cancer [70]. Further research is, however, required since the possibility of an association carries public health implications for the developing countries.

Summary and conclusions

Prostate cancer is a frequent cancer in old men, increasing with age through the most advanced years. Descriptive epidemiology has highlighted the wide geographical variation in prostate cancer occurrence and the large increases taking place in the reported incidence of the disease worldwide. Even if age-specific incidence rates remain stable, the problem of prostate cancer seems sure to increase in absolute terms simply because of the ageing of the population. Life expectancy at birth in many western countries is still increasing and half of boys born today can expect to reach the age of 80 years. This has major implications for the future burden of prostate disease, including cancer. Assuming no change in the age-specific risk of contracting prostate cancer, the number of cases of prostate cancer in the EC countries among men aged 65 and over will increase from 79 000 in 1990, to 92 000 in 2000, 102 000 in 2010, reaching 120 000 in 2020 – an increase of 50% in 30 years. Comparative figures for Canada reveal increases from 6500 cases in 1990 rising to 12 000 cases in 2020. These estimates are based entirely on applying 1980 incidence rates to available population projections: the presence of a temporal trend in risk will only serve to increase these numbers further.

There is, however, new evidence that the risk of dying from prostate cancer has remained unchanged in many countries throughout this century [6]. The increasing availability of TURP and the extensive use of currently available diagnostic modalities (PSA, TRUS and needle biopsies) may have resulted in a considerable increase in detection of otherwise clinically asymptomatic prostate cancers. The detection of latent prostate cancers may expose a large number of patients with this usually non-fatal disease to the risks of surgical treatment, probably with little if any improvement in clinical outcome [16, 71].

It is widely accepted that prostate cancer has important environmental determinants and that a large proportion of cases should be preventable. However, current knowledge of risk factors for prostate cancer is poor and avoidable causes have not yet been identified with any degree of certainty. Scientific intuition tells us that the 'causes' of prostate cancer are hormonal but at the present time there is no consistent evidence of any primary endocrine disturbance that is necessarily implicated in the aetiology of prostatic cancer.

From examination of the available analytical studies, there appears to be a dietary component to prostate cancer risk involving saturated fat intake and particularly intake of meat and (perhaps) milk: this may relate to the hormonal milieu. In view of the putative aetiological role of lifestyle factors, and notably fat consumption, on prostate cancer risk, it is somewhat surprising that there have not been very large and obvious increases in the underlying risk of fatal prostate cancer among cohorts born since the early decades of this current century. The situation in Japan, the usual paradigm of diet-related cancer risks, is most informative in this respect. The lack of any notable increase among successively younger birth cohorts, who are the most likely to have westernized their diet, argues strongly against any important impact of increasing fat consumption on the risk of fatal prostate cancer. This is a situation similar to that of colorectal cancer and breast cancer in the same population.

The role of carotenoids and retinoids remains unclear at the present time, with the suggestion of an increased risk associated with an increased intake still a cause for some concern. The possible protective roles of vitamin D and vitamin E are emerging as of potential interest and should at least be priorities for further research.

Although a large number of different occupations have been associated with an increased risk of prostate cancer, the only fairly consistent finding is that of the increased risk associated with occupation in agriculture. However, the increased risk is proving to be unspecific and not related to exposure to animals, cereals or other types of farming. Recent evidence suggests that the specific factor may be exposure to herbicides and this should be followed up as soon as possible.

There is a likelihood of important genetic effects in prostate cancer which will require international cooperation to help unravel. There is at the present time little evidence that having a vasectomy or BPH leads to an increased risk of prostate cancer. There is no consistent evidence suggesting an association of prostate cancer risk with cigarette smoking, alcohol consumption, coffee consumption or sexually transmitted diseases and prostate cancer risk [9].

Despite this knowledge of such a litany of risk factors, there is little action that can be recommended at the present time to reduce the risk of prostate cancer through alteration of lifestyle factors. Given the ageing population and the arrival early next century of the post Second World War baby boomers at ages where prostate cancer begins to assume public health significance, it is clear that the absolute numbers of cases of prostate cancer will continue to increase and, in the absence of any successful intervention – whether treatment, primary prevention or from screening – so too will the absolute number of deaths from this condition.

Chemoprevention and screening appear to be priority alternatives to alteration of risk through alteration of risk factors. Screening deserves urgent evaluation through randomized trials [21], the search for prostate cancer families should be an urgent research priority and the striking protective effect involving vitamin E should be followed up as a matter of considerable urgency.

Acknowledgements

Dr Pavel Napalkov is supported by a Pfizer fellowship in urological epidemiology. This work was conducted within the framework of support from the Associazione Italiana per la Ricerca sul Cancro (Italian Association for Cancer Research).

References

1 Parkin DM, Muir CS, Whelan S, Gao YT, Ferlay J, Powell J (eds) *Cancer Incidence in Five Continents*, vol VI. IARC scientific publication number 120. Lyon: 1992 IARC.

2 Boring CC, Squires TS & Tong T: Cancer statistics. *CA Cancer J Clin* 1994; **44**: 7–26.

3 Jenson OM, Esteve J, Moller H & Renard H. Cancer in the European Community and its member states. *Eur J Cancer* 1990; **26**: 1167–1256.

4 Alexander FE & Boyle P. The rise in prostate cancer: myth or reality? In: *The Epidemiology of Prostate Diseases*, Garraway MJ, ed. Edinburgh: Churchill Livingstone, 1995.

5 Boyle P. Prostate cancer 2000: evolution of an epidemic of unknown origin. In *Prostate Cancer 2000*, Denis L, ed. Heidelberg: Springer-Verlag, 1994, pp. 5–11.

6 Boyle P, Evstifeeva T, Maisonneuve P, Macfarlane GJ & Pagano F. Temporal trends in prostate cancer mortality: is the risk rising? In *Proceedings of the Second International Consensus on Urological Disease*. Cockett AB, Denis L, Aso Y *et al.*, eds. Oxford: Oxford University Press (in press).

7 Boyle P, Maisonneuve P & Smans M. Epidemiology of urological cancers. In: *Textbook of Genito-Urinary Surgery*, Hendry WF, ed. (in press).

8 Haenszel W & Kurihara M. Studies of Japanese migrants: I. Mortality from cancer and other diseases among Japanese in the United States. *J Natl Cancer Inst* 1968; **40**: 43–68.

9 Boyle P & Zaridze DG. Risk factors for prostate and testicular cancer. *Eur J Cancer* 1993; **29A-7**: 1048–1055.

10 Parkin DM, Laara E & Muir CS. Estimates of the worldwide frequency of 16 major cancers in 1980. *Int J Cancer* 1988; **41**: 184–197.

11 Brody J. Prospects for an aging population. *Nature* 1985; **315**: 463–466.

12 Breslow N, Chan CE, Dhom G *et al.* Latent carcinoma of prostate at autopsy in seven areas. *Int J Cancer* 1977; **20**: 680–688.

13 McNeal JE. The prostate gland: morphology and pathobiology, *Monogr Urol* 1988; **9**: 36–54.

14 Epstein JI, Walsh PC & Brendler CB. Radical prostatectomy for impalpable prostate cancer: the Johns Hopkins experience with tumours found on transurethral resection (stages T1a and T1b) and on needle biopsy (stage T1c). *J Urol* 1994; **152**: 1721–1729.

15 Severson RK. Have transurethral resections contributed to the increasing incidence of prostatic cancer? *J Natl Cancer Inst* 1990; **82**: 1597–1598.

16 Woolf HS. Public health perspective: the health policy implications of screening for prostate cancer. *J Urol* 1994; **152**: 1685–1688.

17 Murphy WM, Dean PJ, Brasfield JA & Tatum L. Incidental carcinoma of the prostate. *Am J Surg Pathol* 1986; **10**: 170–174.

18 Staszewski J. & Haenszel W. Cancer mortality among the Polish-born in the United States. *J Natl Cancer Inst* 1965; **35**: 291–297.

19 Griffiths K & Khoury S (eds) *Primer on Molecular Control of Prostate Growth*. Whitehouse Station, NJ: Merck, 1994.

20 Coleman M, Esteve J, Damiecki P, Arslan A & Renard H. Trends in cancer incidence and mortality. International Agency for Research on Cancer (IARC) Scientific Publication 121, IARC, Lyon, 1993.

21 Boyle P & Alexander FE. Screening for prostate cancer: principles, methods and evaluation. *Urology* (in press).

22 DeCarli A, La Vecchia C. Age, period and cohort models: a review of knowledge and implementation in GLIM, *Riv di Stat Appl* 1987; **20**: 397–410.

23 Boyle P, Alexander FE, Luchini L & Bishop T. Aetiology of prostate cancer. In: *The Epidemiology of Prostate Diseases*, Garraway MJ. ed. Edinburgh: Churchill Livingstone, 1995.

24 World Health Organization, 1992.

25 Handley MR & Stuart ME. The use of prostate specific antigen for prostate cancer screening: a managed care perspective. *J Urol* 1994; **152**: 1689–1692.

26 McNeal JE, Villers AA, Redwine EA, Freiha FS & Stamey TA. Histologic differentiation, cancer volume, and pelvic lymph node metastasis in adenocarcinoma of the prostate. *Cancer* 1990; **66**: 1225.

27 Maeda O, Saiki S, Kinouchi T *et al.* Clinical study for incidental prostatic carcinoma.*Acta Urol Jpn* 1991; **37**: 135–139.

28 Chodak GW, Thisted RA, Gerber GS *et al.* Results of conservative management of clinically localized prostate cancer, *New Engl J Med* 1994; **330**: 242.

29 Kearse WS Jr, Seay TM & Thompson IM. The long-term risk of development of prostate cancer in patients with benign prostatic hyperplasia: correlation with stage A1 disease. *J Urol* 1993; **150**: 1746–1748.

30 Lu-Yao GL & Greenberg ER. Changes in prostate cancer incidence and treatment in the United States. *Lancet* 1994; **343**: 251–254.

31 Macfarlane GJ, Boyle P, Evstifeeva TV, Robertson C & Scully C. Rising trends of oral cancer mortality worldwide. The return of an old public health problem. *Cancer Causes Control* (in press).

32 Holman CDH, James IE, Segal MR & Armstrong K. Recent trends in mortality from prostate cancer in male populations of Australia and England and Wales. *Br J Cancer* 1981; **44**: 340–348.

33 Schroeder F & Boyle P. Screening for prostate cancer: necessity or nonsense? *Eur J Cancer* 1993; **29**: 656–661.

34 Labrie F, Simard J, Belanger A, Luu-The V & Labrie C (1994). Molecular biology of the intracrine steroidogenic enzymes in the human prostate. In: *Sex Hormones and Anti-hormones in Endocrine Dependent Pathology: Basic and Clinical Aspects*, Motta M & Serio M, eds. Amsterdam: Elsevier, 1994, pp. 77–92.

35 Calais da Silva F. The role of somatostatin prostate cancer. In: *Sex Hormones and Antihormones in Endocrine Dependent Pathology: Basic and Clinical Aspects*, Motta M & Serio M, eds. Amsterdam: Elsevier 1994, pp. 209–217.

36 Griffiths K, Harper ME, Eaton CL, Turkes A & Peeling WB. Endocrine aspects of prostate cancer. In: *Prostate Cancer 2000*, Denis L, ed. Heidelberg: Springer-Verlag 1994, pp. 21–39.

37 Rotkin ID. Studies in the epidemiology of prostatic cancer: expanded sampling. *Cancer Treat Rep* 1977; **61**: 173–180.

38 Schuman LM, Mandel J, Blackard C, Bauer H, Scarlett J & McHugh R. Epidemiologic study of prostate cancer: preliminary report, *Cancer Treat Rep* 1977; **61**: 181–186.

39 King M, Diamond E & Lilienfeld AM. Some epidemiological aspects of cancer of the prostate. *J Chronic Dis* 1963; **16**: 117–153.

40 Lancaster HO. The mortality in Australia from cancer peculiar to the male. *Med J Aust* 1972; **2**: 41–44.

41 Hill P, Wynder EL, Garnes H & Walker ARP. Environmental factors, hormone status and prostatic cancer. *Prev Med* 1980; **9**: 657–666.

42 Wynder EL, Mabuchi K & Whitmore WF. Epidemiology of cancer of the prostate. *Cancer* 1971; **28**: 344–360.

43 Giovannucci E, Rimm EB, Colditz GA *et al.* A prospective study of dietary fat and risk of prostate cancer. *J Natl Cancer Inst* 1993; **85**: 1571–1579.

44 Mills P, Beeson L, Philips R & Fraser G. Dietary habits and breast cancer incidence

among Seventh Day Adventists. *Cancer* 1989; **64**: 582–590.

45 LeMarchand L, Kolonel L, Wilkens LR, Myers BC & Hirohata T. Animal fat consumption and prostate cancer: a prospective study in Hawaii. *Epidemiology* 1994; **5**: 276–282.

46 Hsing A & Comstock GW. Serological precursors of cancer: serum hormones and risk of subsequent prostate cancer. *Cancer Epidemiol Biomarkers Prev* 1993; **2**: 27–32.

47 The α-Tocopherol, β-Carotene Cancer Prevention Study Group. The effect of vitamin E and β-carotene on the incidence of lung cancer and other cancers in male smokers. *N Engl J Med* 1994; **330**: 1029–1035.

48 Schwartz GG & Hulka BS. Is vitamin D deficiency a risk factor for prostate cancer? (Hypothesis) *Anticancer Res* 1990; **10**: 1307–1312.

49 Corder EH, Guess HA, Hulka B *et al.* Vitamin D and prostate cancer: a prediagnostic study with stored data. *Cancer Epidemiol Biomarkers Prev* 1993; **2**: 467–472.

50 Lew EA & Garfinkel L. Variations in mortality by weight among 750 000 men and women. *J Chron Dis* 1979; **32**: 563–576.

51 Talamini R, La Vecchia C, De Carli A *et al.* Nutrition, social factors and prostatic cancer in a Northern Italian population. *Br J Cancer* 1986; **53**: 817–821.

52 Van der Gulden JWJ, Kolk JJ & Verbeek ALM. Socioeconomic status, urbanization grade, and prostate cancer. *Prostate* 1994; **25**: 59–65.

53 Morrison H, Savitz D, Semenciw R *et al.* Farming and prostate cancer mortality. *Am. J. Epidemiol.* 1993; **137**: 270–280.

54 Dosemeci M, Hoover RN, Blair A *et al.* Farming and prostate cancer among African-Americans in the south-eastern United States. *J. Natl. Cancer Inst.* 1994; **86**: 18–19.

55 Steele R, Lees REM, Kraus AS & Rao C. Sexual factors in the epidemiology of cancer of the prostate. *J Chronic Dis* 1971; **24**: 29–37.

56 Cannon L, Bishop DT, Skolnick M, Hunt S, Lyon JL & Smart CR. Genetic epidemiology of prostate cancer in the Utah Mormon genealogy. *Cancer Surv* 1982; **1**: 47–63.

57 Carter BS, Bova GS, Beaty TH *et al.* Hereditary prostate cancer: epidemiologic and clinical features. *J Urol* 1993; **150**: 797–802.

58 Gronberg H, Damber L & Damber J-E. Studies of genetic factors in prostate cancer in a twin population. *J Urol* 1994; **152**: 1484–1489.

59 Anderson DE & Badzioch MD. Breast cancer risks in relatives of male breast cancer patients. *Cancer* 1993; **72**: 114–119.

60 Easton D. *et al.* Personal communication.

61 Spurr NK, Kelsell DP, Black DM *et al.* Linkage analysis of early-onset breast and ovarian cancer families, with markers on the long arm of chromosome 17. *Am J Hum Genet* 1993; **52**: 777–785.

62 Bishop DT & Hall NR. The genetics of colorectal cancer. *Eur J Cancer* 1994; **30A**: 1946–1956.

63 Armenian HK, Lilienfeld AM, Diamond EL & Bross IDJ. Relation between benign prostatic hyperplasia and cancer of the prostate: a prospective and retrospective study. *Lancet* 1974; **ii**: 115–117.

64 Greenwald P, Kirmss V, Polan AK & Dick VS. Cancer of the prostate among men with benign prostatic hyperplasia. *J Natl Cancer Inst* 1974; **53**: 335–340.

65 Simons BD, Morrison AS, Young RH & Verhoek-Oftedahl W. The relation of surgery for prostate hypertrophy to carcinoma of the prostate. *Am J Epidemiol* 1993; **138**: 294–300.

66 Hammarsten J, Andersson S, Holmen A, Hogstedt B & Peeker R. Does transurethral resection of a clinically benign prostate gland increase the risk of developing clinical prostate cancer? A 10-year follow-up study. *Cancer* 74: 2347–2351.

67 Guess HA. Is vasectomy a risk factor for prostate cancer? *Eur J Cancer* 1993; **29A**: 1055–1060.

68 Hayes RB, Pottern LM, Greenberg *et al.* Vasectomy and prostate cancer in US blacks and whites. *Am J. Epidemiol* 1993; **137**: 263–269.

69 Der Simonian R, Clemens J, Spirtas R & Perlman J. Vasectomy and prostate cancer risk: methodological review of the evidence. *J Clin Epidemiol* 1993; **46**: 163–172.

70 Howards SS. Possible biological mechanisms for a relationship between vasectomy and prostate cancer. *Eur J Cancer* 1993; **29A**: 1060–1062.

71 Schwab L. Experts sharply divided on prostate cancer screening. *J Natl Cancer Inst* 1991; **83**: 535–536.

2/Is the Behaviour of Prostate Cancer Understood?

D.G. Bostwick

Introduction

There is a need to separate prostate cancers which will progress from those that will not within the expected life span of the patient. However, in order to create such stratification of patients for therapy, an understanding of the behaviour of prostate cancer is necessary. At present, the outcome for an individual patient with cancer cannot be determined with certainty, although considerable progress has been made in this regard in the past decade. This chapter examines the pathological factors derived from needle biopsies and prostatectomy specimens which provide the greatest predictive accuracy. A brief review of pathological anatomy, tissue sampling methods and the putative premalignant lesion prostatic intraepithelial neoplasia is included as pertinent regarding the behaviour of prostate cancer.

Pathological anatomy

The prostate arises during the third month of gestation as a series of epithelial buds within the urogenital sinus. The stroma plays an inductive role in this process by converting testosterone to dihydrotestosterone [1].

The adult prostate is composed of three distinct zones – the peripheral zone, central zone and transition zone (Table 2.1) [2]. The peripheral zone contains about 70% of the volume of the normal prostate, and is the commonest site of prostatic intraepithelial neoplasia (PIN) and carcinoma. Digital rectal examination of the prostate often includes a description of the left and right lobes based on palpation of an indentation in the midline, the median furrow, which divides the peripheral zone into left and right halves. The central zone contains about 25% of the volume of the prostate, forming a cone-shaped area which includes the base of the prostate and encompasses the ejaculatory ducts. The transition zone contains the smallest volume of the normal prostate, about 5%, but may become massive in size due to benign prostatic hyperplasia (BPH). The central zone and peripheral zone are often referred to together as the outer prostate or non-transition zone, whereas the transition zone and anterior fibromuscular stroma are often referred to together as the inner prostate.

Table 2.1 Zonal anatomy of the prostate: implications for disease.

	Central zone	Transition zone	Peripheral zone
Tissue-sampling techniques			
Transurethral resection	Poor	Good	Poor
Needle biopsy	Variable	Poor	Good
Fine-needle aspiration	Variable	Poor	Good
Involvement with pathological processes			
Atrophy	Infrequent	Variable	Frequent
Nodular hyperplasia	Rare	Frequent	Rare
Prostatitis	Infrequent	Variable	Frequent
Infarcts	Rare	Frequent	Rare
Atypical adenomatous hyperplasia	Rare	Frequent	Rare
Prostatic intraepithelial neoplasia	Infrequent	Infrequent	Frequent
Carcinoma	Infrequent	Frequent	Frequent

The capsule of the prostate consists of an inner layer of smooth muscle and an outer covering of collagen, with marked variability in the relative amounts in different areas. At the apex, the glandular elements become scant and the capsule is ill-defined, composed of a mixture of fibrous connective tissue, smooth muscle and striated muscle. Also, there is no sharp line of demarcation of the prostate and the striated muscle of the anterior abdominal wall. As a result, the prostatic capsule cannot be regarded as a well-defined anatomical structure with constant features.

Needle core biopsy

The introduction of the automated spring-loaded 18-gauge needle core biopsy gun in the last decade began a new era in the sampling of the prostate for histological diagnosis. The main disadvantage of the 18-gauge biopsy is that it provides less than half the amount of tissue per needle core for pathological examination than the traditional 14-gauge biopsy.

Transurethral resection

The region of the prostate sampled by transurethral resection (TURP) and needle biopsy tend to be different [2]. TURP specimens consist of tissue from the transition zone, urethra, periurethral area, bladder neck and anterior fibromuscular stroma. Studies of radical prostatectomies performed after TURP reveal that the resection does not usually include tissue from the central or peripheral zones, and not all of the transition zone is removed. Most needle biopsy specimens consist only of tissue from the peripheral zone, seldom including the central or transition zones.

Well-differentiated cancer found incidentally in TURP chips usually represents cancer that has arisen in the transition zone. These tumours are frequently small and may be completely resected by TURP. Poorly differentiated cancer in TURP chips usually represents part of a larger tumour that has invaded the transition zone after arising in the peripheral zone.

Radical prostatectomy

The completeness of pathological sectioning of prostatectomies can affect the determination of pathological stage [3–6]. One study compared the results of limited sectioning (sections of palpable tumour and two random sections of apex and base) with complete sectioning (whole-organ step sectioning procedure), and found a significant increase in positive surgical margins (12% versus 59%, respectively) and pathological stage with the complete approach [5]. Also, the presence and extent of extraprostatic extension in clinical stage T2 cancer (and hence clinical staging error) were related to the number of prostate slices submitted. The Cancer Committee of the College of American Pathologists has published guidelines for examination of specimens removed from patients with prostate cancer, including TURP and radical prostatectomies [7].

Complete and careful submission of tissue for histological evaluation allows the following:

1 unequivocal orientation of specimen and tumour (left, right; transition zone, peripheral zone; anterior, mid, posterior; apex, base, etc.);
2 thorough evaluation of the extent and location of positive surgical margins;
3 thorough assessment and quantitation of the extent and location of capsular perforation and seminal vesicle invasion;
4 quality control data for the surgeon, particularly in regard to surgical margins in nerve-sparing prostatectomy;
5 postoperative measurement of tumour volume for correlation with imaging studies, etc.;
6 complete evaluation of tumour for grading (percentage poorly differentiated cancer, etc.);
7 fulfilment of all recommendations of the Cancer Committee of the College of American Pathologists [7];
8 comparison of results with published prostatectomy studies.

Association of benign prostatic hyperplasia and prostate cancer

There are a number of similarities between BPH and cancer (Fig. 2.1) [8]. Both display a parallel increase in prevalence with patient age according to autopsy studies, although cancer lags by 15–20 years. Both require androgens for growth and development, and both may respond to androgen deprivation treatment. Most cancers arise in prostates with concomitant BPH, and cancer is found incidentally in a significant number of transurethral prostatectomy specimens (10% of specimens). BPH may be related to prostate cancer arising in the transition zone, perhaps in association with certain forms of hyperplasia, but BPH is not a premalignant lesion nor a precursor of carcinoma (see Chapter 1 for a discussion on epidemiology).

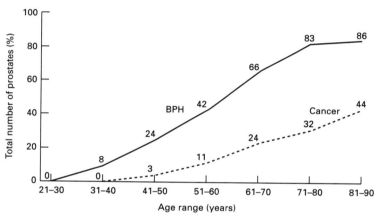

Fig. 2.1 Age-specific prevalence of benign prostatic hyperplasia (BPH) and cancer in autopsy specimens from human prostates. From Bostwick *et al.*, [8] with permission.

Prostatic intraepithelial neoplasia: clinical significance

PIN is considered the most likely precursor of invasive carcinoma [9]. This microscopic finding is characterized by epithelial proliferation within pre-existing ducts and acini, with cytological changes mimicking cancer, including nuclear and nucleolar enlargement (Fig. 2.2). PIN coexists with cancer in more than 85% of cases, but retains an intact or fragmented basal cell layer, unlike cancer which lacks a basal cell layer. Studies to date have not determined whether PIN remains stable, regresses or progresses, although the implication is that it can progress.

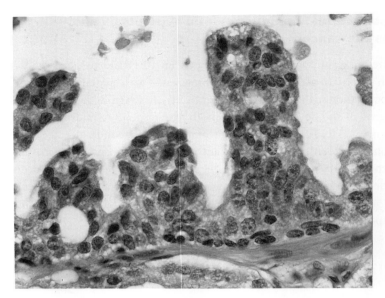

Fig. 2.2 High-grade prostatic intraepithelial neoplasia. Note nuclear and nucleolar enlargement.

The continuum which culminates in high-grade PIN and early invasive cancer is characterized by progressive basal cell layer disruption, loss of markers of secretory differentiation, nuclear and nucleolar abnormalities, increasing proliferative potential, variation in DNA content and allelic loss (Fig. 2.3). Clinical studies suggest that PIN predates carcinoma by 10 years or more, with low-grade PIN first appearing in men in their 30s.

The incidence and extent of prostatic intraepithelial neoplasia and cancer increase with patient age

The incidence and extent of PIN appear to increase with the age of the patient according to most studies. Sakr *et al.* [10] studied the prostates of young men at autopsy, and found the onset of PIN in men in their 20s and 30s (9 and 22% frequency, respectively) which preceded the onset of carcinoma by more than 10 years (Fig. 2.4). Most foci of PIN in young males were low-grade, with increasing frequency of high-grade PIN with advancing age. The prevalence of PIN was similar in blacks and whites.

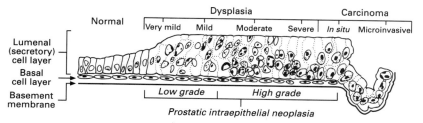

Fig. 2.3 Morphological continuum from normal prostatic epithelium through increasing grades of prostatic intraepithelial neoplasia (PIN) to early invasive carcinoma, according to the disease continuum concept. Low-grade PIN (grade 1) corresponds to very mild to mild dysplasia. High-grade PIN (grades 2 and 3) corresponds to moderate to severe dysplasia and carcinoma-*in situ*. The precursor state ends when malignant cells invade the stroma; this invasion occurs where the basal cell layer is disrupted. Notice that the dysplastic changes occur in the superficial (luminal) secretory cell layer, perhaps in response to luminal carcinogens. Disruption of the basal cell layer accompanies the architectural and cytological features of high-grade PIN, and appears to be a necessary prerequisite for stromal invasion. The basement membrane is retained with high-grade PIN and early invasive carcinoma. Modified from Bostwick and Brawer, [11] with permission.

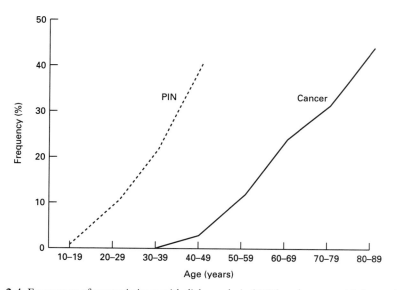

Fig. 2.4 Frequency of prostatic intraepithelial neoplasia (PIN) and cancer with increasing age. There is a parallel increase in the frequency of PIN and cancer, according to serially sectioned autopsy prostates, although PIN appears to predate cancer by more than 10 years. Data on PIN from Sakr *et al.*, [10] data on cancer curve from Bostwick *et al.*, [8].

Clinical importance of prostatic intraepithelial neoplasia

The clinical importance of PIN is based on its strong association with prostatic carcinoma. Because PIN has a high predictive value as a marker for adeno-carcinoma, its identification in biopsy specimens warrants further search for concurrent invasive carcinoma. This is especially true for high-grade PIN; when this lesion is identified, close surveillance and follow-up biopsy appear to be indicated.

To examine the predictive value of high-grade PIN, Davidson *et al.* [12] conducted a retrospective case-control study of needle biopsies from 100 patients with high-grade PIN and 112 without PIN which were matched for clinical stage, patient age, and serum prostate-specific antigen (PSA). Ade-nocarcinoma was identified in 35% of subsequent biopsies from cases with PIN, compared with 13% in the control group (Fig. 2.5). The likelihood of finding cancer was greater in patients with PIN undergoing more than one follow-up biopsy (44%) than in those with only one biopsy (32%). High-grade PIN, patient age and serum PSA level were jointly highly significant predictors of cancer, with PIN providing the highest risk ratio (14.93; 95% confidence intervals 5.6–39.8). No other candidate predictor was found to be significant, including patient race, digital rectal examination findings, transrectal ultra-sound results, amount of PIN on biopsy and architectural pattern of PIN. Other studies have reported a high predictive value of PIN for cancer [9].

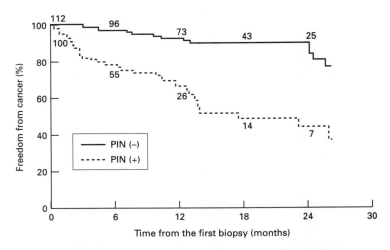

Fig. 2.5 Freedom from cancer from time of first biopsy according to the presence or absence of high-grade prostatic intraepithelial neoplasia (PIN). From Davidson *et al.*, [13] with permission.

These data underscore the strong association of PIN and adenocarcinoma and indicate that vigorous diagnostic follow-up is needed.

High-grade PIN is encountered in up to 16% of contemporary 18-gauge needle biopsies [14] (Fig. 2.6). When PIN is identified, all tissue should be embedded and made available for examination; serial sections of suspicious foci may be useful. Select antikeratin antibodies such as 34β-E12 (high-molecular-weight keratin) may be used to stain tissue sections for the presence of basal cells, recognizing that PIN retains an intact or fragmented basal cell layer, whereas cancer does not. Unfortunately, needle biopsy specimens often fail to show the suspicious focus on deeper levels.

Biopsy remains the definitive method for detecting PIN and early invasive cancer, but non-invasive methods are being evaluated. By transrectal ultrasound, PIN may be hypoechoic, indistinguishable from carcinoma, although these findings have been refuted [9]. Transrectal ultrasound-directed biopsy allows localization of the needle and tissue being sampled. Repeat biopsy has been suggested by some authors if the first attempt is unrevealing. If all procedures fail to identify carcinoma, close surveillance and follow-up are indicated. Follow-up is suggested at 3–6-month intervals for 2 years, preferably with repeat biopsy [9]. Most authors agree that the identification of PIN should not influence or dictate therapeutic decisions.

PIN also offers promise as an intermediate end-point in studies of chemoprevention of prostatic carcinoma. Recognizing the relatively slow

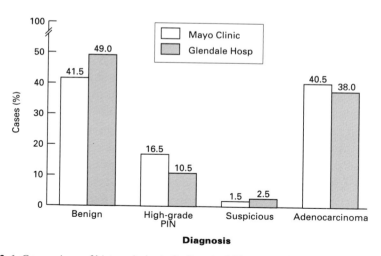

Fig. 2.6 Comparison of histopathologic findings in 200 consecutive contemporary 18-gauge needle biopsies from Mayo Clinic (Rochester, Minnesota) and Glendale Hospital (Glendale, California). From Bostwick and Dundore [15], with permission.

growth rate of prostate cancer and the considerable amount of time needed in animal and human studies for adequate follow-up, the non-invasive precursor lesion PIN is a suitable intermediate histological marker to indicate high likelihood of subsequent cancer [9].

Prostate-specific antigen expression in prostatic intraepithelial neoplasia

PIN has little or no influence on serum PSA level and does not cause clinically suspicious elevations [10]. Some studies have found a positive correlation of PSA and PIN, but this is probably the result of the confounding influence of cancer volume on serum PSA. There is decreased immunohistochemical expression of PSA in PIN when compared with normal epithelium and cancer. Because PIN is a histopathological abnormality involving intact acini, cytoplasmic secretory products such as PSA would be expected to empty into the lumen rather than the stroma and blood vessels, and a strong correlation of PSA and PIN would not be expected.

Is peripheral zone cancer different from transition zone cancer?

Cancer usually arises in the peripheral zone of the prostate, with transition zone origin accounting for about 24% of all cases. However, the majority of incidental (stages T1a and T1b) cancers arise in the transition zone, probably due to selective sampling of this area by TURP, including 75% of stage T1a and 79% of stage T1b cancers. We rarely have difficulty in finding at least a small focus of residual cancer in radical prostatectomy specimens after TURP, although extensive sectioning is sometimes needed. For large tumours, determining the site of origin may be difficult. Most transition zone cancers arise in foci adjacent to BPH, with one-third actually originating within BPH nodules. Transition zone cancer tends to be multicentric.

There appear to be significant morphological and biological differences between cancers originating in different anatomical sites in the prostate (Table 2.2) [8]. Transition zone cancer is better differentiated than cancer in the peripheral zone, accounting for the majority of cases of Gleason pattern 1 and 2 cancer. The volume of this low-grade tumour tends to be smaller than its counterpart arising in the peripheral zone, although frequent exceptions are noted. Further, most cases of transition zone cancer display a distinctive columnar clear cell pattern which is rarely observed in peripheral zone cancer. Finally, there is decreased stromal fibrosis in transition zone cancer and a lower incidence of cribriform pattern.

The favourable prognosis of clinical stage T1a and T1b cancer may be due to the confinement of transition zone cancer to the site of origin. The compressed fibromuscular stroma at the boundary of the transition zone acts as a relative barrier to tumour extension, and malignant glands frequently fan out along the boundary before invasion into the peripheral and central zones. These tumours preferentially cluster at the apex, similar to peripheral zone cancer, but are less likely to extend beyond the prostate. Invasion into the anterior fibromuscular stroma is occasionally seen with small-volume transition zone cancer, but complete perforation only occurs with large tumours, probably due to resistance of the thickened muscular stroma at this site. Only 25% of cases of transition zone cancer display capsular perforation or anterior fibromuscular stromal invasion, and this usually occurs in anterolateral and apical directions where the distance to the capsule is short. The risk of spread to the seminal vesicles is significantly less than with peripheral zone cancer.

Pathological significance of tumour volume

Serial measurements of PSA suggest that prostatic adenocarcinoma has a constant log–linear growth rate, with mean PSA doubling times of 2.4 years for localized adenocarcinoma and 1.8 years for metastatic adenocarcinoma [17, 18]. Higher Gleason grades are associated with faster doubling times.

Tumour volume is therefore considered to be a significant and powerful prognostic factor in prostate cancer. Current technology is imprecise in determining tumour volume preoperatively, but progress is being made which may soon make such measurements feasible. Future staging of early prostate cancer will probably rely on image-based tumour volume rather than on palpability by digital rectal examination. Preoperative assessment of volume may also provide the urologist with the likelihood of positive surgical margins. None the less, at present, this is experimental and not of practical value.

Preoperative prediction of tumour volume

For tumour volume to be clinically useful, it must be able to be measured preoperatively. Most studies of tumour volume have been static pathological studies of prostatectomy specimens. There is limited accuracy of current diagnostic and biopsy modalities (digital rectal examination, transrectal ultrasound, magnetic resonance imaging, serum PSA concentration, needle biopsy and transurethral resection) in predicting tumour volume prior to radical prostatectomy.

Current staging of palpable organ-confined cancer relies on digital rectal

Table 2.2 Prostatic carcinoma: comparison based on anatomical site of origin.*

	Transition zone cancer	Peripheral zone cancer
Incidence		
Stage A1	75%	
Stage A2	79%	
All stage A	78%	
All stages	24%	70%
Origin		
In or near BPH	Yes	No
Near apex	Yes	Yes
Detection rate by TURP	78%	
Pathological features		
Tumour volume	Usually small	Small to large
Tumour pattern	Alveolar–medullary	Tubular–scirrhous
Tumour grade (Gleason)	Usually 1 or 2	Usually 2, 3 or 4
Clear cell pattern	Most cases	Rare
Stromal fibrosis	Uncommon	Common
Associated putative premalignant changes	AAH or PIN	PIN
Aneuploidy	6%	31%
Clinical behaviour		
Extracapsular extension	11%	44%
Site of extracapsular extension	Anterolateral and apical	Lateral
Average tumour size with extracapsular extension	4.98 cm^3	3.86 cm^3
Risk of seminal vesicle invasion	0%	19%
Risk of lymph node metastases	Low	High

* Central zone cancers (5–10% of total) were excluded.
BPH, benign prostatic hyperplasia; TURP, transurethral resection of the prostate; AAH, atypical adenomatous hyperplasia; PIN, prostatic intraepithelial neoplasia.

examination to separate unilateral and bilateral tumours or small and large tumours (tumour diameter less than or greater than 1.5 cm). However, digital rectal examination is inaccurate in measuring tumour size and pathological stage. In a study of radical prostatectomy specimens at the Mayo Clinic, we found considerable overlap of cancer volume in clinical stages T2a+b and T2c, with tumours measuring up to 41 and 43 cm^3, respectively. Also, the problem of interobserver variability with digital rectal examination reported in the literature is substantial. These data suggest that a modality other than digital rectal examination is needed for accurate preoperative assessment of tumour extent and volume.

Transrectal ultrasound (TRUS) allows detection of non-palpable cancers and ensures accurate guided biopsy of many suspicious lesions; however, up to 30% of cancers may be missed by TRUS. The current minimum size threshold of detection for 7 MHz transducers is about 7 mm in diameter (4 mm lateral resolution), but most tumours that small will be overlooked (7 mm diameter is about 0.2 cm^3 in volume if a perfect sphere). Shinohara *et al.* [19] visualized only 19% of tumours less than 10 mm by TRUS, and found that size was underestimated by a mean diameter of 5.8 mm despite a significant positive correlation between TRUS tumour size and pathological size ($r = 0.83$, linear regression). Lee *et al.* [20] identified only 13% of tumours with a mean diameter of 7.3 mm after correlation of TRUS with serially sectioned radical prostatectomy specimens. They concluded that tumours detected by TRUS are not small and clinically innocuous, but rather should be considered significant.

TRUS offers promise for preoperative measurement of tumour volume, but controlled studies are needed to address this issue. A recent prospective study found that TRUS was imperfect in preoperative staging of palpable prostate cancer (64% sensitivity, 46% specificity), and was not accurate for volume determination [21]. TRUS-based tumour volume measurement also lacks standardization; for example, which method of measurement is best – mean or maximum diameter? Which volume calculation should be used – ellipsoid (width × height × length × 0.532) or some other? How does one deal with multifocal tumours – measure only the dominant focus or add the dimensions of all foci? Lee *et al.* [22] proposed a TRUS staging system based on tumour volume (average tumour dimension): UA ⩽ 1.0 cm; UB1 = 1.0–1.5 cm; and UB2+ > 1.5 cm. Further advances in ultrasound technology such as colour Doppler and three-dimensional imaging offer promise, but are not currently practical for measuring tumour extent or volume.

Several studies have found a positive correlation between serum PSA concentration and tumour volume, and preoperative PSA determination may be useful for estimating tumour volume, although it is inexact (Fig. 2.7) [16]. The additive and confounding effect of BPH limits the usefulness of PSA in estimating preoperative tumour size and extent. As cancer enlarges, it usually becomes less differentiated and loses some of its capacity for PSA production. PSA concentration increases with increasing Gleason grade, but when tumour volume is held constant, PSA concentration actually decreased (PSA declined as Gleason grade increased). This finding was probably due to less production of PSA *per cell* in higher-grade tumours (Fig. 2.8).

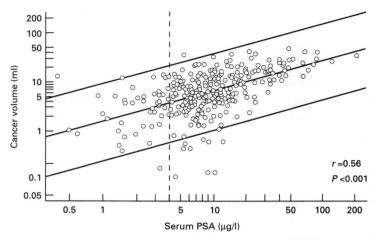

Fig. 2.7 Preoperative serum prostate-specific antigen (PSA) and its relationship to prostate cancer volume in 311 patients treated with radical retropubic prostatectomy. Parallel lines indicate 95% confidence limits for prediction of cancer volume; vertical line indicates upper limit of normal serum prostate-specific antigen value. From Blackwell *et al.*, [16] with permission.

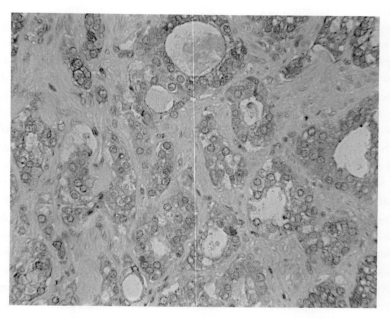

Fig. 2.8 Immunoreactivity of prostate-specific antigen in moderately differentiated cancer. Note heterogeneity of staining.

The combination of serum PSA and TRUS enhances the accuracy of preoperative tumour volume prediction. Lee *et al.* [22] calculated the predicted PSA concentration (TRUS gland volume × 0.20 ng/ml per gram = polyclonal PSA), subtracted this value from the serum PSA and considered the excess PSA unaccounted for by gland volume to be due to tumour; they then found tumour size by dividing 'excess' PSA by that expected to be produced by cancer, based on the assumptions of 3.0 ng/ml per gram cancer, 9 ng/ml 'excess' PSA per 3 cm^3 tumour volume and 3 cm^3 per 1.5 cm average TRUS diameter. These authors reported that this approach significantly increased the specificity and positive predictive value of PSA and allowed better preoperative differentiation of BPH and cancer than PSA alone.

Wolf *et al.* [24] also combined serum PSA and TRUS, but further enhanced the accuracy of preoperative tumour staging by considering a third variable – tumour grade. They calculated the 'expected' PSA level for each patient as follows: K × volume of TRUS hypoechoic area + 0.07 ng/ml × TRUS gland volume; K was 2.1 ng/ml if the Gleason score was greater than or equal to 7, and 4.2 if the score was less than 7. This PSA formula allowed preoperative prediction of stage in 48 men undergoing radical prostatectomy with 84% sensitivity, 82% specificity, 94% positive predictive value and 83% accuracy.

What is the predictive value of needle biopsy tumour volume?

The ability of needle biopsy to predict tumour volume in the prostate is uncertain. We [25] undertook a retrospective study of 162 patients with prostate cancer and compared the tumour burden on needle biopsy with matched step-sectioned whole-mounted radical prostatectomies. Linear regression analysis revealed a weak correlation of the amount of tumour on needle biopsy and prostatectomy ($r = 0.39$). Further, low tumour burden on needle biopsy did not appear predictive of low-volume prostate cancer, whether measured as a percentage of biopsy cores involved, percentage of cancer area in biopsy cores, millimetres of cancer in the entire biopsy, or millimetres of cancer per core. Patients with less than 30% of cores involved had a mean volume of 6.06 cm^3 (range 0.19–16.8 cm^3), indicating that the amount of tumour on transrectal needle biopsy was a poor predictor of tumour volume and should not influence therapeutic decisions. This study was limited by the variability in needle biopsy sampling, with the number of cores ranging from 1 to 18 (mean 5.7), but is probably reflective of current urological practice.

Other investigators have used systematic sextant biopsy and found a much stronger correlation of tumour burden in core biopsies with lymph node metastases. Hammerer *et al.* [26] found positive lymph node metastases in 52 of 57 patients (91% specificity) and 10 of 14 patients (71% sensitivity) when cancer replaced two core biopsies and 80% of a third from the sextant sample. They noted that the addition of grade to tumour volume further improved the sensitivity and specificity of this procedure. Terris *et al.* [27] developed algorithms to increase the accuracy of preoperative volume estimates by combining serum PSA level with TRUS volume as measured by 2 mm axial step sections, biopsy Gleason grade, and amount of cancer in systematic sextant biopsies; they found an excellent correlation ($r^2 = 0.76$) for organ-confined cancer and noted that digital rectal examination added no additional information to the multiple regression analysis.

The cumulative data suggest that systematic sextant biopsies may be useful in estimating tumour volume, but less vigorous methods of sampling are not effective. However, these methods are not adequate for use in individual patients, according to Terris *et al.* [27].

What is the predictive value of cancer volume in TURP specimens?

Current staging systems separate non-palpable TURP-detected cancers into stages T1a and T1b based upon a variety of methods, including counting positive chips, estimating the area of cancer, estimating the volume of cancer, calculating the ratio of benign to malignant chips, calculating the ratio of malignant to total grids (area) and counting cancer foci [3]. The lack of a universal standard for substaging non-palpable tumours has hampered progress.

However, even if a standard for substaging is established, it would not resolve the significant problem of clinical understaging by TURP. The sensitivity of TURP in detecting stage A carcinoma is only 28%, and up to 60% of patients with stage T1a tumours who undergo repeat TURP have residual cancer, with 26% of these being upstaged [3]. Also, the presence and amount of residual tumour cannot be predicted from the TURP specimen. Christensen *et al.* [28] found that 10 of 39 men (26%) with clinical stage T1b carcinoma had higher final pathological stage (8 were stage T3, 2 were stage N+), and all had residual cancer. Interestingly, they found that the final pathological stage correlated with tumour volume and Gleason grade in both TURP and radical prostatectomy specimens. The aggregate results challenge the utility of examining TURP specimens to stage prostate cancer; a volume-based prognostic index has recently been proposed as a possible adjunct or replacement [29].

How does tumour volume correlate with pathological stage?

As tumour volume increases, the likelihood and extent of capsular perforation increase, according to virtually every report addressing this issue [23, 30]. A recent review of the literature found a 10% probability of capsular perforation in tumours measuring about $0.5 \, cm^3$, rising to a level of 50% probability at $6.0 \, cm^3$ (Fig. 2.9). We found capsular perforation or seminal vesicle invasion in 41% of prostatectomies, with a positive correlation with tumour volume. The strong association of tumour volume and capsular perforation has been consistently identified in numerous reports despite variations in methods of volume quantitation and differences in definitions of capsular perforation.

As tumour size increases, the likelihood and extent of seminal vesicle invasion also increase. Cumulative evidence from numerous studies shows a 10% probability of seminal vesicle invasion in tumours measuring about $4.0 \, cm^3$, rising to 50% at $10.0 \, cm^3$ (Fig. 2.9).

Small prostate cancers rarely metastasize, and there is a strong positive correlation of tumour volume and lymph node metastases. According to a recent review, there is a 10% probability of metastases in tumours measuring about $5.0 \, cm^3$, rising to 50% at $13.0 \, cm^3$. McNeal *et al.* [30] studied 209 prostatectomy specimens from patients with clinically localized tumours, and found no metastases in 125 patients with tumours less than $4.0 \, cm^3$, while

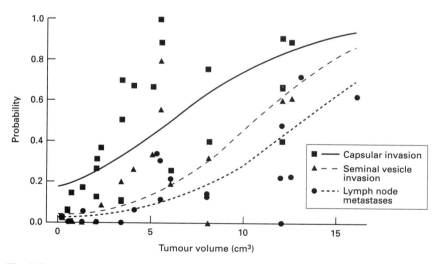

Fig. 2.9 Correlation of tumour volume with probability of capsular invasion, seminal vesicle invasion and metastases. Data are derived from a literature review of nine published studies of serially sectioned totally embedded prostates. From Bostwick *et al.*, [23] with permission.

those with tumours between 4.0 and $16.0\,\text{cm}^3$ had a 21% incidence of metastases, and those with tumours larger than $16.0\,\text{cm}^3$ had a 62% incidence of metastases. Other reports have confirmed the positive correlation of tumour size and metastases, including autopsy studies and clinical studies of stages T1 and T2. We found that cancer volume is predictive of pelvic lymph node metastases, although no significant difference was found between unilateral and bilateral nodal involvement.

Can tumour volume predict survival?

The relationship between tumour volume and patient survival is uncertain. Despite the limited data concerning tumour volume and survival, there is a strong relation of volume with other known predictors of survival such as capsular perforation, seminal vesicle invasion and lymph node metastases. If these are considered as surrogates of patient survival pending results of long-term follow-up studies, then tumour volume will probably be found to be useful in predicting patient survival. Mukamel *et al.* [31] have shown that these factors are significant in predicting tumour recurrence and progression.

Tumour volume and the growth rate of prostatic carcinoma

The volume of low-grade latent prostate cancer is an important marker for the risk of tumour progression, according to Whittemore *et al.* [32]. They combined data from the Surveillance, Epidemiology, and End Results (SEER) programme of the National Cancer Institute with autopsy data from their own institution and showed that the transformation of low-grade to high-grade cancer was proportional to tumour volume, but independent of patient age and race. They predicted that, on average, 2.4 of 100 men with $1.0\,\text{cm}^3$ of low-grade cancer will present with high-grade cancer within 7 years. This hypothesis explains the disparity in the incidence of clinical cancer and autopsy cancer, as well as the disparity in the steep rise in clinical incidence of cancer and the slow rise of latent career prevalence.

Progression of cancer at all body sites is related to cancer volume, with the probability of metastasis increasing with increasing tumour volume, presumably due to greater number of mitotic figures creating genetic instability and tumour heterogeneity. Lowe and Listrom [33] showed that prostate cancer volume and grade are proportional to the probability of progression.

Summary and conclusions

It is essential to separate preoperatively patients with clinically significant and insignificant prostate cancer (those that will progress and those that will not within the expected life span of the patient). However, current methods cannot assess the behaviour of prostate cancer with a sufficient level of accuracy to predict the outcome for an individual patient, limiting the ability to stratify patients effectively for therapy. Pathological factors derived from needle biopsies and prostatectomy specimens provide the greatest predictive accuracy, including tumour grade, volume, serum PSA concentration and clinical stage. Additional factors may improve the predictability of prostate cancer extent and behaviour.

References

1 Chung LWK. Implications of stromal–epithelial interaction in human prostate cancer growth, progression and differentiation. *Semin Cancer Biol* 1993; **4**: 183–192.
2 McNeal JE & Bostwick DG. Anatomy of the prostate: implications for disease. In: *Pathology of the Prostate*. Bostwick DG, ed. New York: Churchill Livingstone, 1990, pp. 1–14.
3 Bostwick DG, Myers RP & Oesterling JE. Staging of prostate cancer. *Semin Surg Oncol* 1994; **10**: 60–73.
4 Hall GS, Kramer CE & Epstein JI. Evaluation of radical prostatectomy specimens: a comparative analysis of sampling methods. *Am J Surg Pathol* 1992; **16**: 315–324.
5 Haggman M, Norberg M, de la Torre M *et al.* Characterization of localized prostatic cancer: distribution, grading and pT-staging in radical prostatectomy specimens. *Scand J Urol Nephrol* 1993; **27**: 7–13.
6 Humphrey PA & Vollmer RT. Intraglandular tumor extent and prognosis in prostatic carcinoma: application of a grid method to prostatectomy specimens. *Hum Pathol* 1990; **21**: 799–804.
** 7 Henson DE, Hutter RVP & Farrow GM. Practice protocol for the examination of specimens removed from patients with carcinoma of the prostate gland: a publication of the cancer committee, College of American Pathologists. *Arch Pathol Lab Med* 1994; **118**: 779–783.
** 8 Bostwick DG, Cooner WH, Denis L, Jones GW, Scardino PT & Murphy GP. The association of benign prostatic hyperplasia and cancer of the prostate. *Cancer* 1992; **70**: 291–301.
** 9 Bostwick DG. High grade prostatic intraepithelial neoplasia (PIN): the most likely precursor of prostate cancer. *Cancer* 1993; **75**: 1823–1836.
10 Sakr WA, Haas GP, Cassin BJ, Pontes JE & Crissman JD. The frequency of carcinoma and intraepithelial neoplasia of the prostate in young male patients. *J Urol* 1993; **150: 379–385.

* Reference of special interest.
** Reference of outstanding merit.

Chapter 2

11 Bostwick DG & Brawer MK. Prostatic intra-epithelial neoplasia and early invasion in prostate cancer. *Cancer* 1987; **59**: 788–794.

*12 Davidson D, Bostwick DG, Siroky M *et al.* Prostatic intraepithelial neoplasia is predictive of adenocarcinoma. *Mod Pathol* 1994; 7: 72A.

13 Davidson D, Bostwick DG, Qian J *et al.* Prostatic intraepithelial neoplasia is a risk factor for adenocarcinoma: Predictive accuracy in needle biopsies. *J Urol* 1995; **154: 1295–1299.

14 Bostwick DG, Qian J, Frankel K. The incidence of high grade prostatic intraepithelial neoplasia in needle biopsies. *J Urol* 1995; **154**: 1791–1794.

15 Bostwick DG & Dundore PD. *Prostate Needle Biopsy Interpretation.* London: Chapman & Hall, 1996 (in press).

16 Blackwell KL, Bostwick DG, Myers RP, Zincke H & Oesterling JE. Combining prostate specific antigen with cancer and gland volume to predict more reliably pathological stage: the influence of prostate specific antigen cancer density. *J Urol* 1994; **151**: 1565–1570.

17 Hanks GE, D'Amico A, Epstein BE & Schultheiss TE. Prostatic-specific antigen doubling times in patients with prostate cancer: a potentially useful reflection of tumor doubling time. *Int J Rad Oncol Biol Phys* 1993; **27**: 125–127.

18 Schmid HP, McNeal JE & Starney TA. Observations on the doubling time of prostate cancer. The use of serial prostate-specific antigen in patients with untreated disease as a measure of increasing cancer volume. *Cancer* 1993; **71**: 2031–2040.

19 Shinohara K, Scardino PT, Carter SSC & Wheeler TM. Pathologic basis of the sonographic appearance of the normal and malignant prostate. *Urol Clin N Am* 1989; **16**: 675–691.

20 Lee F, Torp-Pedersen S, Littrup PJ *et al.* Hypoechoic lesions of the prostate: clinical relevance of tumor size, digital rectal examination, and prostate-specific antigen. *Radiology* 1989; **170**: 29–32.

*21 Rifkin MD, Zerhouni EA, Garsonis CA *et al.* Comparison of magnetic resonance imaging and ultrasonography in staging early prostate cancer: results of a multi-institutional cooperative trial. *N Engl J Med* 1990; **323**: 621–627.

22 Lee F, Littrup PJ, Loft-Christensen L *et al.* Predicted prostate specific antigen results using transrectal ultrasound gland volume. *Cancer* 1992; **70** (suppl): 211–220.

23 Bostwick DG, Graham SD Jr, Napalkov P *et al.* Staging of early prostate cancer: a proposed tumor volume-based prognostic index. *Urology* 1993; **41**: 403–409.

24 Wolf JS Jr, Shinohara K & Narayan P. Staging of prostate cancer. Accuracy of transrectal ultrasound enhanced by prostate-specific antigen. *Br J Urol* 1992; **70**: 534–541.

*25 Cupp MR, Bostwick DG, Myers RP & Oesterling JE. The volume of prostate cancer in the biopsy specimen cannot reliably predict the quantity of cancer in the radical prostatectomy specimen on an individual basis. *J Urol* 1995; **153**: 1543–1548.

26 Hammerer P, Huland H & Sparenberg S. Digital rectal examination, imaging, and systematic-sextant biopsy in identifying operable lymph node-negative prostatic carcinoma. *Eur Urol* 1992; **22**: 281–287.

*27 Terris MK, Haney DJ, Johnstone IM, McNeal JE & Stamey TA. Prediction of prostate cancer volume using prostate-specific antigen levels, transrectal ultrasound, and systematic sextant biopsies. *Urology* 1995; **45**: 75–80.

28 Christensen WN, Partin AW, Walsh PC & Epstein JI. Pathologic findings in clinical stage A2 prostate cancer. Relation of tumor volume, grade and location to pathologic stage. *Cancer* 1990; **65**: 1021–1027.

*29 McNeal JE, Bostwick DG, Kindrachuk RA *et al.* Patterns of progression in prostate cancer. *Lancet* 1986; **1**: 60–63.

30 McNeal JE, Villers AA, Redwine EA, Freiha FS & Stamey TA. Capsular penetration in prostate cancer. Significance for natural history and treatment. *Am J Surg Pathol* 1990; **14**: 240–247.

31 Mukamel E, deKernion JB, Dorey F & Hannah J. Significance of histological prognostic indicators in patients with carcinoma of the prostate. *Br J Urol* 1990; **65**: 46–51.

32 Whittemore AS, Keller JB & Betensky R. Low-grade, latent prostate cancer volume: predictor of clinical cancer incidence? *J Natl Cancer Inst* 1991; **83**: 1231–1235.

33 Lowe BA & Listrom MB. Incidental carcinoma of the prostate: an analysis of the predictors of progression. *J Urol* 1988; **140**: 1340–1344.

3/Induction and Growth of Prostate Cancer

F.K. Habib

Introduction

Prostate cancer is now the commonest diagnosed tumour and the second leading cause of cancer death amongst the male population in the Western world. In the UK alone 7500 men died of the disease in 1986 and the death figure has risen to 9900 in 1988. As long as our understanding of the natural history of this disease remains incomplete then unfortunately this alarming trend will go on increasing unabated.

The disease exhibits an improved prognosis when discovered early but most frequently the cancer has already spread and there is no effect of treatment at that stage [1]. Indeed 5 year survival rates for patients with prostate cancer range from 88% for those with localized disease to 29% for those with metastatic disease. One limiting factor in our efforts to diagnose the disease is the absence of sufficient knowledge about the prostate in both its normal and neoplastic states. An understanding of the molecular events associated with normal development and differentiation should open the way for a better view of the cellular mechanisms leading to neoplastic transformation; these should provide the necessary tools for the future treatment of this all too common and life threatening condition.

Foetal prostate – hormonal aspects

As a result of the elegant studies undertaken by Cunha and his coworkers [2] new evidence establishing the importance of mesenchymal and stromal cells in prostatic development, growth and cyto-differentiation has been provided. Analysis of recombinant tissue consisting of urogenital sinus mesenchyme from wild-type mice and epithelium from the urinary bladders of testicular feminization mice (Tfm) has shown that in the developing prostate of the foetus and neonate it is the mesenchyme that is the actual target and mediator of androgenic effects upon the epithelium: androgen-dependent events are expressed in Tfm epithelial cells which are devoid of nuclear androgen binding sites, while the associated wild-type stromal cells have androgen receptors. Similarly mature prostatic epithelial cells lacking androgen receptors can

50

express a typical growth response following androgenic stimulation. Thus, the proliferative effect of androgens upon prostatic epithelium is not a direct effect mediated by intraepithelial androgen receptors but rather it appears to be elicited directly via regulatory influences from androgen-positive stromal cells. Microdissection and autoradiographic analysis of the recombinant tissue demonstrates important regional heterogeneities in ductal organization both between and within the lobes of the mouse prostate. So far three main regions have been identified; the proliferative region at the tip of the duct, the secretory region in the distal and intermediate segments, which accounts for approximately 90% of the ductal system, and the non-secretory cells located in the proximal region of the duct and immediately adjacent to the urethra [3–5]. Surrounding the ductal regions are the stromal/fibroblast components of the prostate which support the epithelial outgrowth. Although the process that induces ductal morphogenesis is androgen-sensitive, differences exist in the response to the androgens, depending on the region of the ductal system: the luminal epithelial cells of the intermediate segments of the ducts are androgen-sensitive and their secretory activity is dependent on the availability of the steroid, whereas the luminal epithelial cells of the proximal region are androgen-independent [6]. The results of *in vitro* studies with human primary epithelial cells are also consistent with the concept of indirect androgen action and with the possible existence of androgen-independent growth inducing activity of mesenchymal origin [7].

Further support for the importance of stroma/epithelial interactions in the growth and maintenance of the prostate comes from the studies of McNeal [8] who found that the primary lesion of benign prostatic hypertrophy (BPH) was not the formation of stromal nodules but a glandular budding and branching mechanism which gave rise to new alveoli in the prostatic zone. It should also be noted that the stroma surrounding the ducts also manifest regional heterogeneity as far as the distribution of small muscle cells are concerned: in prostatic stroma of the distal segments there is only a single layer of small muscle cells surrounding the epithelial cells whereas in the proximal region there are as many as four to five layers. Prostatic fibroblasts, on the other hand, would appear to be evenly distributed throughout the stroma of the ductal system. It is therefore possible that the regional heterogeneity and androgen responsiveness is due to the regional variation in the distribution of prostatic fibroblast in smooth muscle [9]; this in turn might regulate the relative expression of the androgenic pathways within the prostate. It is also worth noting that the stroma/epithelial interactions in the gland are influenced also by the nature of extracellular matrices that underlie the epithelial cells in the gland. Indeed, some of the earlier reports failed to establish the presence of basal epithelial cells in the hormone-responsive secretory regions of the prostate ductal system. However these same studies demonstrated continuous layers of basal cells intertwined between the stromal compartment and the luminal epithelial cells of the androgen insensitive proximal region of the duct [6]. It is not evident whether the interaction of the stromal/epithelial cells with basement membrane components including collagen 4, laminin, fibronectin and heparin sulphate proteoglycans could possibly account for the differences in androgen-sensitivity amongst the different regions of the ductal system. Such inter cellular dependence highlights a tight interactive circuit that influences growth and proliferation and demonstrates the complexity of the events which are responsible for the development of prostate cancer. However, the importance of the stroma in controlling prostatic morphogenesis is further underlined by the recent experiments showing that the transfection of *ras* plus *myc* oncogenes into urogenital mesenchyme promotes malignant conversion of the epithelial component [10]. This transformation to the neoplastic state is also accompanied by a change in the metabolic profiles of the gland.

Growth inhibitory factors in normal prostate compared to those in benign prostatic hypertrophy and prostate cancer

Human prostate requires a continuous supply of testosterone for its growth-development, differentiation and function. Removal of the source of these androgens by surgical or medical castration causes prostatic involution. The subsequent administration of exogenous androgens results in regrowth of the prostate gland but only to its original size [11]. This suggests that factors other than the systemic ones might possibly be involved in the development and maintenance of the gland. Attempts will therefore be made to identify some of these factors and to highlight their role in the induction of prostate cancer.

Testosterone and 5-α reductase

On entering the prostate gland, testosterone metabolizes to dihydrotestosterone (DHT) in a reaction catalysed by the nuclear membrane bound steroid 5-α reductase enzyme. The conversion of testosterone into DHT is essential both for the formation of the complete male phenotype during embryogenesis and for androgen-mediated growth of secondary sex organs such as the prostate [12]. Single gene defects that impair this conversion lead to pseudohermaphroditism in which 46 X,Y males have male internal urogenital tracts but female external genitalia [13]. In man, two separate genes encoding two steroid 5-α reductase isoenzymes with 50% sequence homology, designated type I and type II have been cloned [14–15]. The type I enzyme which maps to chromosome 5 has a neutral basic pH optimum and is expressed mainly in non-genital skin and liver. Type II enzyme, located on chromosome 2, is predominantly associated with prostate and genital skin and has an acidic pH optimum. The mechanism regulating 5-α reductase gene expression is unusual. In rat prostate, DHT induces expression of its own steroid 5-α reductase which is secondary to enhancement of 5-α reductase mRNA levels [16]. This in turn increases DHT synthesis thereby triggering a positive developmental cascade resulting in a feedforward control of prostatic growth. It is not clear whether a similar mechanism is found in human prostate tissue, the little evidence available suggests that the controlling mechanism might be different in the human gland: treatment of a group of BPH patients with 5-α reductase inhibitors inhibited the 5-α reductase activity of the gland but appeared not to reduce the expression of the gene itself [17]. Furthermore, no one has so far elucidated the exact distribution of the 5-α reductase in the human prostate but the initial studies on the mRNA expression employing reverse transcription-polymerase chain reaction (RT-PCR) suggests that the type I and type II were found in both stromal and epithelial cells and this was also confirmed by Northern blot analysis [18]. In some of the earlier studies it was also demonstrated that 5-α reductase (type I and type II) mRNA levels were markedly lower in BPH affected subjects than in young adult men and old normal subjects [18]. This was attributed to the lower epithelium/stroma ration in BPH patients when compared to men with normal prostate and to the preferential location of the 5-α reductase in the epithelial compartments of the prostate gland. However, our own studies have found the 5-α reductase isoenzymes were invariably located in the epithelial and stromal compartments of the gland and their ratios varied not only from patient to patient but also in different regions within the same gland. We also reported a loss of 5-α reductase activity in prostate cancer but the causes for this down-regulation in 5-α reductase activity is not clear and we are, at present, investigating the possibility of mutational changes in the gene for the type I and type II 5-α reductase enzymes. Significantly the 5-α reductase in prostate cancer patients mirrors the hormone sensitivity of the gland. In a retrospective study involving 19 patients with prostate cancer, it was found that those patients who failed to respond to endocrine therapy, showed little or no 5-α reductase activity whereas the bulk of the responders exhibited significantly higher enzyme activity [19]. If indeed the 5-α reductase isoenzyme controls the sensitivity of the prostate gland to hormones then genetic manipulation might also open the way for a new approach to override the resistance of the tumour cell to endocrine therapy.

Androgen receptors

The formation of DHT/androgen receptor complexes is crucial to the biological pathways concerned with both growth regulation and synthesis of secretory proteins [20]. Binding of DHT to androgen receptors releases the DNA binding domain of the receptor protein, enabling it to associate with the genome, thereby modulating the transcription of specific genes and the regulation of particular biological responses. Although testosterone also binds to the androgen receptor, the importance of DHT to the action of androgen in the human prostate is highlighted by the fact that no development of prostate occurs in males with inherited 5-α reductase deficiency syndrome [21].

The presence of androgen receptors is essential but not, in itself, sufficient to maintain androgen responsiveness. Both abnormal growth and the development of hormonal unresponsiveness can occur in the presence of androgen receptors [22]. Nevertheless, regulation of many of the proliferative and secretory pathways in the prostate is mediated through steroid receptor complexes that interact with defined sequences near or within affected gene 'hormone-responsive elements' (HRE). The binding of the hormone receptor to HRE controls the efficiency of the transcription process which in turn, modulates the activity of specific androgen-responsive genes leading either to stimulation or inhibition of protein synthesis. The precise mechanism(s) and requirements of the interaction between androgen receptors and the responsive gene are not fully understood. Interestingly, androgens can also down-regulate, in an autologous fashion, the levels of androgen receptor transcripts. This is believed to be a factor in the gradual transition of the prostate to a hormone-refractory state [23]. The protein product arising from the translation of the androgen receptor mRNA transcripts exist as two different isoforms which migrate as a closely spaced doublet of a 110–112 kD on a polyacrylamide gel electrophoresis. Most receptors are present in the larger of the two forms; however it is evident that both will bind hormone and undergo transformation to a nuclear binding form.

The intracellular distribution of androgen receptors has been the subject of considerable controversy for many years [24], but with the introduction of monoclonal antibodies this issue has now been resolved. Immunohisto-chemical analysis of normal and hyperplastic prostate has identified the nucleus of epithelial and stromal cells as the specific site for androgen-receptor proteins [25]. In normal prostates, uniform staining of epithelial-cell nuclei was observed, whereas hyperplastic tissues revealed heterogenous staining. Furthermore, the proportion of androgen-receptor positive cells was found to be far greater in the epithelium than in the stroma for both normal and benign tissues which might account for the high levels of DHT in the epithelium of hyperplastic cells. Interestingly, androgen receptor content was significantly higher in well-differentiated adenocarcinoma compared to moderately and poorly differentiated cancers and this in a sense confirmed the earlier findings of this laboratory demonstrating high androgen receptor concentrations in patients with metastasis who had escaped hormonal therapy [26]. Of immediate relevance to these earlier reports are the recent findings showing that distant metastasis from prostate carcinoma express also androgen-receptor proteins [27]. Although very little is known about the structure of the androgen receptor in prostate cancer metastasis, analogy with the mutant androgen receptor detected in the lymph node derived prostate cancer cell line, LNCaP, suggests that there may be a point mutation in the metastasized cells which could account for their elevated receptor levels. In the case of LNCaP, the mutation changes amino acid 876 threonine (ACT) to alanine (GCT). This promotes a shift in the specificity of the androgen receptor of this cell line thereby prompting an increased preference for other steroid hormones; this characteristic is not associated with androgen receptors in normal cells [28]. It is possible that a similar mutation is present in the androgen receptor of the metastasizing prostate cell and this might render the secondaries responsive to other steroid androgens besides DHT. The mutated androgen receptor could also be activated by antiandrogens during androgen ablation therapy and this might account for the mechanism responsible for tumour progression as seen in patients following 'hormone escape'.

It is also uncertain whether it is possible to reverse the hormonal status of androgen-insensitive prostate cancer by introducing an androgen receptor gene to the cell. To test this possibility, an expression vector carrying androgen receptor cDNA was transfected into DU145 cells to determine the growth characteristics of this cell line in response to androgens and antiandrogen treatment [29]. Surprisingly, exposure of the transfected cells to androgens prompted a reduction in cell growth and a loss of characteristic associated with the malignant phenotype. These findings might have important implications to the future treatment of both androgen-dependent and independent prostate cancer.

There is also increasing evidence that substances other than androgens might have a role in the stimulation and suppression of androgen receptor mediated gene transcription [30]. A number of polypeptide growth factors such as insulin-like growth factor-1, keratinocyte growth factor and epidermal growth factor stimulate androgen-receptor dependent reporter gene activity; these effects might be mediated via the second messenger cyclic AMP which in turn enhances androgen effects [31].

Chapter 3

Peptide growth factors

The failure of androgens to induce a direct mitotic effect on epithelial cells of the prostate has encouraged researchers to explore alternative mechanisms. Recently, attention has focused on a group of peptide growth factors actively involved in intracellular signalling between epithelial and stromal elements. These processes are mediated through intra/inter cellular spaces whereupon the growth factors act locally either in a paracrine or autocrine fashion. Unlike classical endocrine hormones, each growth factor may be synthesized by a variety of tissues, both adult and embryonic and is thought to be released by many if not all cells in culture. Growth factors have a wide range of biological activities and are considered to be multi-functional agents [32].

Much of the earlier work on growth factors in the human prostate concentrated on the epidermal growth factor (EGF) family because of high concentrations of EGF found in prostate fluid. EGF is also a potent mitogen for primary culture of human prostate epithelial cells. The EGF peptide induces a stimulatory effect via a 170 kD receptor which is expressed in 90% of normal and BPH tissue but the concentrations may be different in the two tissue types whereas in the majority of prostate cancer EGF receptors were negative [33]. In BPH tissue, the receptors are confined to the basal or basement membrane site of glandular epithelial cells and are not present in the fibroblastic/stroma cell populations [34]. The reduced sensitivity of prostate cancer cells to EGF coincides with the development of a hormone refractive tumour, a phenomenon which may be linked to autologous production of other growth factors. In an attempt to investigate androgen-sensitive prostate cancer cell growth [35] PC-3 prostate cancer cells, which express little or no endogenous androgen receptors, were stably transfected with a normal human androgen receptor cDNA expression vector to provide a useful model for delineating the relationship between EGF-receptor pathway and androgen sensitivity in prostate cancer cells. The results suggested the dihydrotestosterone increased both EGF receptor number and receptor ligand affinity and that these effects correlated with increased EGF binding and an enhanced mitogenic response to EGF. Whether similar responses are manifested in the human prostate has not been demonstrated so far even though the down-regulation of EGF receptor as reported in prostate cancer takes place at a time when 5-α reductase activity of the gland is at its lowest. Nevertheless, a pattern of events is emerging whereby metabolism of testosterone to DHT by the fibroblast/stroma compartment initiates secretion of EGF which, in turn, acts in a paracrine fashion on epithelial cells to stimulate their growth. However, because of the interdependence between stroma and epithelium, it is possible that *in vivo* these proliferative effects are further amplified through interaction with other growth factors. In this respect the role of the trans-forming growth factor (TGF)-β families is of particular interest because of their reported implication on the pathogenesis of prostate disease [36]. The actions of TGF-β may be stimulatory or inhibitory depending on the cell types, growth conditions, state of differentiation and on the presence of other growth factors. TGF-β was found to be inhibitory to both epithelial cells and fibroblast stroma though the latter was found to be far more sensitive to the presence of TGF-β [37]. In addition TGF-β is known to modulate cellular responses to other growth factors. Recent studies in our laboratory have demonstrated that the inhibitory action of TGF-β on fibroblasts was totally reversed and stimu-lation was induced following co-supplementation of the primary culture growth medium with exogenous EGF [37]. Interestingly, the synergistic action of TGF-β with EGF had no effect on epithelial cells even though EGF receptors were located exclusively on epithelium. Whether the differential action of these two growth factors is manifested in the physiological system must be an intriguing possibility not least because the proliferation of the fibroblast/stroma cells at the expense of the epithelium could lead to devel-opment of BPH. In some systems, TGF-β induces its effects on the target cell by means of specific receptors but these have so far not been quantified in human prostate tissue even though the presence of these receptors had been demonstrated in rat prostate cancer cells. Indeed, the receptors in rat prostate are up-regulated during the active phase of prostatic cancer regression impli-cating TGF-β as an important factor in prostate cell growth following androgen withdrawal [38]. TGF-β was also found to regulate the production of FGF by fibroblasts [39]. Although several members of the FGF family have been identified, only basic FGF (bFGF) and acidic FGF (aFGF) have been implicated in prostate growth [40]. More recent experiments involving a third member of the FGF family, heparin binding growth factor-3 (HBGF-3) suggest that this growth factor might be involved in prostate growth. A new DNA construct was engineered into a mouse genome. This construct con-tained the *int*-2 gene which is associated with HBPG-3 production and was found to enlarge the prostate gland of the animal in a manner similar to human BPH [41]. There are also reports showing that aFGF mRNA is abundant in the rat prostate epithelium but those peptides disappear as the animal matures. However, the expression of aFGF mRNA in the slow-growing androgen responsive Dunning R3327PAP prostate carcinoma appears to be specific to the mesenchymal cells of the tumour leading to speculation that mesenchyme-derived aFGF supports the growth of the malignant epithelium in a paracrine fashion [42]. The production of α-FGF in the prostate was also found to be under hormonal control since castration reduced the level of this growth factor; these were subsequently returned to baseline levels after the administration of exogenous testosterone. Thus, there may be a role for FGF intervention in BPH and cancer as an adjunct to hormonal therapy but more studies are needed to clarify the nature of these interactions within the prostate.

Keratinocyte growth factor (KGF) is a fourth member of the FGF family. KGF is produced by fibroblast cells and induces a mitogenic activity on cultures of normal prostate epithelium [43]. This peptide mediates its effects via the same class of receptors as the other members of the FGF family but their sites of expression have not been localized.

Sites of action by intracellular pharmacological agents

Over the last decade we have witnessed a great surge in our understanding of mammalian cell biology with specific application to malignant transformation. This information is providing new insights into the mechanism of control in both the normal and cancer cells. Efforts are now being directed towards examining alternative approaches to the treatment of prostate cancer and new agents are being developed and tested for future application to the management of this disease. Even so, prostate cancer treatment has witnessed very little change since the early days of Professor Charles Huggins and hormone therapy still remains the only effective systemic treatment of any value.

In the previous section, an account was given of the role of growth factors in the development of prostate. However the progression to androgen independence may also occur via a mechanism in which the cells obtain the ability to respond to growth factors and autonomously produced growth factor receptors. Much effort has been geared towards exploiting this phenomenon and new agents that inhibit the influence of growth factors in the prostate cell have been developed with a view to stifling the progression of hormone resistant prostate cancers. Amongst the new generation of chemotherapeutic agents, are a number of new drugs with reported antagonistic effects towards a host of endogenous growth factors and of these, two have so far been used with a variable degree of success in the treatment of prostate cancer.

Suramin

Suramin is a hexasodium salt of 8,8'-(carbonylimin) bis-1,3,5-naphthalene-sulfonic acid which was shown to reverse the malignant transformation of fibroblasts caused by the simian sarcoma virus. The simian sarcoma virus transforms cells by virtue of expressing v-sis. The v-sis product has extensive homology with platelet derived growth factor (PDGF), binds to the PDGF receptor and transforms cells through an autocrine mechanism. Suramin binds to both the v-sis gene product and PDGF thereby blocking the interaction of either peptide with the PDGF receptor [44]. Suramin was also shown to act as an anti-cancer drug through its action as an antagonist of key cytokines [45]. The administration of suramin results in accumulation of heparin sulphates which inhibit the growth of human prostatic carcinoma cell lines [46]. Furthermore, suramin inhibits lysosomal enzymes including hyaluronidase, nucleic acid polymerases, protein kinase C, glycolysis and induces the differentiation of a number of cancer cell lines. A major drawback to suramin administration relates to its capacity to bind tightly to plasma proteins and this has led to some reservations about whether it would be active *in vivo*. There are a number of on-going clinical trials on hormone refractive prostate cancer employing suramin and the early signs indicate that the effectiveness of the drug is limited dramatically by the extent of disease [46] but the results are sufficiently promising to warrant continuation of the trials.

Somatostatin

Somatostatin is a naturally occurring cyclic tetradecapeptide which inhibits the release of growth hormone. Administration of somatostatin agonists to humans resulted in a marked decline of circulating growth hormone and IGF-1 levels [47]. However the clinical usefulness of somatostatin has been limited in the past by its extremely short plasma half-life. This was overcome by the development of long-acting somatostatin analogues which provide clinically useful agents for treatment of hormone-producing tumours. The exact mechanism of the anti-tumour effects of somatostatin is not known and its role in prostate physiology has not been well defined; besides brain, the prostate is the tissue with the highest concentration of somatostatin [48]. Somatostatin agonists have exhibited anti-tumour activity against prostatic carcinoma in combination with luteinizing hormone releasing hormone agonist and this was far more effective in inhibiting tumour growth than either agent alone [49]. The action of somatostatin analogues might be mediated via inhibition of the proliferative activity of prolactin on the prostate [50]. However, in recent clinical trials somatostatin agonists yielded unequivocal results when given to patients with advanced prostate cancer but this might have been the consequence of sub-optimal dosages and more aggressive usage of the agent will have to be considered [51].

Naturally other pharmacological agents are being developed and many of these will focus on the large array of growth factors acting on the prostate. Recently attention has focused on mechanisms associated with tissue homeostasis; these require a balance between cell proliferation and cell death. Any shift in the equilibrium between these two fundamental processes would lead to drastic changes in the physiological development of the normal prostate cell. Previously, much attention has been directed to processes associated with cell growth in human prostate tissue and little attention has been devoted to understanding the pathways responsible for cell death. This state of knowledge is being rectified and several laboratories are attempting to identify the genes responsible for the induction of apoptosis in the human prostate. Once these have been characterized and mechanisms identified, then this will open the way for another class of pharmaceutical agents directed at slowing down the growth of the tumour.

Programmed cell death and control of intracellular Ca^{2+}

The death of a cell can occur through several biochemically and morphologically distinct pathways. One pathway is necrotic cell death, elicited by any of a large variety of factors that lead to increased plasma membrane permeability with the resultant osmotic lysis of the cell and its internal membranes. In necrotic cell death, the cell has a passive role in initiating cell death. In contrast, there is a second pathway for cell death termed programmed cell death or apoptosis in which the cell actively participates in the initiation of its own death.

In programmed cell death, specific intracellular signals induce the cell to undergo an active, energy dependent process. Fragmentation of DNA is an early event that irreversibly commits the cell to die and occurs before changes in plasma and internal membrane permeability. In many systems, DNA fragmentation results from activation of the Ca^{2+}/Mg^{2+} dependent endonuclease which is present within the cell nucleus. This, in turn, selectively hydrolyses DNA at sites located between nucleosomal units and induces a stereotypical nucleosomal ladder of DNA fragments [52]. Endonuclease activation is thought to be triggered by sustained elevation in the intracellular free Ca^{2+} concentration initiated early in apoptosis.

Biochemical and morphological studies have demonstrated that involution of the normal prostate after castration is not the result of necrotic cell death but is an active process brought about by the initiation of a series of specific biochemical steps that lead to the programmed cell death of androgen-dependent glandular epithelial cells [53]. As with other systems in which programmed cell death occurs, there is initial fragmentation of genomic DNA followed by irreversible morphological changes which are histologically characteristic of apoptosis including: chromatic condensation, nuclear disintegration, cell surface blebbing and eventually cellular fragmentation into a cluster of membrane-bound apoptotic bodies.

Studies have demonstrated that not only rat prostatic cells but also human androgen-dependent prostate cancer cells activate the pathway of programmed cell death after androgen ablation. Unfortunately, approximately 60% of cases of prostate cancer are non-organ confined at the time of initial diagnosis and are therefore not candidates for curative surgery. These patients eventually require systemic androgen ablation therapy. Nearly all men with prostate cancer treated by androgen ablation respond initially, demonstrating that at least a proportion of their cancer cells are androgen responsive. However, almost all of these patients eventually relapse to a state unresponsive to further anti-androgen therapy, no matter how aggressive their secondary treatment. The epithelial cells of these tumours do not undergo apoptosis under such circumstances. It has been proposed that it is the proliferation of these cells that leads to tumour relapse and eventually death from the disease. Subsequent studies have demonstrated that androgen-dependent tumours can be induced to undergo programmed cell death through administration of cytotoxic drugs [38]. However, in the human prostate a high proportion of tumours are slow growing and contain a high proportion of non-proliferative androgen-independent cells which renders them refractive to cytoxic drugs. Recently, it has been shown that repression of Ca^{2+} levels in androgen-dependent cells following androgen ablation leads to the inhibition of the apoptotic process [54]. It was therefore suggested that the use of Ca^{2+} ionophores could lead to an elevation of intracellular Ca^{2+} by 3–6-fold above basal levels and this may induce programmed cell death in cells within 48–72 hours. Clearly manipulation of intracellular Ca^{2+} concentrations offers exciting new alternatives in the treatment of androgen-dependent prostate cancer and one foresees, in the coming years, substantial developments in this direction.

Angiogenesis and adherence factors

Angiogenesis is the formation of new capillaries from the existing vascular network and is essential to tumour growth [55]. Indeed without such a blood supply, tumours can not grow to more than 3 mm in diameter. Regulation of angiogenesis is effected by numerous 'angiogenic' peptides many of which have pleotropic effects. Two recently identified growth factors, vascular endothelial growth factor (VEGF) and platelet derived endothelial cell growth factor (PDEGF) have attracted particular attention since they are specific for endothelium [56]. This has been directly proven both by blocking the tumour-secreted angiogenic factor VEGF with antibodies and by introducing dominant negative VEGF receptors in endothelial cells to interfere with receptor signalling [57]. Angiogenesis is not only essential for the expansion of the primary tumour but is also required for growth of established metastasis at distant sites. Inhibition of vascularization or lack of an angiogenic phenotype for these metastases might explain how some tumour cells remain dormant. Whilst the quantification of angiogenesis in invasive breast carcinoma and bladder cancer is predictive of metastasis and survival no one has so far evaluated the biological role of tumour angiogenesis in both early and advanced prostate cancer.

Besides angiogenesis, the other step of particular relevance to the success of the metastatic process is the depletion in the levels of adhesion molecules at the primary sites. This leads to the loss of cell to cell contact and prompts the invasion by the tumour cell of the secondary organs. Of particular relevance to the prostate are the family of E-cadherin and fibronectin molecules whose expression in the primary prostate tumour is significantly down-regulated with the increasing invasiveness of the prostate tumour [58, 59]. In parallel with the loss of adhesion molecules at the primary site of the prostate, metastasis is also stimulated because of enhanced adhesion, chemotaxis or growth at the secondary sites. Adhesion molecules such as laminin and fibronectin are thought to be major determinants of site specific metastasis [60]. However the mechanism by which human prostate tumour cells induce new bone formation have yet to be determined.

Conclusions

Studies on experimental and human cancers have demonstrated that the proliferation of normal cells is regulated by growth-promoting proto-oncogenes and counter-balanced by growth-constraining tumour suppressor genes. Alteration in the activities of these genes will initiate a cascade of molecular and cellular events resulting in the progressive transformation of normal cells to full malignancy. In prostate cancer, our understanding of these processes remains unresolved. However, it is known that allelic loss is common in chromosomes 16q and 10q and that the region 11p11.2–13.3 may contain a metastasis suppressor gene. 11p13 is the chromosomal site of the oncogene Ha-*ras* which has a low mutation frequency in prostate cancers [61], but whether this is a contributory factor is unknown. Of the known tumour suppressor genes which may have associations with prostate cancer only p53 and *bcl*-2 show correlation with progression. However, within a complex multi-focal tumour, genetic mutations can not easily be related to progression [62]. There is also the important question of how the loss of hormone responsiveness in prostate cancer relates to the mutational inactivation of tumour suppressor genes. This is an area of active investigation. It is hoped that a fundamental understanding of the basic molecular events leading to the transformation of normal cells and the progression of urological tumours might provide the clinician with new tools in the diagnosis, prognosis and therapy of prostate cancer.

References

1 Carter HB & Coffey DS. The Prostate: an increasing medical problem. *The Prostate* 1990; **1**: 39–48.
** 2 Cunha GR, Donjacour AA, Cooke PS *et al.* The endocrinology and development biology of the prostate. *Endocrine Rev* 1987; **8**: 338–362.
3 Sugimura Y, Cunha GR & Donjacour AA. Morphogenesis of ductal networks in the mouse prostate. *Biology of Reprod* 1986; **34**: 961–971.
4 Lee C, Sensibar JA, Dudek SM, Hiipakka RA & Liao S. Prostatic ductal system in rats: regional variation and morphological and functional activities. *Biology of Reprod* 1990; **43**: 1079–1086.
* 5 Tenniswood MP, Montpetit ML, Leger JG, Wong P. Pineault JM & Rouleau M. Epithelial/stromal interactions and cell death in the prostate. In: *The Prostate as an Endocrine Gland*. Farnsworth WE & Ablin RJ eds. Bocca Raton, Florida: CRC Press, 1990, pp 187–207.
** 6 Rouleau M, Leger G & Tenniswood M. Ductal heterogeneity of cytokeratins, gene expression and cell death in the rat ventral prostate. *Mol Endocrin* 1990; **4**: 2003–2013.
7 Peehl DM & Stamey TA. Serum free growth of adult human prostate epithelial cells. *In Vitro Cell Devel Biol* 1986; **22**: 82–90.
8 McNeal JE. Origin and evolution of benign prostatic enlargement. *Invest Urol* 1978; **15**: 340–345.
9 Griffiths K, Akaza H, Eaton CL *et al.* Regulation of prostatic growth. In *The 2nd International Consultation on Benign Prostatic Hyperplasia (BPH)*. Cockett K, Aso Y, Chatelain G *et al.* eds. Paris: SCI Press, 1994, pp 49–75.
10 Thompson TC, Truong LD, Timme TL *et al.* Transforming growth factor $\beta1$ as a biomarker for prostate cancer. *J Cell Biochem* 1992; **16H** (suppl): 54–61.
11 Bruchovsky N, Lesser B, Vandoorn E & Craven S. Hormonal effects on cell proliferation in rat prostate. *Vitam Horm* 1975; **33**: 61–102.
12 Griffin CE & Wilson JD. Disorders of the testis and the male reproductive tract. In *Williams Textbook of Endocrinology*. Wilson JD & Foster DW, eds. 8th edn, Philadelphia: W B Saunders, 1992, pp 799–851.
13 Thigpen AE, Davis DL, Milatovich A *et al.* Molecular genetics of 5 alpha reductase II deficiency. *J Clin Invest* 1992; **90**: 799–809.
*14 Jenkins EP, Andersson S, Imperato-McGinley J, Wilson JD & Russell DW. Genetic and

* Reference of special interest.
** Reference of outstanding merit.

pharmacological evidence for more than one human steroid 5 alpha reductase. *J Clin Invest* 1992; **89**: 293–300.

15 Andersson S & Russell DW. Structural and biochemical properties of cloned and expressed human rat steroid 5 alpha reductases. *Proc Natl Acad Sci USA* 1990; **87**: 3640–3644.

*16 George FW, Russell DW & Wolfson JD. Feed-forward control of prostate growth; dihydrotestosterone induces expression of its own biosynthetic enzyme, steroid 5 alpha reductase. *Proc Natl Acad Sci USA* 1991; **88**: 8044–8047.

17 Habib FK, Ross M, Tate R, *et al.* Unpublished results.

18 Bonnet P, Reiter E, Bruyninx M *et al.* Benign prostatic hyperplasia and normal prostate aging: differences in type I and type II 5 alpha reductase and steroid hormone receptor messenger ribonucleic acid (mRNA) levels but not in insulin-like growth factor mRNA levels. *J Clin Endocrin Metab* 1993; **77**: 1203–1208.

19 Habib FK & Chisholm GD. Management of advanced prostate cancer: The biological basis of endocrine treatment. In *Urological Dilemma and Developments*. Bloom JG, ed. New York: Wiley & Sons, 1991, pp 191–201.

20 Montgomery BJ, Young CWF, Bilhartz DL *et al.* Hormone regulation of prostate specific antigen (PSA) glycoprotein in the human prostate adenocarcinoma cell line LNCaP. *The Prostate* 1992; 21: 63–73

*21 Imperato-McGinley J, Gautier T, Ziminsky T *et al.* Prostate visualisation studies in male homozygous and heterozygous for 5 alpha reductase deficiency. *J Clin Endocrin Metab* 1992; **75**: 1022–1026.

22 Diamond DA & Barrack AR. The relationship of androgen receptor levels of androgen responsiveness in the Dunning R-3327 rat prostate tumour sublines. *J Urol* 1994; **132**: 821–827.

23 Tilley WD, Wilson CM, Marcelli M & McPhaul MJ. Androgen receptor gene expression in human prostate carcinoma cell lines. *Cancer Res* 1900; **50**: 5382–5386.

24 Habib FK. Prostate mechanism of normal and abnormal metabolism. In: *Scientific Foundation of Urology*. Chisholm GD & Fair WR, eds. 3rd edn. London: Heinneman Medical Books, 1990, pp 358–365.

25 Chodak GW, Cranc DM, Libertad AP *et al.* Nuclear localisation of androgen receptor in heterogeneous samples of normal, hyperplastic and neoplastic human prostate. *J Urol* 1992; **147**: 798–803.

*26 Habib FK, Odoma S, Busuttil A & Chisholm GD. Androgen receptors in cancer of the prostate: Correlation with the stage and grade of the tumour on receptor content. *Cancer* 1986; **57**: 2351–2356.

27 Hobisch A, Culig Z, Radmayr C, Bartsch G, Klocker H & Hittmair A. Distant metastases from prostatic carcinoma express androgen receptor protein. *Cancer Res* 1995; **55**: 3068–3072.

*28 Brinkman AO. Androgen receptor of abnormalities. *J Steroid Biochem Mol Biol* 1991; **40**: 349–352.

29 Grant ES, Batchelor KW & Habib FK. The androgen-independence of primary epithelial cell cultures of the prostate is associated with a down-regulation of androgen receptor gene expression. *The Prostate* (in press).

30 Culig Z, Hobisch A, Cronauer MV *et al.* Androgen receptor activation of prostate tumour cell lines by insulin-like growth factor I, keratynosite growth factor and epidermal growth factor. *Cancer Res* 1994; **54**: 5474–5478.

31 Ikonen T, Palvimo JJ, Kallio PJ, Reinikainen P & Janne OA. Stimulation of androgen-

regulated transactivation by modulators of protein phosphorylation. *Endocrinology* 1994; **135**: 1359–1366.

32 Sporn MB & Roberts AB. Peptide growth factors are multi-functional. *Nature* 1988; **332: 217–219.

33 Maddy SQ, Chisholm GD, Busuttil A & Habibi FK. Epidermal growth factor receptors in human prostate cancer: correlation with histological differentiation of the tumour. *Br J Cancer* 1989; **60**: 41–44.

*34 Maddy SQ, Chisholm GD, Hawkins RA & Habib FK. Localization of epidermal growth factor receptors in the human prostate by biochemical and immunocytochemical methods. *J Endocrin* 1987; **112**: 147–153.

35 Brass AL, Bernard J, Batai BL, Salvi D & Rukstalis DB. Androgen up-regulated epidermal growth factor receptor expression in binding affinity PC3 cell lines expressed in the human androgen receptor. *Cancer Res* 1995; **55**: 3197–3123.

36 Foster CS. Structural and functional aspects of transforming growth factor β in prostate cancer and other human malignancies. *Human Pathol* 1993; **24**: 1–3.

*37 McKeehan W. Growth factor receptors and prostate cell growth. In *Cancer Surveys*. Issacs JT, ed. New York: Cold Spring Harbor Laboratory Press, 1991, pp. 165–173.

38 Kyprianou N & Isaacs JT. Expression of transforming growth factor beta in the rat ventral prostate during castration induced programme cell death. *Mol Endocrin* 1989; **3**: 1515–1522.

39 Storey MT, Baeten LA, Molter MA & Lawson RK. Influence of androgen in transforming growth factor beta on basic fibroblast growth factor levels in human prostate derived fibroblast cell cultures. *J Urol* 1990; **143**: 241A.

40 Gelman AP. Oncogenes and growth factors in prostate cancer. *J Natl Inst of Health Res* 1991; **3**: 62–64.

41 Muller WJ, Lee FS, Dickson C, Peters G, Pattengale P & Leder P. The int-2 gene product acts as an epithelial growth factor in transgenic mice. *EMBO J* 1990; **9: 907–913.

42 Thompson TC. Growth factors and oncogene in prostate cancer. *Cancer Cells* 1990; **2**: 345–354.

43 Yan G, Fukabori Y, Nikolaropoulos S, Wang F & McKeehan WL. Heparin binding keratinocyte growth factor is a candidate stromal to epithelial cell andromedin. *Mol Endocrin* 1992; **6**: 2123–2128.

44 Williams LT, Treble PM, Lavin MF & Sunday ME. Platelet derived growth factor receptors form a high affinity state in membrane preparations: Kinetics and affinity cross-linking studies. *J Biol Chem* 1984; **259**: 5287–5294.

45 Stein CA, La Rocca RV, Thomas R, McAtee M & Myers CE. Suramin: an anti-cancer drug with unique mechanism of action. *J Clin Oncol* 1989; **7**: 499–508.

46 Myers CE, Tripel J, Sartor O, Cooper M, Ranson M, Toko T & Linehan MW. Anti-growth factor strategies. *Cancer* 1993; **71**: 1172–1178.

47 Katz MD & Erstad BL. Octreotide, a new somatostatin analogue. *Clin Pharma* 1989; **8**: 255–273.

48 Sasaki AYK. Immunoreactive somatostatin in the male reproductive tract system in humans. *J Clin Endocrin Metab* 1989; **68**: 996–999.

*49 Schally AV. Oncological application of somatostatin analogues. *Cancer Res* 1988; **48**: 6977–6985.

*50 Rana A, Habib FK, Halliday P *et al.* A case for synchronous reduction of testicular androgen, adrenal androgen and prolactin for the treatment of advanced carcinoma of the prostate. *Eur J Cancer* 1995; **31A**: 871–875.

51 Carteni G, Biglietto M, Tucci A & Pacilio G. Sandostatin, a long acting somatostatin analogue in the treatment of advanced metastatic prostate cancer. *Eur J Cancer* 1990; **26**: 186.

52 Wiley AH, Kerr JFR & Currie AR. Cell death: The significance of apoptosis. *Int Rev Cytol* 1980; **68: 251–306.

53 Kyprianou N & Isaacs JT. An activation of programme cell death in the rat central prostate after castration. *Endocrin* 1988; **122**: 552–562.

54 Martikinen P, Kyprianou N, Tucker RW & Isaacs JT. Programme cell of non-proliferating androgen independent prostate cancer cells. *Cancer Res* 1991; **51**: 4693–4700.

*55 Folkman J. What is the evidence that tumours are angiogenesis dependent? *J Natl Cancer Inst* 1990; **82**: 4–6.

56 Bicknell R & Harris AL. Novel growth regulatory factors in tumour angiogenesis. *Eur J Cancer* 1991; **27**: 781–785.

57 Millauer B, Shawver LK, Plate KH, Risau W & Ullrich A. Glyoblastoma growth inhibited *in vivo* by a dominant negative FLK-1 mutant. *Nature* 1994; **367**: 576–579.

*58 Giroldi LA & Schalken JA. Decreased expression of the intracellular adhesion molecule E-cadherin in prostate cancer: Biological significance and clinical implications. *Cancer Metastat Rev* 1993; **12**: 29–37.

59 Schalken JA, Ebeling SB, Isaacs JT, Treiger B, Bussemakers MG, de gong M & Van der Ven W. Down modulation of fibronection messenger RNA in metastasising rat prostatic cancer cells revealed by differential hybridisation analysis. *Cancer Research* 1988; **48**: 2042–2046.

*60 Zetter BR. The cellular basis of site specific tumour metastasis. *New Eng J Med* 1990; **322**: 605–612.

61 Carter BS, Epstein J & Isaacs WB. Ras gene mutation in human prostate cancer. *Cancer Res* 1990; **50**: 6830–6832.

62 Sakr WA, Macoska GA, Benson P *et al*. Allelic loss in locally metastatic, multisampled prostate cancer. *Cancer Res* 1994; **54**: 3273–3277.

4/The Biology of Metastatic Prostate Cancer

M. Hussain

Introduction

A significant increase in the diagnosis of prostate cancer has resulted from intensified screening efforts and expansion of the ageing male population. Localized stage disease is now contributing to an increasing percentage of all diagnosed prostate cancer cases. While one might logically assume that diagnosis of earlier-stage disease should result in an overall survival improvement, data from surgical series coupled with recent observations on the presence of detectable circulating and bone marrow micrometastatic prostate cancer cells in patients with clinically localized prostate cancer raise concern regarding the potential curability of certain subsets of patients, particularly those with pathologically advanced local/locoregional disease with local therapy only. While improved understanding of the metastatic biology of prostate cancer provides the basis for designing more effective treatment strategies, the former has been hampered by limited ability to establish suitable human cell lines as well as *in vivo* and *in vitro* models. Therefore, observations regarding the biology of prostate cancer metastases would be derived from clues provided by the primary tumour together with years of follow-up.

Clinically, prostate cancer has a diverse behaviour with an intriguing progression and dissemination pattern. Despite a low doubling time and relatively low blood flow to bone, cancer cells have the tendency to metastasize preferentially to bone, where they develop a more rapid growth rate relative to the primary prostate cancer [1]. It has been well-established that pathological characteristics of primary prostate tumours can identify subsets of patients who are destined for systemic relapse; specifically these are tumour size, capsular penetration, seminal vesicle involvement, nodal metastases, margin positivity and tumour grade [2, 3]. Although considered as the primary clinical determinants of the disease's natural history, these factors collectively have not been predictive of prognosis at an individual level. Interest in improving the ability to prognosticate better outcome has led to the investigation of a variety of markers, most of which are related to the primary tumour in the prostate. Date on DNA ploidy, nuclear morphology, genetic instability, alteration in cell adhesion, enhanced angiogenesis and increased cellular motility, while not firmly established, appear to characterize more usefully the metastatic biology of a particular tumour [4].

While the importance of growth factors, cytokines, autocrine–paracrine regulatory mechanisms and stromal–epithelial interactions are recognized, interest has developed in the presence of neuropeptides or neuroendocrine differentiation in primary prostate cancer in relation to tumour growth, prognosis and treatment. Studies suggest that neuroendocrine differentiation occurs with relatively high frequency (frequency is increasing owing to better and more sensitive staining methods) and is associated with higher stage, higher grade, hormonal resistance and worse survival [5, 6].

As our understanding of this disease is evolving, it is clear that its biology is determined not only by the constitution of the tumour cells but also by the microenvironment surrounding these cells and the interaction between the two. The microenvironment, both at the primary and metastatic site, appears to be crucial for the cancer cells to thrive. At the metastatic site, in line with the 'seed and soil' hypothesis, recent experimental models suggest that bone stromal cells are capable of facilitating the growth of prostate cancer cells through paracrine and autocrine mechanisms. A variety of growth factors are implicated, for example, fibroblast growth factor (heparin-binding) was shown to be a potent growth stimulus for the formation of LNCaP tumours, stimulating angiogenesis and acting as chemotactic factor for mesenchyme-derived cells; insulin-like growth factors (IGF) and cytokines (interleukin-6: IL-6) also appear to play a stimulatory role in prostate cancer cell growth [7–9]. There is also evidence to suggest the presence of a paracrine interaction between prostate-specific antigen (PSA; secreted from prostate cancer cells) and IGFs (produced by bone stromal cells). PSA is able to digest IGF-binding protein, thus causing the release of IGF from its latent complex [10]. The latter may be one of the mechanisms responsible for the autonomous growth of androgen-independent prostate cancer cells [7]. Experimentally, an androgen-independent phenotype was derived from the interaction of the LNCaP cells with bone fibroblasts, suggesting that, perhaps, clinically such an interaction may be one of the factors fostering progression to androgen independence [11].

The natural history of metastatic disease

Micrometastatic disease

The presence of systemic micrometases at the time of initial diagnosis of prostate cancer is suggested by the outcome of several surgical series indicating that approximately 30% of patients with organ-confined prostate cancer and

60–80% of patients with extraprostatic disease will develop a relapse at 10 years despite potentially curative local therapy [2, 12–16]. Their presence is further supported by recent data using a sensitive molecular (reverse transcriptase polymerase chain reaction: RT-PCR) assay to detect PSA-RNA in the peripheral blood or bone marrow of patients with clinically localized prostate cancer. Preliminary reports indicate that 10–35% of patients with localized prostate cancer have detectable circulating prostate cancer cells and 20% of patients with pathologically organ-confined prostate cancer and 65% of patients with extraprostatic disease had micrometastases in bone marrow [17–20]. While the prognostic value of these observations has yet to be confirmed prospectively they are in line with the anticipated relapse rate of organ-confined and extraprostatic cancers.

PSA has been one of the most useful tumour markers in specifically predicting early prostate cancer relapse following local therapy despite lack of objective evidence for a relapse. Approximately 90% of patients have undetectable serum PSA within 1 month after radical prostatectomy and 90% have PSA levels in the normal range 12 months after radiation therapy [21]. Increasing PSA level after radiation therapy or a detectable level after surgery almost uniformly implies a systemic relapse or persistent disease. Accumulating data on rising PSA have altered our concepts of potential cure from prostate cancer following primary therapy and are shedding light with regard to the varying biology of this disease. D'Amico and Hanks [21] investigated PSA doubling time (DT) as a means of predicting clinical progression following primary radiation therapy. PSA DT was found to be a constant, i.e. signifying an exponential increase in the PSA value, and had a linear correlation with the interval to clinical relapse after PSA failure. Using this model the authors could delineate patients with aggressive tumour biology as having a PSA DT < 3.8 months versus a relatively indolent tumour biology where PSA DT is ⩾ 3.8 months.

Metastatic disease

Suppression of androgenic stimuli has remained the primary therapeutic strategy for metastatic prostate cancer. This has been achieved through primary gonadal suppression with or without an antiandrogen. While the issue remains somewhat controversial, data from two large randomized studies (NCIINT-0036 and EORTC-30853) indicate the superiority of the combined therapy approach; however, this is modest with only about 6 months' prolongation in median survival [22]. The inability of androgen deprivation (combined or monotherapy) to eradicate permanently all cancer cell populations, which is a prerequisite for the cure of a tumour, is evident by the pattern of a high initial response rate followed by progression of virtually all patients to androgen independence. While there is some variability in the course of the disease, the median survival of patients with hormone-refractory prostate cancer has remained dismal at about 40 weeks. We recently reported on patients' characteristics, disease course and outcome through the analysis of five phase II South West Oncology Group studies that evaluated a variety of chemotherapeutic agents in patients with hormone-refractory prostate cancer [23]. The focus was whether there were response or survival advantages to the continuation of androgen deprivation therapy in patients with hormone-refractory prostate cancer. Eighty-four per cent of the 205 evaluated patients were orchidectomized and 50% had more than one hormonal manipulation. The median survival durations for the non-orchidectomized patients (who were required to discontinue exogenous hormone therapy) and the orchidectomized patients were 6 and 7 months, respectively ($P = 0.73$). In a univariate analysis, orchidectomy patients had a significantly longer median time from diagnosis to first hormone therapy (1.1 versus 0.1 years), were more likely to have had chemotherapy initiated ≥ 2 years from diagnosis (75 versus 56%), had a lower incidence of liver metastases (16 versus 30%), and had a lower likelihood of being black (8 versus 18%). Absence of liver metastases, haemoglobin level ≥ 10 g/dl, acid phosphatase < 1.2 IU/l, response to chemotherapy and ≥ 2 years from initial hormone treatment were statistically significant factors for survival. Although retrospective, this analysis indicated that intrinsic biological factors seem to contribute to disease course and rate of progression and that as hormone-refractory prostate cancer approaches end-stage, there does not appear to be a beneficial effect to androgen withdrawal, suggesting that these patients not only have androgen-independent but also androgen-insensitive tumours. The lack of significant response rates to chemotherapy, while disappointing, is not surprising. The latter is a reflection of the nature of hormone-refractory prostate cancer with high tumour burden increasing the odds for multiple drug resistance mechanisms.

Mechanisms of tumour progression

The exact aetiology of the progression to androgen independence and hormone-refractory phenomenon in humans remains poorly understood; however, experimental data on the androgenic regulation of the prostate and prostate cancer have been instructive in that there appears to be a gradual and systematic shift in reliance on endocrine controls to paracrine and eventually autocrine controls.

Androgen effects on the target tissue occur via interaction with cellular receptor proteins to stimulate tissue-specific gene transcription, cellular metabolism and cell growth. In normal prostate three distinct phases are observed. A growth phase results from the stimulation of the undifferentiated cells to undergo DNA synthesis and proliferation. As a normal size is achieved, the growth phase is followed by a shutdown of further DNA synthesis and proliferation through negative regulatory mechanisms. The glandular size is maintained as long as androgens are present. The third phase ensues upon androgen withdrawal with rapid regression in the glandular size to basal levels due to the activation of a process of cellular suicide termed programmed cell death or apoptosis [24]. In prostate cancer these regulatory mechanisms are altered with a gradual loss of hormonal regulation. Androgens stimulate prostate cancer cells to undergo DNA synthesis and cellular proliferation but this growth phase is not checked by negative regulation. Androgen deprivation, therefore, will lead to inhibition of DNA synthesis and cellular proliferation and will induce active cell death. A tumour with these features is considered androgen-dependent, a condition akin clinically to hormone-naïve prostate cancer. The continued lack of androgenic exposure causes further loss in regulatory effects so that growth is still stimulated by androgens but the tumour cells lose their apoptotic potential, resulting in an androgen-sensitive but independent tumour, a situation clinically akin to early phases of hormone-refractory prostate cancer. Ultimately, with additional progression, control over DNA synthesis is lost, resulting in an androgen-independent and insensitive tumour which is a situation that is clinically comparable to end-stage hormone-refractory prostate cancer [24]. It has been proposed that this progression phenomenon may represent either an adaptation to an environment lacking androgen, a clonal selection secondary to androgen withdrawal, or a combination of both, thus indirectly implicating androgen deprivation as a mechanism for eventual progression despite an apparent clinical response.

Recent experimental data suggest that a series of events do occur, causing a systematic transition of prostate cancer through a spectrum of androgen dependence, androgen sensitivity and ultimately androgen insensitivity and that these events occur at basic levels of cellular control, specifically at a tumour stem cell and molecular levels. Data implicating tumour stem cells are primarily derived from the Shionogi mammary carcinoma [25]. This particular tumour model has a strong resemblance to human prostate cancer in its growth and response patterns to androgen withdrawal. Upon transplanting the parent tumour into a male mouse, it grows with a short doubling time, undergoes almost complete regression in response to castration and recurs in an androgen-independent state. Using this model it was determined that androgen withdrawal leads to alteration in the stem cell ratio of the tumour cell population. During the initial apoptotic or regression phase, following castration, elimination of differentiated tumour cells ensues, together with a significant reduction in the number of tumorigenic stem cells. Progression, however, was associated with a 20-fold increase in the proportion of total stem cells and a massive 500-fold increase in the proportion of the androgen-independent stem cells over what was measured in the precastration parent tumour [25]. These data would suggest that progression to androgen independence may occur as a result of stem cells losing their apoptotic potential secondary to lack of androgen-induced differentiation. Furthermore, these data would also suggest that a critical number of androgen-independent prostate cancer cells must be achieved prior to progression becoming clinically evident.

At a molecular level, androgen withdrawal results in the expression of two sets of genes in the prostate: those involved in the active cell death of the androgen-dependent cell population and those involved in the avoidance of death in the surviving androgen-independent population. Testosterone-repressed prostate message-2 (TRPM-2, clusterin), *bcl*-2 and its interaction with Bax, p53, c-*myc* are examples of the intense genetic activity associated with the apoptotic process [22]. TRPM-2 (clusterin) appears to inhibit the complement-induced cytolysis of epithelial cells and as such may stabilize cell membranes. *bcl*-2 expression is associated with extension of cellular viability by overriding mechanisms of programmed cell death. *bcl*-2 interactions with a variety of proteins such as Bax determines whether cellular death or survival is the outcome of an apoptotic stimulus. The expression of *bcl*-2 has been associated with the androgen-independent phenotype of prostate cancer recurrences with most androgen-dependent tumours exhibiting undetectable levels of *bcl*-2. *bcl*-2 also appears to be a factor in determining chemotherapy responsiveness in cancer cell lines [26], thus, implicating *bcl*-2 in both the androgen-independent progression of prostate cancer and, in part, accounting for the chemoresistance of hormone-refractory prostate cancer. c-*myc*, an essential regulator of cellular proliferative ability, is also involved in the programmed cell death process. In the presence of critical factors or absence of others, c-*myc* will take the cell into a particular pathway. For example, the simultaneous expression of *bcl*-2 appears to overcome the ability of c-*myc* to induce apoptosis [22].

Implications for future therapy strategies

The last 50 years' experience with hormone deprivation using either mono- or combination therapy for metastatic prostate cancer clearly indicates that it would be unlikely to improve survival of these patients significantly if we only continue with the current approach of trying to maximize androgen deprivation. This notion is supported by experimental data which collectively suggest that androgen withdrawal and activation of the process of programmed cell death are associated with the triggering of complex processes with changes at stem cell, molecular and growth factor levels limiting and counteracting the damaging effects of androgen deprivation. In a sense, these represent survival mechanisms with the purpose of self-preservation. Furthermore, considering the data on disease-free survival following local therapy [2, 12–16], it would be logical to proceed to develop future therapeutic strategies in two directions. The first should be to develop adjuvant systemic therapy aimed at prevention or elimination of micrometastases in patients with pathologically localized prostate cancer who are determined to be at a high risk for future relapse. Potential agents would include hormonal therapy, chemotherapy (cytotoxic, antiangiogenic) and chemohormonal therapies. While limited, available data from National Prostate Cancer Project (NPCP) trials [27] with estramustine would suggest a potential advantage to this approach. The second therapy strategy should target patients with clinically metastatic disease.

In reviewing the clinical data on metastatic disease it is obvious that there are two groups of patients – good- and poor-prognosis subsets [22, 28]. The former includes patients who have a high clinical response to androgen deprivation with sustained PSA nadirs in the normal range and superior survival, while the latter is represented by patients who do not achieve an adequate response or have short-lived responses and are destined to have poor survival. These facts, coupled with the currently available observations on mechanisms of progression, would suggest that we need not lump all metastatic disease patients for therapy purposes but rather design clinical trials for metastatic disease, taking into account patients' risk profile. This logic leads to two attack strategies. One is based on the premise that androgen replacement prior to the initiation of progression may cause the stem cells to differentiate and regain apoptotic potential, therefore become androgen-dependent and amenable to further hormonal manipulation. This provides the basis for intermittent androgen deprivation (IAD). Data supporting the role of IAD are twofold. Experimentally, IAD has retarded progression to androgen independence by threefold as compared with a one-time castration [28]. Using the Dunning R3327H prostatic adenocarcinoma, Trachtenberg failed to demonstrate significant growth reduction with intermittent hormone therapy [29]. These observations underscore the importance of using IAD in androgen-dependent tumours. Because the Dunning R3327H prostate adenocarcinoma is androgen-sensitive but not androgen-dependent (does not undergo apoptotic regression secondary to androgen withdrawal, it would not be expected to exhibit an improved outcome with IAD. Therefore, clinically this approach is likely to benefit patients who achieve a sustained response to androgen deprivation which is indicative of the hormonal dependence of their tumour.

Clinically, there are preliminary encouraging data in support of IAD. Klotz *et al.* [30] reported on the use of intermittent diethylstilboestrol (DES) in 20 patients with advanced prostate cancer, citing Noble's observations and reduction of side-effects as the rationale. Seventeen patients had documented bony metastasis. Median induction duration was 10 months. When therapy was interrupted, 12 of 20 progressed with a median of 8 months (1–24 months). All of the 12 patients responded promptly to retreatment with hormones. Of the 10 patients who became impotent on treatment, 9 resumed sexual activity during therapy interruption. No apparent adverse effects on survival were noted.

Using a combination of luteinizing hormone releasing hormone agonist and antiandrogen, Goldenberg *et al.* [31] tested the feasibility of IAD in 47 patients with prostate cancer. Mean follow-up time was 125 weeks. Of these patients, 14 were D2, 10 were D1, 11 were C, 2 were B2, 2 patients had stage A2 and 8 patients had local and PSA progression following primary radiation therapy. On average, treatment was continued for at least 6 months. Therapy was interrupted when a stable PSA nadir in the normal range ($\leqslant 4.0\,\text{ng/ml}$) was attained. Treatment was resumed when the serum PSA recovered to an arbitrarily chosen value of $10\text{–}20\,\text{ng/ml}$. Cycles of treatment and no treatment were repeated until patients exhibited signs of androgen independence by PSA. The mean percentage time off therapy during the first and second cycles was 41 and 45%. The mean time to achieve a nadir PSA was 20 and 18 weeks for cycles 1 and 2 respectively.

Of significance is the median progression-free and overall survival of the patients with metastatic disease. Seven of the 14 patients with stage D2 disease progressed with a median progression-free survival (by PSA) and median survival of 27 and 42 months, respectively. This outcome compares quite favourably with what is expected, considering that 13 of 14 patients with stage D2 disease were characterized as having widespread metastases and thus a poor prognosis. The off-treatment periods were associated with an improvement in sense of well-being, and recovery of libido and potency in men who reported normal or near-normal sexual function.

In addition to the obvious advantages to IAD, in terms of quality of life and cost of therapy, there is the potential for prolonging the duration of androgen dependence, thus response and, hopefully, survival. Moreover, this approach provides the opportunity for the integration of chemotherapy with hormonal therapy. For example, chemotherapy can be initiated simultaneously or at time of PSA nadirs after maximal debulking to eliminate residual androgen-independent stem cells or at time of testicular recovery to eliminate actively dividing cells. Once feasibility and efficacy are established through larger and randomized trials, this approach will have more applicability for the long-term management of other stages of prostate cancer.

The second attack strategy in treating metastatic prostate cancer focuses on the eradication of androgen-independent stem cells, thus providing the basis for chemohormonal approaches with cytotoxic therapy or therapies that can induce the active cell death process. Experimentally, the intracellular Ca^{2+} and endoplasmic reticulum Ca^{2+} pump have been identified as potential targets for the cell proliferation-independent activation of programmed cell death of the non-proliferating androgen-independent prostate cancer cells [32]. Obviously, of significance is that the latter can occur at any time of the cell cycle, which is the usual limitation of conventional cytotoxic chemotherapy. Inhibiting the expression of the apoptotic blocker genes, such as *bcl*-2, or the expression of autocrine and paracrine growth factors provides legitimate targets for therapy development. In this regard agents like suramin (a hexa-sulphonated naphthylurea with a broad-spectrum effect on cellular biological systems and growth factor-inhibitory effects) or less toxic analogues hold promise.

Conclusion

Prostate cancer exhibits heterogeneity in its natural history and progression. A variety of tumour and host biological-related factors collectively determine the outcome for individual patients. As our understanding of this disease is unfolding, it is evident that clinical trials investigating future therapies must take into account the rapidly accumulating data on mechanisms of progression, must employ therapies that should target both androgen-dependent and independent tumour cells, and must have appropriate patient selection.

References

1 Jacobs SC. Spread of prostatic carcinoma to bone. *Urology* 1983; **21**: 337–344.
2 Schmidt JD, Gibbons RP, Bartolucci A *et al*. Prognosis in stage D1 prostate cancer relative to anatomic sites of nodal metastases. *Cancer* 1989; **64**: 1743–1746.

  * Reference of special interest.
** Reference of outstanding merit.

  * 3 Epstein JI, Carmichael MJ, Pizov G. & Walsh PC. Influence of capsular penetration on progression following radical prostatectomy: a study of 196 cases with long-term follow-up. *J Urol* 1993; **150**: 135–141.

  ** 4 Rinker-Schaeffer CW, Partin AW, Isaacs WB, Coffey DS & Isaacs JT. Molecular and cellular changes associated with the acquisition of metastatic ability by prostatic cancer cells. *Prostate* 1994; **25**: 249–265.

    5 Hoosein NM, Logothetis CJ & Chung LWK. Differential effects of peptide hormones bombesin, vasoactive intestinal polypeptide and somatostatin analog Rc-160 on the invasive capacity of human prostatic carcinoma cells. *J Urol* 1993; **149**: 1209–1213.

    6 di Sant'Agnese PA. Neuroendocrine differentiation in carcinoma of the prostate. *Cancer* 1992; **70**: 254–268.

    7 Hsieh J. Bone-derived growth factors in the promotion of osseous metastasis from prostate cancer. *Cancer Bull* 1993; **45**: 442–447.

    8 Gospodarowicz D, Neufeld G & Schweigerer L. Fibroblast growth factor. *Mol Cell Endocrinol* 1986; **46**: 187–204.

  * 9 Polychronakos C, Janthly U, Lehoux JG *et al.* Mitogenic effects of insulin and insulin-like growth factors on PA-III rat prostate adenocarcinoma cells: characterization of receptors involved. *Prostate* 1991; **19**: 313–321.

  *10 Cohen P, Graves HCB & Peehl DM. Prostate-specific antigen (PSA) is an insulin-like growth factor binding protein-3 protease found in seminal plasma. *J Clin Endocrinol Metab* 1992; **75**: 1046–1053.

  11 Thalmann GN, Anezinis PE, Chang SM *et al.* Androgen-independent cancer progression and bone metastasis in the LNCaP model of human prostate cancer. *Cancer Res* 1994; **54: 2577–2581.

    12 Barzell W, Bean MA, Hilaris BS & Whitmore Jr WF. Total perineal prostatectomy for carcinoma of prostate. *J Urol* 1977; **118**: 278–282.

    13 Paulson DF, Moul JW & Walther PJ. Radical prostatectomy for clinical stage T1-2N0M0 prostate adenocarcinoma: long-term results. *J Urol* 1990; **144**: 1180–1184.

    14 Partin AW, Pound CR, Clemens JQ *et al.* Serum PSA after anatomic radical prostatectomy: the Johns Hopkins experience after 10 years. *Urol Clin North Am* 1993; **20**: 713–725.

    15 Gibbons RP, Correa RJ, Brannen GE & Weissman RM. Total prostatectomy for clinically localized prostate cancer: long-term results. *J Urol* 1989; **141** 564–566.

    16 Schroeder FH & Belt E. Carcinoma of the prostate: a study of 213 patients with stage C tumors treated by total perineal prostatectomy. *J Urol* 1975; **114**: 257–260.

  17 Wood DP, Banks ER, Humphreys S *et al.* Identification of bone marrow micrometastases in patients with prostate cancer. *Cancer* 1994; **74: 2533–2540.

  18 Moreno JG, Croce MC, Fischer R *et al.* Detection of hematogenous micrometastasis in patients with prostate cancer. *Cancer Res* 1992; **52: 6110–6112.

  *19 Katz AE, Olsson CA, Raffo AJ *et al.* Molecular staging of prostate cancer with the use of an enhanced reverse transcriptase-PCR assay. *Urology* 1994; **43**: 765–775.

    20 Seiden MV, Kantoff PW, Krithiva K *et al.* Detection of circulating tumor cells in men with localized prostate cancer. *J Clin Oncol* 1994; **12**: 2634–2639.

  *21 D'Amico AV & Hanks GE. Linear regressive analysis using prostate-specific antigen doubling time for predicting tumor biology and clinical outcome in prostate cancer. *Cancer* 1993; **72**: 2638–2643.

    22 Hussain M & Crawford ED. Androgen deprivation strategies for metastatic prostate cancer. In: *Principles and Practice of Genitourinary Oncology*, 1st edn, Raghavan D, Scher HI, Leibel SA & Lang P, eds. Philadelphia, PA: JB Lippincott, 1994.

*23 Hussain M, Wolf M, Marshall E, Crawford ED & Eisenberger M. Effects of continued androgen deprivation therapy and other prognostic factors on response and survival in phase II chemotherapy trials for hormone-refractory prostate cancer: a Southwest Oncology Group report. *J Clin Oncol* 1994; **12**: 1868–1875.

24 Bruchovsky N, Brown EM, Coppin CM *et al*. The endocrinology and treatment of prostate tumor progression. In: *Current Concepts and Approaches to the Study of Prostate Cancer: Progress in Clinical and Biological Research*, Coffey DS, Bruchovsky N, Gardner WE Jr, Resnick MI & Karr JP, eds. New York: Alan R Liss, 1987, pp 347–387.

25 Bruchovsky N, Rennie PS, Coldman AF *et al*. The effects of androgen withdrawal on the stem cell composition of the Shionogi carcinoma. *Cancer Res* 1990; **50: 2275.

26 Walton MI, Whysong D, O'Connor PM *et al*. Constitutive expression of human *bcl-2* modulates nitrogen mustard and camptothecin induced apoptosis. *Cancer Res* 1993; **53**: 1853–1861.

27 Schmidt JD, Gibbons RP, Murphy GP & Bartolucci A. Adjuvant therapy for localized prostate cancer. *Cancer* 1993; **71**: 1005–1013.

*28 Akakura K, Bruchovsky N, Goldenberg SL *et al*. Effects of intermittent androgen suppression on androgen dependent tumors. *Cancer* 1993; **71**: 2782.

29 Trachtenberg J. Experimental treatment of prostatic cancer by intermittent hormonal therapy. *J Urol* 1987; **137**: 785–788.

30 Klotz LH, Herr HW, Morse MJ & Whitmore WF. Intermittent endocrine therapy for advanced prostate cancer. *Cancer* 1986; **58**: 2546.

*31 Goldenberg SL, Bruchovsky N, Gleave ME *et al*. Intermittent androgen suppression in the treatment of prostate cancer: a preliminary report. *Urology* 1995; **45**: 839–44.

*32 Isaacs JT, Furuya Y & Berges R. The role of androgen in the regulation of programmed cell death/apoptosis in normal and malignant prostatic tissue. *Semin Cancer Biol* 1994; **5**: 391–400.

Part 2
Diagnosis and Evaluation

5/Clinical Decisions taken from Grading of Prostatic Adenocarcinomas

J.I. Epstein

Grading systems

Numerous grading systems exist for the evaluation of prostatic adenocarcinoma. Several grading schemes are worth citing, even though they are utilized almost exclusively by their proponents and their institutions, because of their frequent appearance in the literature. The systems are those of Mostofi [1, 2], Gaeta [3, 4], Mayo Clinic [5] and M.D. Anderson [6]. Two other grading systems are of particular importance because of their widespread use in many institutions as well as in much of the literature.

The Gleason method of histological grading has been recommended as a common reference system by the prostate cancer working group operating under the auspices of the National Cancer Institute for histological grading which should accompany any other grading system being presented in the literature [7–10]. The Gleason system is based on the glandular pattern of the tumour as identified at relatively low magnification (Fig. 5.1). In contrast to some of the other proposed systems for grading prostate carcinoma cytological features play no role in the grade of the tumour.

Those who offer different grading systems, especially Gaeta and Mostofi, object that the Gleason system considers only the glandular pattern without accounting for cytological features such as nuclear anaplasia [1, 3]. In the majority of cases, nuclear features and glandular differentiation are not independent variables. Tumours with well-formed glands usually have bland nuclei, while undifferentiated tumours without glandular formation have greater cytological atypia. Although it has been shown that in some cases there is a disparity between the degree of nuclear atypia and the degree of glandular differentiation, an advantage in the predictive value of nuclear features, as compared to that of glandular pattern, has not been demonstrated [11].

We have investigated the use of nuclear morphology in prostate cancer using a computerized image analysis system [12]. Every study that we have performed has shown that, when nuclear shape is measured with a computer, it adds prognostic information to that of the architectural pattern determined by the Gleason system. In our most recent study we looked at a group of 114 men with Gleason sum 6–7 tumours who had a minimum of 8 years' follow-up after

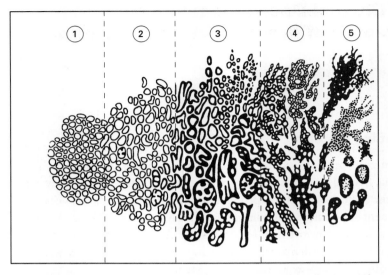

Fig. 5.1 Schematic diagram of Gleason's grading system (see text). After D.F. Gleason.

radical prostatectomy. Although Gleason score (i.e. 6 versus 7) was very predictive of outcome, nuclear roundness as determined on a computer was very powerful and additive to that of Gleason score in predicting outcome. We have found that variability of nuclear shape determines outcome rather than the worst nuclei present within the case. The human eye is not capable of determining nuclear variability accurately in prostate cancer given that there is often a small percentage of cells with nuclear irregularities. We are currently investigating whether this technique can be applied to needle biopsy material as well as attempting to develop more automated systems of calculating nuclear morphometry.

The other most commonly used system is a three-grade system corresponding to tumours that are well, moderately well and poorly differentiated [13, 14]. With the three-grade system, only the predominant grade is recorded. In the uncommon cases where most of the tumour is grade 1 (well-differentiated) or grade 2 (moderately differentiated), and there is a significant amount of grade 3 (poorly differentiated) tumour as a secondary component, its presence is recorded by a note on the report. The disadvantage of the 1, 2, 3 system is that, although Gleason sum 2–4 might be equated with grade 1 tumour, and Gleason sum 8–10 can be regarded as grade 3 tumour, one cannot consider Gleason 5–7 tumour as grade 2. It has been demonstrated that Gleason sum 7 tumour is significantly more aggressive than Gleason sum 5–6 cancers. Whereas some tumours with Gleason score 5–6 may be followed conservatively, most urologists will treat Gleason sum 7 cancers definitively. Using the 1–3 grading scheme, this distinction is lost.

Gleason grading system

Because the Gleason system is based solely on architecture, there exists a simplified schematic illustration of Gleason grading system which can be readily referred to when first learning this system (Fig. 5.1). Both the primary (predominant) and the secondary (second most prevalent) architectural patterns are identified and assigned a grade from 1 to 5, with 1 being the most differentiated and 5 being undifferentiated.

When Gleason compared his grading system with survival rates, it was noted that in tumours with two distinct tumour patterns the observed number of deaths generally fell in between the number expected on the basis of the primary pattern and that based on the secondary pattern [8, 9]. Since both the primary and secondary patterns were considered influential in predicting prognosis, there resulted a combined Gleason grade obtained by the addition of the primary and secondary grade. If a tumour had only one histological pattern, then for uniformity the primary and secondary scores were given the same grade. The combined Gleason grades range from 2 $(1 + 1 = 2)$, which represents tumours uniformly composed of Gleason pattern 1 tumour, to 10 $(5 + 5 = 10)$, which represents totally undifferentiated tumours. A tumour that is predominantly Gleason pattern 3 with a lesser amount of Gleason pattern 5 has a combined Gleason grade of 8 $(3 + 5 = 8)$, as does a tumour that is predominantly Gleason pattern 5 with a lesser amount of Gleason pattern 3 tumour $(5 + 3 = 8)$.

Gleason pattern 1

Gleason pattern 1 tumour is composed of circumscribed nodules of uniform, single, separate, closely packed glands (Fig. 5.2). Although most cases of Gleason pattern 1 tumour have small, benign-appearing nucleoli, there are some cases where numerous large prominent nuclei can be visualized. Because the Gleason system only looks at architecture, the cytological features are not factored into the evaluation of the grade. The glands in Gleason pattern 1 and Gleason pattern 2 tumour tend to be larger than intermediate-grade carcinomas. Typically, both Gleason 1 and Gleason pattern 2 carcinomas have abundant pale eosinophilic cytoplasm. It has been proposed that transition zone cancers be termed clear cell carcinomas [15]. We do not feel that these tumours represent a unique histology, but rather reflect the finding that

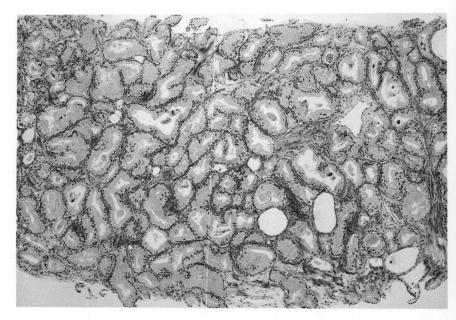

Fig. 5.2 Gleason pattern 1 tumour consisting of uniform, single, separate closely packed glands.

transition zone cancers are frequently low-grade. Carcinomas with pale cytoplasm may also be found in the peripheral zone.

Gleason pattern 2

In Gleason pattern 2, though the tumour is still fairly circumscribed, at the edge of the tumour nodule there can be minimal extension by neoplastic glands into the surrounding non-neoplastic prostate (Fig. 5.3). The glands are more loosely arranged and not quite as uniform as Gleason pattern 1. As with Gleason pattern 1 tumour, the glands are larger than intermediate-grade tumour, fairly uniform in size and shape and have abundant eosinophilic cytoplasm. The finding of Gleason 2 + 2 tumour on needle biopsy is unusual since most peripherally located prostatic carcinomas sampled by needle biopsy are of intermediate or higher grade.

Gleason pattern 3

Gleason pattern 3 tumour infiltrates in and amongst the non-neoplastic prostate, as seen in Fig. 5.3. The glands have marked variation in size and

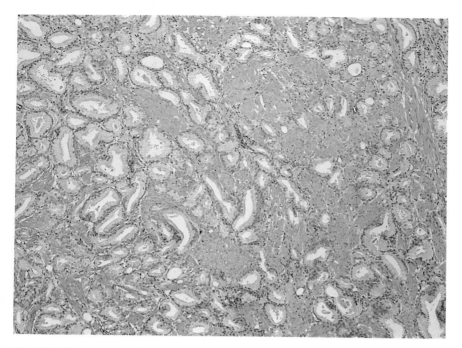

Fig. 5.3 Gleason pattern 2 carcinoma showing a less uniform and looser arrangements of the neoplastic glands as compared to Gleason pattern 1.

shape (Fig. 5.4). Many of the glands are smaller than those seen in Gleason pattern 1 or 2. In contrast to Gleason pattern 4, the glands in Gleason pattern 3 are discrete units. If one can mentally draw a circle around well-formed individual glands, then it is Gleason pattern 3. One should assign a Gleason grade at relatively low power (i.e. 2.5 × or 4 ×); the presence of a few poorly formed glands at high power is still consistent with Gleason pattern 3 tumour. Smoothly circumscribed cribriform nodules of tumour are also classified as grade 3. Almost always when cribriform glands are present, small infiltrating glands of Gleason pattern 3 will be visible as well.

Gleason pattern 4

Gleason pattern 4 glands are no longer single and separate, as seen in patterns 1–3 (Fig. 5.5). The glands appear fused and ill-defined, even at low magnification. In Gleason pattern 4, one may also see large cribriform glands or cribriform glands with an irregular border as opposed to the smoothly circumscribed smaller nodules of cribriform Gleason pattern 3. Another form

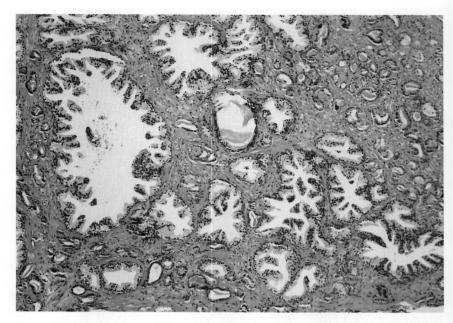

Fig. 5.4 Gleason pattern 3 tumour on needle biopsy showing large variation in size and shape of the neoplastic glands as well as an infiltrative pattern.

of Gleason pattern 4 tumour resembles renal cell carcinoma and is referred to as a hypernephromatoid pattern. It is important to recognize Gleason pattern 4 tumour, since tumours with this pattern have been shown to be associated with a significantly worse prognosis than those with pure Gleason pattern 3 [16, 17].

Gleason pattern 5

Gleason pattern 5 tumour shows no glandular differentiation, composed of solid sheets (Fig. 5.6) cords or single cells. Solid nests of tumour with central comedonecrosis are also classified under Gleason pattern 5. Although cytological features are not taken into account within the Gleason system, it is of interest that within high-grade prostatic carcinomas there is often not as much pleomorphism or mitotic activity as compared to poorly differentiated tumours in other organs such as the bladder. Some men with low-grade cancers will, following several years, develop high-grade tumour [18]. It is unclear whether the residual low-grade cancer progressed or whether there was subsequent development of multifocal more aggressive tumour.

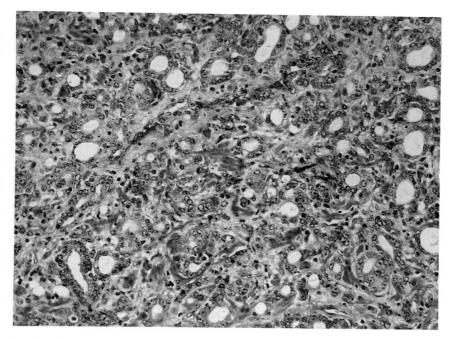

Fig. 5.5 Gleason pattern 4 tumour showing loss of glandular differentiation with only minimal lumen formation.

Application of the Gleason grading system

Some of the practical advantages of the Gleason grading system are that it is easy to learn and apply and is based on low magnification pattern recognition and hence is less time-consuming than grading systems that examine cytological features. Two studies have demonstrated good interobserver and intraobserver reproducibility using the Gleason system with agreements to within one combined Gleason grade of over 80% and 90% respectively [2, 19]. One of the most frequent causes of discordant grading is the grading of tumours that straddle two grades. As shown on Gleason's schematic diagram (Fig. 5.1), there is a gradient of differentiation between the various Gleason patterns such that there may be variability in the grade assigned at the extremes of a particular Gleason pattern. The most critical situation on biopsy material with bridging grades is with tumours that are between a Gleason pattern 3 and 4.

A practical way to approach Gleason grading on needle biopsy material is as follows. If one has well-formed glands on needle biopsy, some of which are relatively small, and there is some variation in gland size, there is an element of

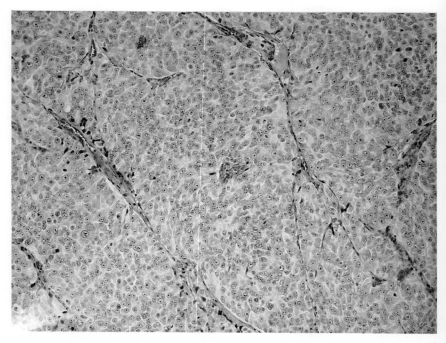

Fig. 5.6 Gleason pattern 5 with large solid nests of tumour.

Gleason pattern 3. In some cases that will be the sole pattern, resulting in the diagnosis of 3 + 3 = 6. In other cases, in addition to seeing well-formed individual glands, one will see areas where the glands start becoming indistinct and it is difficult to outline discrete gland formation. In these cases one is dealing with a tumour towards the more poorly differentiated side of Gleason pattern 3, resulting in a diagnosis of Gleason 3 + 4 = 7. Although there is also subjectivity as whether a tumour is Gleason sum 6 or 5, we have not found this distinction to be critical since the prognosis and treatment of these tumours are similar [16]. Most cases on needle biopsy with mixed Gleason patterns, such as Gleason 3 + 4 = 7, consist of tumours where there are not discrete foci with different patterns, but rather tumours which tend to bridge between two patterns.

The question arises whether one should assign both a primary and secondary pattern to limited adenocarcinoma of the prostate on needle biopsy. How is it possible to assign both a primary and secondary pattern when only a few neoplastic glands are present? There is nothing wrong with assigning only a Gleason pattern rather than a Gleason score in these cases. However, it should be made perfectly clear by the pathologist that he or she is only assigning a pattern and not a score. I have seen several cases where the pathologist signed out a case as Gleason grade 4 which represented Gleason pattern 4 (i.e. high-grade tumour) on needle biopsy. However, the urologist mistook this report to read Gleason sum of 4 (i.e. low-grade tumour). Consequently, I prefer to assign both a primary and secondary pattern even when presented with limited cancer so as not to give rise to any confusion. By assigning Gleason score of 3 + 3 = 6 on a small focus of small glands infiltrating between larger benign glands there can be absolutely no confusion in the urologist's mind as to the grade of the tumour.

Correlation of needle biopsy and prostatectomy

The Gleason grade on biopsy material has been shown to correlate fairly well with that of the subsequent prostatectomy. Two large series comparing radical prostatectomy specimens and their diagnostic biopsies have shown a correlation to within one combined Gleason grade in approximately 73% of cases [20, 21]. Two studies have evaluated the correlation of grade assigned to an 18-gauge needle biopsy with that of the corresponding radical prostatectomy [22, 23]. There was exact concordance in 35–58% of cases, and concordance to within one grade in 74–94%. In one study, only 45% of the tumours diagnosed as Gleason < 7 on needle biopsy revealed Gleason sum < 7 tumour in the radical prostatectomy [23]. In contrast, when Gleason sum ≥ 7 tumour was diagnosed on needle biopsy, 79% were ≥ 7 in the prostatectomy. Undergrading of the needle biopsy is to some extent unavoidable due to sampling error. An error, which is frequently avoidable, is to grade the tumour on biopsy as Gleason sum 2–4 with the subsequent prostatectomy showing predominantly Gleason pattern 3 tumours, resulting in a combined Gleason grade of 6 or sometimes 5 [23]. The tendency to undergrade needle biopsy material results from the minimal amount of tumour often found on needle biopsy and the consequent difficulty in appreciating either the infiltrative nature of the tumour or the variability in size and shape of the neoplastic glands – features that are characteristic of a Gleason pattern 3. A feature of Gleason pattern 3 tumour that may be more readily identifiable on limited material is that the glands with Gleason pattern 3 are smaller than those of Gleason pattern 1 or 2. Consequently, if the tumour on needle biopsy is composed of small glands or the glands are seen infiltrating between non-neoplastic prostate glands, the tumour may be graded 3 + 3 = 6 even though there may be a few malignant glands present. Low-grade tumours (i.e. combined Gleason grades 2–4) should be assigned only when a tumour is composed of closely packed, larger, open uniform glands with abundant pale cytoplasm. In our own material, we diagnose Gleason sum 2–4 on only 3% of our needle biopsy specimens; this incidence correlates well with our incidence of low-grade carcinoma at radical prostatectomy.

Prognosis

The ultimate value of any grading system is its prognostic ability. Both Gleason's data with 2911 patients and subsequent studies with long-term follow-up have demonstrated a good correlation between Gleason sum and prognosis [8, 24]. When stage of disease is factored in with the grade, prognostication is enhanced. Whatever prognostic parameters we have evaluated, Gleason score has been shown to be predictive. In our data an increase in the Gleason score of the radical prostatectomy specimen is associated with a worsening of all prognostic parameters (Table 5.1).

As shown in Fig. 5.7, prognostication is not needed in patients with Gleason 2–4 tumour or Gleason 8–10 tumour as these patients have either an excellent or dismal prognosis, respectively. What is needed is more refined prognostication in patients with Gleason sum 5–7 tumour. Although patients with Gleason sum 7 tumour do worse than those with Gleason sum 5 and 6, enhanced prognostication in radical prostatectomy specimens can be achieved by factoring in both status of capsular penetration and surgical margins. In patients with Gleason sum 5–6 tumour, patients can be stratified into three groups with different prognoses (Fig. 5.8). Patients with Gleason sum 7 tumour can be stratified into two groups with different risks of progression (Fig. 5.9). However, with Gleason sum 7 tumour it appears that the long-term risk of progression is similar regardless of other pathological parameters. The long-term prognosis appears to be dictated by the high-grade tumour and is not modulated to a great extent by having better risk factors such as more organ-confined disease or negative margins of resection.

Table 5.1 Correlation of Gleason score with pathology at radical prostatectomy.

Pathology	Gleason score			
	5	6	7	8–10
Established capsular penetration	16%	24%	62%	85%
Positive margins	20%	29%	48%	59%
Mean tumour volume	2.2	2.7	5.1	4.0
Seminal vesicle invasion	1%	4%	17%	48%
Lymph node metastases	1%	2%	12%	24%

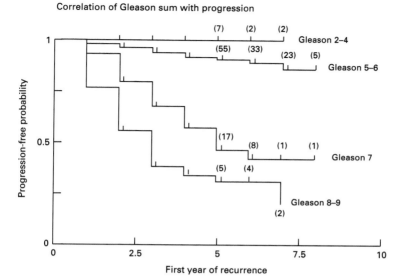

Correlation of Gleason sum with progression

Fig. 5.7 Kaplan–Meier actuarial curves demonstrate the likelihood of having undetectable postoperative serum prostate-specific antigen stratified by Gleason score. The numbers in parentheses represent censored data.

Therapeutic decisions based on the needle biopsy grade

Currently, even at low and high ends of the grading system, therapeutic decisions are rarely made based on the grade of the tumour on biopsy. If one examines the ability of the Gleason system to predict pelvic lymph node metastases (therefore allowing a urologist to forgo a staging lymphade-nectomy in selected cases), there are conflicting data. The incidence of lymph node metastases in patients with combined Gleason grades from 2 to 4 ranges from 0 to 27%, with the average being 12% [25–28]. Those studies showing over 20% incidence of lymph node metastases probably have undergraded many of their biopsy specimens, since their low-grade specimens make up a disproportionate number of the cases of their study. The range in lymph node metastases for combined Gleason grade 5–7 tumour is between 10 and 54%, with an average of 35%. At the high end of the spectrum, with Gleason grade of 8–10, the incidence of lymph node metastases in various studies ranges between 26 and 93%, averaging 61%.

The conflicting results from the various studies are probably due to the effect of clinical stage. Taking into account both the biopsy grade and the clinical stage, the incidence of lymph node metastases ranges from rare (Gleason 2–4 and clinically confined) to 80% (Gleason 8–10 and palpable). In

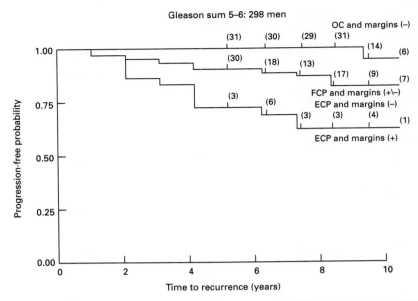

Fig. 5.8 Kaplan–Meier actuarial curves of men with Gleason score 5–6 demonstrate the likelihood of having undetectable postoperative serum prostate-specific antigen stratified by capsular penetration and margin status. The numbers in parentheses represent censored data. OC, organ-confined; FCP, focal capsular penetration; ECP, established capsular penetration; margins (+/−), margins positive or negative.

addition to correlating with lymph node metastases, Gleason grade has also been shown to correlate with capsular penetration, seminal vesicle involvement and tumour volume [17, 27, 29].

The practical significance of the grade assigned to the needle biopsy material is usually not critical in determining the management of the patient. If there is a palpable nodule which appears clinically confined to the gland in a patient who is an operative candidate, then regardless of the grade assigned on the needle biopsy, the patient most likely will be offered a chance of a curative procedure. There are some circumstances where the grade is influential. In patients with combined Gleason grades of 8–10 on needle biopsy we have shown that if the lymph nodes are involved, these men will not benefit from radical surgery, whereas if the nodes are free of tumour a chance of cure following radical prostatectomy is possible [30]. Consequently, in men with Gleason sum 8–10 on biopsy, we will examine all the nodes at the time of surgery and the urologist will abort the prostatectomy if the nodes are positive. If the grade on the biopsy is less than 8, we examine the nodes only on permanent section.

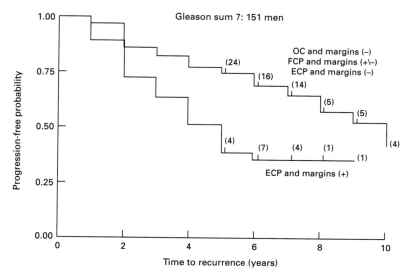

Fig. 5.9 Kaplan–Meier actuarial curves of men with Gleason score 7 demonstrate the likelihood of having undetectable postoperative serum prostate-specific antigen stratified by capsular penetration and margin status. The numbers in parentheses represent censored data. OC, organ-confined; FCP, focal capsular penetration; ECP, established capsular penetration; margins (+/−), margins positive or negative.

The other critical distinction on needle biopsy is between Gleason sum 6 and 7 tumours, when the lesion is non-palpable. Depending on the serum prostate-specific antigen (PSA) level, the extent of tumour on the biopsy, and the age of the patient, some urologists will follow conservatively men with limited Gleason sum 5–6 tumours [31]. Gleason sum 7 tumours, however, are almost always treated with definitive therapy.

Grade on transurethral resection specimens

There are several differences concerning grade on transurethral resection (TURP) material. The potential for having discrete areas of different grades more frequently comes about when grading tumour on TURP given the greater amount of tumour sampled. Lower-grade prostatic adenocarcinoma (Gleason patterns 1 and 2) tends to be located more within the central regions of the prostate and is usually sampled by TURP.

Incidental adenocarcinoma of the prostate found on TURP is divided into those tumours which are relatively low-volume and low-grade (stage T1a), or high-volume and/or high-grade (stage T1b) [32]. The definition of stage T1a disease is controversial. Some authors require that stage T1a disease consists only of low-grade tumours (Gleason sum $\leqslant 4$), while others allow that tumour to be low- or intermediate-grade tumour. In our data, as long as the tumour occupied $\leqslant 5\%$ of the specimen, there was no difference in the progression rate at 8 years following diagnosis whether the Gleason sum was $\leqslant 4$ or 5–6 [33]. Consequently, the distinction between low-grade adenocarcinoma and Gleason sum 5–6 is not critical in our minds in substaging patients with incidental cancer found on TURP. However, the finding of Gleason sum 7 or greater tumour on TURP is critical in that these patients have a higher risk of progression and should be classified as having stage T1b disease.

Future goals

The two major criticisms of the Gleason grading system are its reproducibility and relative inaccuracy in predicting prognosis in patients with Gleason sums 5–7. Ultimately, development of a computer-assisted image analysis program which will quantify architectural pattern would be a major advancement in the grading of prostate cancer. This would provide an objective architectural grading system rather than the subjective ones currently in use.

Although Gleason sum 7 tumours do worse than Gleason sums 5 and 6, there is still significant room for enhanced prognostication within these grades. Enhanced prognostication is now attainable in radical prostatectomy specimens using pathological stage, status of capsular margins and nuclear morphometry. Work is needed to validate these findings on needle biopsy specimens and develop new prognosticators that can help in determining which tumours need definitive therapy and which can be followed expectantly.

References

1 Mostofi FK. Grading of prostatic carcinoma. *Cancer Ther Rep* 1975; **59**: 111–117.
2 Harada M, Mostofi FK, Corle DK, Byar DP & Trump BF. Preliminary studies of histologic prognosis in cancer of the prostate. *Cancer Treat Rep* 1977; **61**: 223–224.
* 3 Gaeta JF, Asiriwatham JE, Miller G *et al*. Histologic grading of primary prostatic cancer. In New Approach to an Old Problem. *J Urol* 1980; **123**: 689–693.
4 Gaeta JF. Glandular profiles and cellular patterns in prostatic cancer grading: National Prostatic Cancer Project System. *Urology* 1981 (suppl); **17**: 33–37.
5 Utz DC & Farrow GM. Pathologic differentiation and prognosis of prostatic carcinoma. *JAMA* 1969; **209**: 1701–1703.
6 Brawn PN, Ayala AG, Von Eschenbach AC, Hussey DH & Johnson DE. Histologic grading study of prostatic adenocarcinoma: the development of a new system in comparison with other methods – a preliminary study. *Cancer* 1982; **49**: 525–532.

* Reference of special interest.

7 Gleason DF, Mellinger GT, and the Veterans Administration Cooperative Urological Research Group. Prediction of prognosis for prostatic adenocarcinoma by combined histologic grading and clinical staging. *J Urol* 1974; **111**: 58–64.

* 8 Gleason DF and The Veterans Administration Cooperative Urological Research Group. Histologic grading and clinical staging of prostatic carcinoma. In: *Urologic Pathology: The Prostate*, Tannenbaum M, ed. Philadelphia: Lea & Febiger, 1977, pp. 171–197.

9 Mellinger GT, Gleason D & Bailar J. The histology and prognosis of prostatic cancer. *J Urol* 1967; **97**: 331–337.

10 Gardner WA Jr, Coffey D, Karr JP *et al*. Nomenclature of prostatic carcinoma. *Arch Pathol Lab Med* 1987; **111**: 898.

11 Gaeta JF, Englander, LC & Murphy GP. Comparative evaluation of the National Prostatic Cancer Treatment Group and Gleason systems for pathologic grading of primary prostatic cancer. *Urology* 1986; **27**: 306–308.

12 Partin AW, Steinberg GD, Pitcock RV *et al*. Use of nuclear morphometry, Gleason histologic scoring, clinical stage and age to predict disease-free survival among patients with prostate cancer. *Cancer* 1992; **70**: 161–168.

13 Catalona WJ, Stein AJ & Fair WR. Grading errors in prostatic needle biopsies: relation to the accuracy of tumour grade in predicting pelvic lymph node metastases. *J Urol* 1982; **127**: 919–922.

14 Fowler JE Jr & Whitmore WF Jr. The incidence and extent of pelvic lymph node metastases in apparently localized prostatic cancer. *Cancer* 1981; **47**: 2941–2945.

15 McNeal JE, Redwine EA, Freiha FS & Stamey TA. Zonal distribution of prostatic adenocarcinoma. Correlation with histologic pattern and direction of spread. *Am J Surg Pathol* 1988; **12**: 897–906.

*16 Epstein JI, Pizov G & Walsh PC. Correlation of pathologic findings with progression following radical retropubic prostatectomy. *Cancer* 1993; **71**: 3582–3593.

*17 McNeal JE, Villers AA, Redwine EA, Freiha FS & Stamey T. Histologic differentiation, cancer volume, and pelvic lymph node metastasis in adenocarcinoma of the prostate. *Cancer* 1990; **66**: 1225–1233.

18 Brawn PN. The dedifferentiation of prostate carcinoma. *Cancer* 1983; **52**: 246–251.

19 Bain GO, Koch M & Hanson J. Feasibility of grading prostatic carcinomas. *Arch Pathol Lab Med* 1982; **106**: 265–267.

20 Garnett JE, Oyasu R & Grayhack JT. The accuracy of diagnostic biopsy specimens in predicting tumour grades by Gleason's classification of radical prostatectomy specimens. *J Urol* 1984; **131**: 690–693.

21 Mills SE & Fowler JE. Gleason histologic grading of prostatic carcinoma. Correlations between biopsy and prostatectomy specimens. *Cancer* 1986; **53**: 346–349.

*22 Spires SE, Cibull ML, Wood DP Jr, Miller S, Spires SM & Banks ER. Gleason histologic grading in prostatic carcinoma. Correlation of 18-gauge core biopsy with prostatectomy. *Arch Pathol Lab Med* 1994; **118**: 705–708.

*23 Bostwick DG. Gleason grading of prostatic needle biopsies. Correlation with grade in 316 matched prostatectomies. *Am J Surg Pathol* 1994; **18**: 796–803.

24 Sogani PC, Israel A, Lieberman PH, Lesser ML & Whitmore WF. Gleason grading of prostate cancer: a predictor of survival. *Urology* 1985; **25**: 223–227.

25 Catalona WJ & Stein AJ. Accuracy of frozen section detection of lymph node metastases in prostatic carcinoma. *J Urol* 1982; **127**: 460–461.

26 Donahue RE, Mani JH, Whitesel JA *et al*. Pelvic lymph node dissection: guide to patient

management in clinically locally confined adenocarcinoma of prostate. *Urology* 1982; **20**: 559–565.

*27 Oesterling JE, Brendler CB, Epstein JI, Kimball AW & Walsh PC. Correlation of clinical stage, serum prostatic acid phosphatase, and pre-operative Gleason grade with final pathologic stage in 275 patients with clinically localized adenocarcinoma of the prostate. *J Urol* 1987; **138**: 92–98.

28 Smith JA, Seaman JP, Gleidman JB & Middleton RG. Pelvic lymph node metastases from prostatic cancer: influence of tumour grade and stage in 452 consecutive patients. *J Urol* 1983; **130**: 290–292.

29 Fowler JE & Mills SE. Operable prostatic carcinoma: correlations among clinical stage, pathological stage, Gleason histologic score, and early disease-free survival. *J Urol* 1985; **133**: 49–52.

30 Sgrignoli AR, Walsh PC, Steinberg GD, Steiner MS & Epstein JI. Prognostic factors in man with stage D1 prostate cancer: identification of patients less likely to benefit from radical surgery. *J Urol* 1994; **152**: 1077–1081.

31 Epstein JI, Walsh PC, CarMichael M & Brendler CB. Pathological and clinical findings to predict tumour extent of non-palpable (stage T1c) prostate cancer. *JAMA* 1994; **271**: 368–374.

32 Cantrell BB, Deklerk DP, Eggleston JC, Boitnott JK & Walsh PC. Pathological factors that influence prognosis in stage A prostatic cancer: the influence of extent versus grade. *J Urol* 1981; **125**: 516–520.

*33 Eble JN & Epstein JI. Stage A carcinoma of the prostate. In: *Pathology of the Prostate, Seminal Vesicles, and Male Urethra*, Roth LM, ed. New York: Churchill Livingstone, 1990; pp. 61–82.

6/Prostate-Specific Antigen in the Early Detection of Prostate Cancer

M.P. Chetner and M.K. Brawer

Introduction

Adenocarcinoma represents a major cause of morbidity and death in most western nations. In the USA it is the most common non-cutaneous malignancy and the second most common cause of cancer-related mortality, second only to carcinoma of the lung [1]. While it is widely recognized that the histological incidence far exceeds clinically manifest disease, the fact remains that approximately one in three men who are diagnosed with prostate cancer will die from it [2].

There exists impetus from clinicians, health policy makers, legislators and, most importantly, our patients to reduce prostate cancer deaths, which, even after adjusting for the ageing of the population, are increasing [3]. Certainly the most appealing method of lowering the death from any malignancy is to reduce the incidence. In general this requires understanding of the pathogenesis of the cancer and, despite significant strides, we are a long way from understanding the aetiology of prostate cancer. Nevertheless, a number of chemopreventive approaches to achieve a reduction in cancer incidence are underway, with a variety of malignancies, including prostate. Under the auspices of the National Cancer Institute (NCI), the Prostate Cancer Prevention Trial (PCPT), in which men are randomized to receive either finasteride or placebo for 7 years, is actively accruing patients [4]. All men at the completion of the study will undergo biopsy. This trial will involve 18 000 men across the USA and has enrolled approximately 75% of the required participants.

The second approach to reduction of cancer mortality is to improve therapy. Significant strides have certainly been made, not only in radical prostatectomy, but in radiation therapy with respect to morbidity of treatment. Moreover, new therapeutic approaches such as neoadjuvant hormonal therapy, followed by radiation therapy or radical prostatectomy, cryotherapy and use of new isotopes for brachytherapy are also under investigation. The fact remains, however, that the main cause of prostate cancer mortality is progression following hormonal ablation. Few, if any, real advances have been made in this setting. It is likely that therapeutic methods for reduction of prostate cancer mortality must await effective immunotherapeutic, gene therapeutic or other approaches to advanced systemic disease.

In the absence of clear evidence that prostate cancer incidence can be reduced and lack of effective therapy for advanced disease, most investigators as well as clinicians in general have focused their attention on early detection – that is, identifying more men at a stage when their cancer is curable with conventional modalities.

Current available tests for early detection of prostate cancer

Advanced prostate cancer may present with clinical signs and symptoms to alert the clinician. Bone pain from metastatic deposits and constitutional symptoms such as weight loss, anorexia and weakness are characteristic of advanced stage disease. Men with early-stage prostate cancer often have little in the way of disease-specific signs and symptoms. Clinical signs and symptoms of concurrent benign prostatic hyperplasia (BPH) are extremely prevalent in the ageing male population. In this circumstance, suspicion of a potential malignant diagnosis originates from an abnormal digital rectal examination (DRE) and abnormal levels of prostate-specific antigen (PSA) or an abnormal transrectal ultrasound (TRUS). An abnormality on these examinations should prompt the clinician to confirm his or her suspicion of cancer with a prostate needle biopsy.

Digital rectal examination

This examination has been the standard method of detection for prostate cancer [5, 6]. About half of the abnormal DREs in Jewett's classic study actually demonstrated cancer in the biopsy specimen [5]. This illustrates the lack of specificity of an abnormal DRE. A compilation of 10 needle biopsy series [7] plus a review of 15 series compiled by Sika and Lindquist illustrates the lack of specificity and sensitivity of DRE. Among almost 5000 patients with abnormal DREs, prostate cancer was identified in 39%. The identification of prostate cancer patients ranged between 18 and 100%.

DRE is a subjective examination. Clinicians vary in their ability to recognize subtle abnormalities, resulting in a wide variation in cancer detection rates. Several trials have allowed an assessment of DRE in terms of detection rates and positive predictive value. The cancer detection rates have ranged from 0.1 to 25.2% and positive predictive values range from 17 to 31%. Table 6.1 provides a summary of prostate cancer detection by DRE.

It is well-recognized that a man can have a normal DRE and still harbour a significant volume of prostate cancer. Gann *et al.* have shown that men with

Table 6.1 Results of prostate cancer screening by digital rectal examination.

Authors	No. of cancers/no. of patients screened (%)	Positive predictive value
Catalona *et al.* [30]	146/6630 (2.2)	146/683 (21.4)
Cooner *et al.* [10]	203/807 (25.2)	203/470 (43.2)
Chodak and Schoenberg [77]	36/2131 (1.7)	36/144 (25.0)
Faul [78]	1951/1 500 000 (0.1)	1951/11 308 (17.3)
Gilbertsen [79]	75/5856 (1.3)	
Jenson *et al.* [80]	36/4367 (0.8)	
Lee *et al.* [11]	10/784 (1.3)	10/29 (34.5)
McWhorter *et al.* [81]	4/34 (1.8)	4/8 (50.0)
Mettlin *et al.* [45]	33/2425 (1.4)	33/118 (28.0)
Mueller *et al.* [82]	312/11 523 (2.7)	122/312 (39.1)
Thompson *et al.* [6]	17/2005 (0.8)	17/65 (26.2)
Vihko *et al.* [83]	6/771 (0.8)	6/27 (22.2)
Waaler *et al.* [84]	1/480 (0.2)	1/16 (6.25)

normal rectal examinations may have clinically detectable carcinoma within 4–5 years [8].

A number of reports demonstrate finding prostate cancer in men with normal rectal examinations. For example, in our series we detected prostate cancer in 40 of 224 men (18%) with completely normal rectal examinations [9]. Twenty-four of 181 men (13%) with asymmetric glands on rectal examination had a positive biopsy. In contrast, among men with palpable nodules or obvious induration suggestive of cancer on DRE, 189 of 596 men (32%) had biopsy-proven adenocarcinoma of the prostate [9].

Transrectal ultrasound

TRUS is the most utilized modality for imaging the prostate and adjacent tissue. It is widely available and provides excellent visualization. Many authors have reported a significant increase in the detection rate of cancer when TRUS was compared to DRE [10, 11] (Table 6.2).

Lee and associates advanced our understanding of prostate ultrasound when they identified that the commonest appearance of prostate cancer by TRUS was a hypoechoic peripheral zone lesion [12].

Despite its utility in imaging and particularly in guiding needle biopsy, TRUS lacks sensitivity and specificity and is relatively expensive. Often non-palpable and isoechoic cancer is detected contralateral to the index lesion when systematic sector biopsies are employed. For example, Carter *et al.* reported that 25 or 59 patients (42%) had contralateral cancer that was not identified at

Table 6.2 Results of prostate cancer screening by transrectal ultrasound.

Authors	No. of cancers/no. of subjects screened (%)	Positive predictive value
Catalona *et al.* [30]	153/1167 (13.1)	153/540 (28)
Cooner *et al.* [10]	263/1807 (14.6)	263/835 (31.5)
Devonec *et al.* [85]	42/213 (19.7)	42/132 (31.8)
Fritzsche *et al.* [86]	41/228 (18.0)	41/121 (33.9)
Hunter *et al.* [87]	29/508 (5.7)	29/119 (24.4)
Lee *et al.* [11]	20/748 (2.7)	20/64 (31.3)
McWhorter *et al.* [81]	7/34 (20.6)	7/12 (58.3)
Mettlin *et al.* [45]	44/2425 (1.8)	44/290 (15.2)
Perrin *et al.* [88]	11/666 (1.7)	11/162 (6.8)
Ragde *et al.* [89]	50/765 (6.5)	50/138 (36.2)
Rifkin *et al.* [90]	3/8 (37.5)	3/112 (2.7)

the time of ultrasound in a series that looked at postprostatectomy pathological specimens [13]. In a review of systematic sector TRUS-guided biopsies in 1001 patients, we noted that 23 of 253 patients (9.1%) in whom cancer was detected by biopsy had only isoechoic cancer [9].

TRUS also appears to lack specificity. Although cancer often appears as a hypoechoic peripheral zone lesion on TRUS, in our series only 16% of these lesions were malignant [9]. A number of other histological findings can produce a hypoechoic lesion of TRUS, including normal histology, inflammation, infarct and prostatic intraepithelial neoplasia [12].

TRUS-guided prostatic needle biopsy (PNB) provides the best method for sampling the prostate to confirm the histological diagnosis. Several authors have demonstrated the superiority of TRUS/PNB over digitally guided biopsies [14–16]. Hodge *et al.* [17] found that over half (23 of 43 patients: 53%) of the men who had negative digitally guided biopsies had cancer demonstrated on ultrasound-guided biopsy. Brawer and Nagle found carcinoma in 11 of 22 patients (50%) with ultrasound-guided biopsies when the initial digitally guided biopsies had been negative [15]. In a similar fashion, Rifkin *et al.* found positive biopsies when previously performed digitally guided biopsies had been negative [16].

Prostate-specific antigen

The recognition in the 1970s that PSA was elevated in most men with adenocarcinoma of the prostate prompted a number of investigators to begin to look at the feasibility of using this analyte for early detection or screening.

Several recent reviews of this most important of all tumour markers may be found [18–22].

The use of PSA in an early detection or screening approach was initially suspect owing to the multiple reports suggesting that significant elevation of PSA may be found in men with BPH (Table 6.3). Because histological evidence of BPH is found in all men over age 50 – the likely screening population – it was theorized that this would make the specificity of PSA inadequate.

Table 6.3 Serum prostate-specific antigen (PSA) in patients with histologically confirmed benign prostatic hyperplasia (%).

Authors	Assay	PSA > 4.0%	PSA > 10.0%
Ercole *et al.* [91]	Tandem-R	75 (21)	10 (3)
Ferro *et al.* [92]	Tandem-R		13 (33)
Hudson *et al.* [93]	Tandem-R	35 (21)	3 (2)
Stamey *et al.* [40]	Pros-Check	70 (88)	

We became interested in the issue of whether BPH could indeed induce elevation of serum levels of PSA. In a series of men undergoing simple prostatectomy we measured PSA preoperatively [23]. In 34 of 81 patients in this study a Hybritech PSA > 4.0 ng/ml preoperatively was found. We could identify incidental carcinoma, intraepithelial neoplasia or acute inflammation. It appeared that significant pathological entities, in addition to BPH, were most commonly associated with elevation in a serum PSA level.

We have investigated the relationship of the prostatic luminal cell where PSA is elaborated to the capillary bed (to which it must attain access for it to be detectable in the serum detection; Fig. 6.1). Using immunohistochemical as well as electron microscopic techniques, we have demonstrated disruption in some of the barriers between the site of PSA elaboration and the capillary bed in invasive carcinoma as well as prostatic intraepithelial neoplasia [24–27]. Further, it seems likely that tissue destruction that may be associated with acute inflammation may also be associated with barrier disruption, confirming our findings in the clinical study.

The first efforts to examine the role of PSA in early detection or screening came from investigators who measured PSA but did not make therapeutic decisions with regard to the elevation. For example, Cooner *et al.* evaluated men referred to him with DRE and TRUS and biopsied those who had an abnormality on the latter [10]. Table 6.4 demonstrates the results. We also examined a referral population and measured PSA prior to biopsy. Biopsy in our series was performed under ultrasound guidance; however, the indication

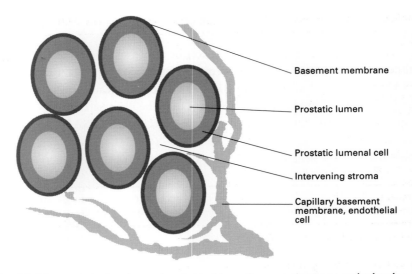

- Basement membrane
- Prostatic lumen
- Prostatic lumenal cell
- Intervening stroma
- Capillary basement membrane, endothelial cell

Fig. 6.1 The prostatic duct lumen in relationship to the prostatic stroma and related capillary bed.

Table 6.4 Prostate-specific antigen performance in carcinoma detection in patients undergoing ultrasound-guided prostate biopsy.

Authors	n	CAP n (%)	Sensitivity	Specificity	PPV
Cooner *et al.* [10]	835	263 (32)	80	61	48
Brawer and Lange [94]	246	79 (32)	65	69	50

PPV, positive predictive value; CAP, carcinoma of prostate.

for biopsy was an abnormality on DRE and no specific ultrasound abnormality was required for biopsy. These data are also shown in Table 6.4. A Hybritech PSA > 4.0 ng/ml provided a positive predictive value (PPV) in the series by Cooner *et al.* [10] of 48% and 50% in our own. As shown in Table 6.5, several authors studying patients derived from mixed referral or screening populations have observed a 30–50% PPV for the Hybritech Tandem assay, irrespective of the indication for biopsy.

The first two studies to examine the role of PSA alone as an early detection or screening test were those reported by Catalona *et al* [28] and our own group [29]. Table 6.6 demonstrates the yield of these studies, including an elaboration of the initial report of Catalona *et al.* [28], a multicentre PSA-based trial [30], as well as our own initial [31] and as serial studies [32, 33]. As is shown, impressive PPVs are observed and serial monitoring of patients with an initial normal PSA who cross over thresholds on subsequent examination still has impressive yields for carcinoma.

Table 6.5 Positive predictive value (PPV) for prostate-specific antigen > 4.0 ng/ml.

Authors	Year	Population	No. Bx.	PPV
Babaian and Camps [95]	1991	Mixed	67	31.3
Bazinet *et al.* [43]	1994	Referral	565	37.0
Brawer and Lange [31]	1989	Referral	188	54.2
Brawer *et al.* [29]	1992	Screening	105	30.5
Catalona *et al.* [96]	1992	Screening	112	33.0
Catalona *et al.* [28]	1993	Screening	1325	37.1
Catalona *et al.* [30]	1994	Screening	686	31.5
Cooner *et al.* [97]	1988	Referral	96	51.2
Cooner *et al.* [10]	1990	Referral	436	35.0
Mettlin *et al.* [98]	1991	Screening	70	41.4
Rommel *et al.* [44]	1994	Referral	2020	41.0

No Bx, number biopsied.

Table 6.6 Yield from prostate-specific antigen-based screening studies.

Authors	Subjects	PPV	Detection rate observed (%)	Detection rate estimated (%)
Catalona *et al.* [28]	9629	34.4	3.1	
Catalona *et al.* (serial) [28]	9333	41.9	2.1	
Catalona *et al.* [30]	6630	31.5	3.3	4.6
Brawer and Lange [31]	1249	30.5	2.6	4.6
Brawer *et al.* (serial) [32]	701	17.1	2.0	6.7
Brawer *et al.* (serial) [33]	738	18.6	1.8	3.8

PPV, positive predictive value.

PSA as the initial test for men over age 50 provides an excellent carcinoma yield. However, it should be emphasized that PSA alone is inadequate to provide effective early detection or screening. This stems from the observation that a number of men with malignancy have PSA values less than 4.0 ng/ml – the most commonly used cut-off for initial testing. In a recent review of our experience at the University of Washington involving patients who have undergone six systematic sector ultrasound-guided biopsies, 21% of those with carcinoma had a PSA less than 4.0 ng/ml [9]. In the multicentre trial reported by Catalona and associates [30], 6630 men were screened with a DRE and a Tandem PSA assay. A total of 264 carcinomas were identified, showing a detection rate of 6 and PPV of 23%. Eighteen per cent of men with carcinoma had normal PSA but an abnormal DRE.

The American Cancer Society (ACS) now recommends a DRE and serum PSA determination on an annual basis for those seeking a cancer prevention check-up. Their recommendation is for testing to begin at age 50 or younger for those with a strong family history of African-Americans [34]. Of the five PSA assays currently approved by the US Food and Drug Administration (FDA) for monitoring established malignancy, only the assays by Hybritech Inc. are approved for early detection or screening.

Clinical and pathological stage of prostate-specific antigen-detected cancer

Not only is PSA determination a useful tool that clinicians can employ to detect prostate cancer, the data indicate that cancers so identified are favourable and tend to be of curable stage both clinically and pathologically. PSA has had a major impact on the presentation of prostate cancer. Lead time bias has allowed for the early detection of disease that presented clinically at some point in the future. Gann *et al.* estimated a mean lead time of 5.5 years, with the sensitivity for detection using a PSA of 4.6 ng/ml of 87%, in what they defined as aggressive cancers [8]. Overall the PSA-based detection rate for all men with prostate cancers was 73%.

Table 6.7 demonstrates the clinical staging of the screening studies reported by Catalona and our own group. Table 6.8 demonstrates pathological staging by these authors. As is readily apparent, most cancers are of favourable stage. Moreover, stage migration following serial testing is appar-

Table 6.7 Clinical stage in prostate-specific antigen screening patients.

Clinical stage	Catalona *et al.* [96] (initial)	Catalona *et al.* [30] (initial)	Catalona *et al.* [28] (initial)	Catalona *et al.* [28] (serial)	Brawer *et al.* [29] (initial)	Brawer *et al.* [32, 33] (serial)
Local	293 (81)	261 (99)	277 (94)	170 (97)	30 (94)	19 (95)
Advanced	7 (19)	3 (1)	17 (6)	5 (3)	2 (6)	1 (5)

Table 6.8 Pathological stage in prostate-specific antigen screening studies.

Pathology	Catalona *et al.* [96] (initial)	Catalona *et al.* [28] (initial)	Catalona *et al.* [28] (serial)	Catalona *et al.* [30] (initial)	Brawer *et al.* [29] (initial)	Brawer *et al.* [32, 33] (serial)
Local	12 (36)	153 (62)	92 (71)	170 (67)	9 (56)	10 (91)
Advanced	21 (64)	91 (38)	37 (29)	84 (33)	7 (44)	1 (9)

ent. This is intuitively obvious, as with the initial testing of a cohort the more aggressive cancers would be more likely to be identified. Following the initial screening experience, those cancers identified would be earlier in their natural history and thus more favourable, both clinically and pathologically.

Smith and Catalona found that, of the men with prostate cancer detected by PSA screening, 97% had clinically localized disease (stage T1, T2) and 69% had pathologically confined disease after surgical staging [35]. Mettlin *et al.* found a similar number of men with locally confined disease [36]. In their review of men screened with PSA who were eventually treated by radical prostatectomy, 62% of them had pathologically confined cancer [36]. We found similar clinical and pathological stages of prostate cancer in men from our screening study [29]. In men with serum PSA values less than 10.0 ng/ml, 75% had pathologically organ-confined disease. Among men with PSA values over 10.0 ng/ml, 57% of men had pathologically organ-confined prostate cancer.

Enhancing the specificity of prostate-specific antigen

As impressive as the performance of PSA is, considerable efforts are underway to improve this tumour marker. Two of the most important parameters with regard to the performance of any diagnostic test are sensitivity – the number of people with a disease who have an abnormal test result – and specificity – the number of people free of disease who have a negative test result. These two statistics are inversely related (Fig. 6.2). In Fig. 6.2 the sensitivity and specificity for various PSA cut-offs among 1920 men undergoing systematic sector biopsy are shown. As is readily apparent, any lowering of the PSA threshold which would achieve improvement in sensitivity of necessity results in a decrease in specificity and vice versa.

Attempts at improving test performance in general will always have to sacrifice sensitivity for improved specificity, or specificity for enhanced sensitivity. In prostate cancer testing, most efforts are underway to improve specificity. This stems from the likelihood that men will be repeatedly tested during their lifetime and thus a false-negative test report may well become a positive test in those with prostatic carcinoma. Thus, a reduction of the sensitivity may be less important. In contrast, false-positive tests are exceedingly costly, both financially and in terms of patient anxiety. An abnormal PSA does not connote a diagnosis of prostatic carcinoma. Rather, it mandates further testing, most commonly ultrasound-guided prostatic biopsy, and thus the costs are compounded with an abnormal test. Reduction of false-positives is achieved by improvements in specificity. Four approaches to improve the

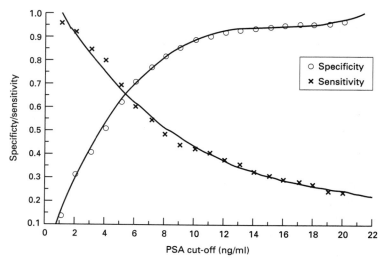

Fig. 6.2 Sensitivity and specificity of PSA detection of prostate cancer at various cut-offs.

performance of PSA are currently under investigation – PSA density (PSAD), age-specific PSA, PSA velocity and PSA forms. Each will be discussed.

Prostate-specific antigen density

As noted, it has been widely reported that BPH is associated with an elevation of serum PSA level. Indeed, Hammerer *et al.* [37] demonstrated that the single greatest predictor of PSA in men with insignificant volumes of prostate cancer was the volume of the transition zone where BPH arises. Our observation cited above that it is not simple BPH but other pathological entities that may cause leakage is not totally at odds with these observations in that a larger prostate would be more likely to harbour foci, perhaps subclinical, of these pathological entities. Nevertheless, the concept of larger benign glands being associated with elevated PSA is well-ensconced in the literature.

This phenomenon has given rise to the concept of PSAD, in which the serum PSA is adjusted for the volume of the gland by deriving the quotient of serum PSA divided by prostate volume. Although first widely promulgated by Benson *et al.* [38, 39] Stamey and associates had previously reported a 10-fold increase of PSA arising from carcinomas as opposed to that derived from BPH [40]. Actually, it was Babaian *et al.* [41] who first clearly demonstrated the relationship between prostatic volume and serum PSA level. Nevertheless, Benson *et al.* made a significant contribution when they provided impressive performance results of PSAD. These authors were able to stratify the majority of patients who did or did not have prostatic carcinoma by dividing the serum PSA by the prostatic volume, as measured initially by magnetic resonance imaging [38] and subsequently by TRUS [39].

We were interested in these observations and, in an attempt to replicate them, we evaluated PSA density based on ultrasound-guided volume [42]. Unfortunately we were unable to reproduce the findings of Benson *et al.* Our receiver operating characteristics curve from this report is shown in Fig. 6.3. As is apparent, PSAD was no better than PSA itself in predicting who did or did not have carcinoma. We attempted to adjust the PSAD by manipulating that PSA that may have emanated from the non-transition zone (Table 6.9).

Certainly a number of explanations are possible as to why we could not reproduce the results of Benson *et al.*, including different patient populations, ultrasound volume techniques, PSA assay variability and statistical analysis employed. We believe that the major factor, however, results from issues of sampling. Figure 6.4 assumes 2 men with equivalent PSA but widely disparate gland volumes. If we assume that within each prostate there is an equal-volume carcinoma that is both isoechoic and non-palpable (T1c), sample considera-

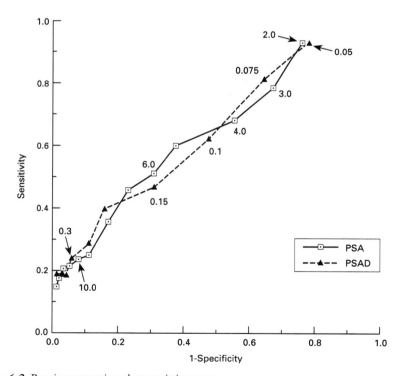

Fig. 6.3 Receiver operating characteristics curve.

Table 6.9 Mean values for all patients stratified by biopsy result.

Variable	Negative (159 patients)	Positive (68 patients)	t-value	Mann–Whitney (Z score)
PSA	5.23 ± 5.04	10.39 ± 11.65	3.51*	3.34*
Gland volume	42.60 ± 25.64	40.54 ± 16.56	0.72	0.41
Peripheral zone volume	28.86 ± 16.95	26.87 ± 11.39	1.03	0.12
Gland density	0.137 ± 0.14	0.290 ± 0.41	2.98**	3.43*
Peripheral zone density				
0.05	0.182 ± 0.21	0.420 ± 0.67	2.89**	3.44*
0.10	0.158 ± 0.20	0.393 ± 0.66	2.87**	3.31*
0.20	0.110 ± 0.20	0.342 ± 0.55	2.82**	3.22*
0.30	0.056 ± 0.21	0.287 ± 0.66	2.82**	3.07*

Gland density refers to the prostate-specific antigen (PSA) density for the entire gland.
$*P < 0.01$
$**\ P < 0.05$.

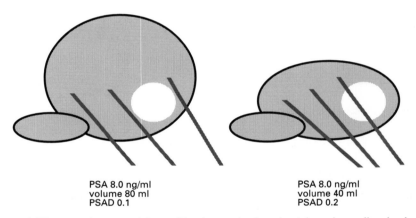

PSA 8.0 ng/ml
volume 80 ml
PSAD 0.1

PSA 8.0 ng/ml
volume 40 ml
PSAD 0.2

Fig. 6.4 The same size cancer is located in a larger gland on the right and a smaller gland on the left. The smaller gland by definition will have a higher PSAD and because of chance sampling the cancer is more likely to be detectable in the smaller gland with the higher PSAD.

tions would suggest that with an equivalent number of biopsies taken from both patients, cancer would more readily be found in the man with the smaller prostate who incidentally has a higher PSAD. While it is true that volume expansion is more a factor of the transition zone as opposed to the peripheral zone (which most clinicians tend to sample preferentially), displacement of the peripheral zone by an expanding transition zone also makes carcinomas more difficult to identify in such glands.

Table 6.10 illustrates five reports from the literature in which PSAD has been investigated. Those by Bazinet *et al.* [43], Benson *et al.* [38] and Rommel *et al.* [44] demonstrate increased stratification using PSAD. However, in each of these cases the glands harbouring malignancy were statistically significantly smaller than those without. In our study [42], as well as that by Mettlin *et al.* [45], there was either no difference in the gland volume, or in the case of Mettlin's experience, the gland was actually larger.

Table 6.10 Prostate-specific antigen (PSA) density.

Author	Biopsy	No.	PSA (ng/ml)	Volume (cm^3)	PSAD
Bazinet *et al.* [43, 99]	Positive	217	21.4 (29.6)*	37.6 (21.4)*	0.63 (0.86)*
	Negative	317	9.1 (8.1)	51.6 (27.3)	0.21 (0.25)
Benson *et al.* [38]	Positive	98	7.0 (1.7)*	28.9 (14.6)*	0.30 (0.15)*
	Negative	191	6.8 (1.8)	40.1 (20.2)	0.21 (0.11)
Rommel *et al.* [44, 100]	Positive	612	15.5 (21.6)*	42.7 (27.2)	0.47 (0.11)*
	Negative	1394	4.9 (4.7)	47.0 (31.6)	0.105 (0.09)
Brawer *et al.* [42]	Positive	68	10.4 (11.7)*	40.5 (16.6)	0.29 (0.41)*
	Negative	159	5.2 (5.0)	42.6 (25.6)	0.14 (0.14)
Mettlin *et al.* [45]	Positive	171	12.0 (16.0)*	38.9 (16.4)*	0.35 (0.5)*
	Negative	650	2.1 (2.3)	33.5 (14.2)	0.08 (0.09)

* $P < 0.05$.
PSAD, prostate-specific antigen density.

We have recently expanded our experience with PSAD calculations among 665 men undergoing systematic sector biopsy. Table 6.11 demonstrates the results. Among 240 men with carcinoma we found that PSAD was useful in identifying those who had cancer in the range of 4.0–10.0 ng/ml. Of note, however – examination of the gland volumes showed that those men with carcinoma had statistically significantly smaller prostates than those without.

Table 6.11 Prostate-specific antigen density (PSAD) revisited.

PSA range (ng/ml)	No. CAP/ben.	Mean PSA CAP/Ben.	Mean PSAD CAP/Ben.	Mean volume (cm^3) CAP/Ben.
< 4.0	59/328	2.3/1.9*	0.08/0.072	32.0/29.6
4.0 < PSA < 10.0	89/271	6.3/6.2	0.20/0.16**	37.9/48.5**
> 10.0	92/66	36.2/29.1	1.15/1.03	41.8/66.0**
0.2–220.0	240/665	16.7/6.4**	0.53/0.20	37.9/40.9

* $P < 0.05$
** $P < 0.01$.
CAP, carcinoma of prostate; Ben, benign.

This adds credibility to our hypothesis that the putative advantage of PSAD may stem largely from sampling.

Age-specific prostate-specific antigen

Another attempt to improve the specificity of PSA is to adjust the cut-off for abnormalities according to the age of the man. It is widely accepted that PSA levels increase with increasing patient age. For example, in our PSA screening series this trend was evident and is demonstrated in Table 6.12. This adjustment may enhance the sensitivity in a younger cohort of men and improve specificity in an older cohort of men. Oesterling *et al.* and Dalkin *et al.* have reported their age-specific cut-offs for the upper limit of normal (defined as the 95th percentile) and their results are shown in Table 6.13 [46, 47]. Catalona *et al.* expressed some concern over age-adjusted PSA cut-off values [48]. Although age-adjusted PSA appears to enhance the specificity in the over-70-year age group, Catalona and colleagues raised concern of a lower rate of organ-confined disease when compared to a cohort of men where a traditional cut-off of 4.0 ng/ml was used. For this reason they recommended that the traditional cut-off of 4.0 ng/ml be maintained. We have shown in a simulation of the use of the age-specific cut-offs recommended by Oesterling versus 4.0 ng/ml that the latter would result in significant reduction in the overall longevity of a screening population [49].

Table 6.12 Prostate-specific antigen versus age.

Age (years)	No. (%)	Mean (ng/ml)	Median (ng/ml)	SD (ng/ml)
50–59	222 (17.8)	1.62	1.0	6.5
60–69	600 (48.0)	2.7	3.8	1.4
70–79	365 (29.2)	3.1	5.0	1.7
>79	62 (5.0)	8.8	11.9	2.2
Totals	1249	2.9	2.2	10.4

After Brawer *et al.* [29]

Table 6.13 Age-adjusted prostate-specific antigen.

Age (years)	Oesterling *et al.* [46]	Dalkin *et al.* [47]
40–49	2.5	
50–59	3.5	3.5
60–69	4.5	5.4
70–79	6.5	6.3

Prostate-specific antigen velocity

Despite its overall impressive performance, it is recognized that a significant number of men with prostate cancer have a normal PSA level. For example, in our series 5 of 79 men (6.3%) with prostate cancer had PSA less than 4.0 ng/ml [50]. Changes in PSA level identified with serial PSA measurements might identify men with cancer and allow for better selection of patients who require biopsy.

Carter *et al.* reported on data from the Baltimore Longitudinal Aging Cohort and identified a significant stratification between men with prostate cancer and those without by using an annual rise in PSA of greater than 0.75 ng/ml per year [51]. This identification of men at risk was particularly evident when the initial PSA was > 4.0 ng/ml. Below this cut-off the sensitivity was significantly reduced [51]. This cohort was followed over a long period of time, with a minimum assay interval of 7 years. A PSA doubling time of 74 ± 13 years at age 60 was identified in the control cohort of men. In the men with BPH the PSA doubling time was between 1.8 and 2.4 ± 0.3 years [52].

Bernier and Roehrborn [53] and Porter *et al.* [54] also reported on data which followed patients longitudinally with serial PSA measurements. Neither report indicated a significant advantage of PSA velocity in identifying prostate cancer. These studies, however, are handicapped by the relatively short time interval between PSA determinations owing to biological variation which may mask the actual information obtained. This may be minimized with multiple determinations and longer follow-up.

Prostate-specific antigen forms

A final approach to enhancing the performance of PSA surrounds the issue of PSA forms that are in circulation. It is now known that PSA circulates in three forms: free PSA, PSA complex with α_2-macroglobulin, and the major form of circulating PSA, that complexed with α_1-antichymotrypsin [55–58]. Figure 6.5 demonstrates conceptual models of these three circulating forms. Free PSA has five epitopes available for antibodies, including those employed in conventional serum assays. In general, this represents the minority of identifiable PSA in systemic circulation. It is, however, the major component in the seminal plasma. PSA complexed to α_1-antichymotrypsin constitutes approximately 90% of the identifiable PSA in the systemic circulation. Three of the epitopes that are present in free PSA are masked when PSA complexed with α_1-antichymotrypsin. PSA complexed to α_2-macroglobulin has no epitopes available for the current commercially available immunoassays.

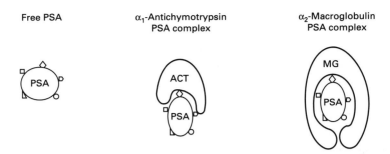

Fig. 6.5 Conceptual models of the three forms of PSA that circulate the bloodstream.

The recognition that free PSA comprised a greater proportion of that in men without malignancy raised the question of whether two identifiable forms could be measured independently and the results compared to enhance detection of carcinoma. Lilja *et al.* [59] reported on 89 men and noted the ratio of free to complexed PSA and compared it to total PSA. Holding the sensitivity at 90% they noted that this ratio afforded specificities of 64–68%, as opposed to 32–33% employing total PSA alone as measured by conventional assays. Multiple investigations are underway currently to investigate this phenomenon more fully.

It is apparent that the majority of circulating PSA is complexed to α_1-antichymotrypsin, although a greater percentage in men without malignancy appears to be in the free form. Stamey *et al.*, using gel chromatography from very well-characterized patients, noted that 88–98% of the PSA in those with cancer was complexed [60]. In 10 patients with BPH with no evidence of carcinoma, 73–84% was complexed. Using an experimental assay that measures free and total PSA we have observed a large range in the percentage free in men both with and without malignancy (Fig. 6.6).

Prostate-specific antigen assay techniques

There are at least 20 different techniques to assay serum levels of PSA available throughout the world. It is critical that the clinician should know which assay has been used on any given patient and then to ensure that the same assay is used on subsequent evaluations. Many assays are different in design and it is difficult to make any correlation between results of different assays.

One of the most widely used assay in North America is the Tandem-R (Hybritech). This is a solid-phase radioimmunometric assay which uses murine monoclonal antibodies to identify the epitopes of the PSA molecule [61]. The first antibody is fixed in a solid phase and extracts the antibody from the serum.

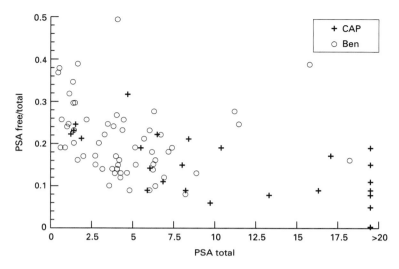

Fig. 6.6 This depicts the wide variation of free PSA measured in men with both benign and malignant prostate disease, using an experimental assay for free PSA.

The second antibody is radiolabelled and binds to the fixed PSA antigen–antibody complex. The analytic sensitivity for the Tandem-R assay is 0.1–0.2 ng/ml [62]. The clinical sensitivity, which is the lowest measure that can regularly discriminate from a true 'zero' reading, is reported to range between 0.1 and 0.6 ng/ml [62]. Most labs report an undetectable level at less than 0.2 ng/ml [63].

The Tandem-E assay (Hybritech) is similar to the Tandem-R assay but instead of using a radiolabelled second antibody it uses an enzyme labelled second antibody (alkaline phosphatase) to measure PSA. This immunoenzymatic assay has the same analytical and clinical sensitivities as the Tandem-R assay but has the advantage of not involving any radioactivity.

The Pros-Check assay (Yang Laboratories) is a radioimmunoassay based on competitive protein binding. It uses polyclonal rabbit anti-PSA antibodies which have the potential disadvantage of inherent instability. The analytical sensitivity of this assay is 0.1–0.2 ng/ml and the clinical sensitivity is 0.2–0.3 ng/ml [64].

The IMx assay (Abbott Laboratories) is a radioimmunometric assay. As opposed to the Tandem assay, which uses two mouse monoclonal antibodies, the IMx assay uses a mouse monoclonal antibody to bind the PSA in serum and then uses a radiolabelled goat antimouse polyclonal antibody to bind the PSA antigen–antibody complex. The analytical sensitivity of this assay is 0.03 ng/ml and the clinical sensitivity is 0.2–0.6 ng/ml [65].

There are also several other assays available. The Oris assay is manufactured by a subsidiary of the French Atomic Energy Agency and is a radio-immunoassay using two monoclonal antibodies. Ciba–Corning manufactures automated chemiluminescent immunoassay (ACS) for the measurement of serum levels of PSA utilizing a monoclonal/polyclonal antibody combination.

Few data exist with regard to the correlation of one assay to another. Owing to the likelihood that patients and clinicians may switch among assays, we have begun a series of investigations to compare the results obtained from different manufacturers' kits [66, 67]. We have examined 256 random sera from our archival bank and compared three lots of IMx assay with three lots of Tandem-E assay. All assays were run according to the manufacturers' specifications on one freeze thaw of the archived serum.

We noted significant lot-to-lot variation among the three IMx assays compared to the Hybritech ERA. Between-lot slopes of the former revealed biases ranging from 1.1 to 10.9%, whereas in the latter, the range was from 0.3 to 3.7% proportional bias [66]. This indicates the potential for significant lot-to-lot variability when the Abbott assay is employed.

Figure 6.7 demonstrates variation among the three IMx lots studied compared to three of Tandem in the clinically useful range of 2.0–10.0 ng/ml. Significant scatter was observed, but more importantly the bias was lower in almost every IMx measurement. Figure 6.8 demonstrates the regression over

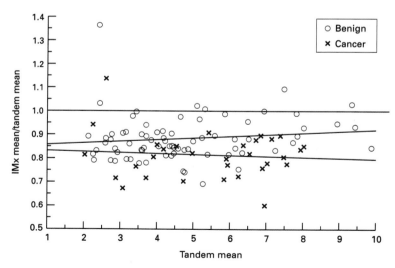

Fig. 6.7 The variation of serum PSA measurement by the IMx method when compared to the Tandem method.

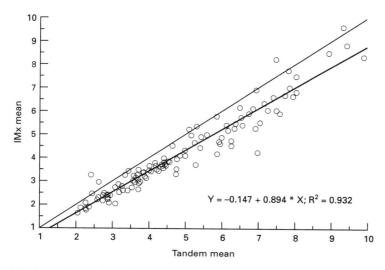

Fig. 6.8 Regression analysis of serum PSA measurements using the Tandem and IMx methods.

the mean Tandem versus mean IMx. A 13% lower reading overall was observed for the IMx.

The clinical relevance of this bias is shown in Fig. 6.9. Using various arbitrary cut-offs for men with an established diagnosis of cancer, there is a stepwise reduction in the percentage of patients that would exceed this

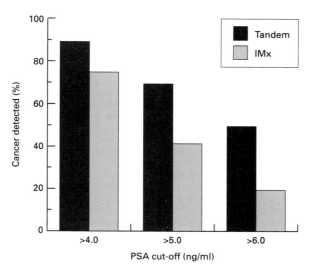

Fig. 6.9 The clinical significance of the variation in PSA assays is highlighted here showing the reduction in prostate cancer detection at increasing serum PSA cut-off values.

threshold. Obviously further work is necessary to confirm these findings; however, it certainly suggests that manufacturers should provide data indicating the yield of carcinoma for their assay so that meaningful comparisons to the more widely studied Hybritech assay can be made.

A comparison has also been made between the Tandem-R assay and the Pros-Check assay [68]. PSA levels as measured by the Pros-Check assay are 1.4–1.8 times higher than the levels measured by the Tandem-R assay. This difference is apparently due to differences in the standards used with each of their respective kits [68]. When similar standards are used as replacements for those found in the kits, the assay results are almost identical.

Unfortunately, no international standard is available for PSA. Under the direction of Dr Thomas Stamey, significant strides have been made in this regard. Recently the second annual Stanford PSA standardization conference was held [69, 70]. Amongst various seminal conclusions generated from this conference was the decision that a standard calibrator determined by mass weight of PSA should be used by various manufacturers to allow direct comparison. It was determined that the calibrator should be comprised of 10% free and 90% complexed PSA. It is hoped that the adoption of such a calibrator by all manufacturers would allow the variability between assays to be minimized.

Screening – yes or no?

It is doubtful that any issue in urological oncology has generated as much controversy as that surrounding the notion of screening for prostatic carcinoma. Indeed, this would appear to be one of the major issues in medicine today, at least as evidenced by the amount of lay press this topic has generated. Our august bodies seemingly are at odds. For example, the Canadian Task Force has recommended against the use of PSA for population-based screening [71]. In contrast, the American Cancer Society [34] has recommended PSA testing.

Physicians with an opportunity to cure disease may impulsively feel that early detection of prostate cancer is beneficial. Unfortunately, we lack any definitive data demonstrating a reduction in mortality as a result of early detection and treatment of prostate cancer. There are numerous reports of long-term follow-up on patients who have received either radical surgery or radical radiotherapy [72, 73]. These are retrospective analyses which demonstrate that disease-specific survival in the prostate cancer patient is equal to age-matched controls [72–74]. However, results of randomized prospective trials of screening and treatment are required before proof of reduction of prostate cancer mortality will be available (see Chapter 19 for a review of screening).

Until such time, we might act on what seems reasonable for a given man. Littrup *et al.* have analysed the benefit and cost of various early detection techniques [75]. By using data from the American Cancer Society–National Prostate Cancer Detection Project they proposed a plausible and potentially cost-effective means for early detection in prostate cancer [76]. Although their report is not conclusive, they suggest that DRE in combination with PSA become an ethical and economic means for early detection. A reduction of test use in the oldest age groups and early institution in high-risk groups where mortality is greatest may result in a net benefit [76].

The cost of screening for prostate carcinoma, both economic, as well as the potential for human suffering, is overwhelming. This is particularly problematic given that no definitive studies can be cited to present proof that early detection and aggressive management will actually be associated with a reduction of prostate cancer mortality. While, as noted, multiple studies are underway to investigate this phenomenon, the conclusions of those studies will not be known for some time.

When clinicians are daily faced with patients seeking testing for prostate cancer, they are often at a loss for what to do. Ultimately it is our belief that the primary care-provider must make the decision as to whether the early detection of prostate cancer is in the individual patient's best interest. In evaluating the parameters such as patient age, current illness, social situation, desires, etc., the primary physician is best suited to counsel the patient regarding the risk-benefit ratio of such testing. If such counselling leads to the decision of the patient to go ahead with screening, then a carefully performed DRE and serum PSA should be measured. If, however, it is conducted that an early diagnosis of prostate cancer will not enhance the quality and quantity of life, then no testing should take place.

References

1 Boring CC, Squires TS, Tong T & Montgomery S. Cancer statistics, 1994. *CA Cancer J Clin* 1994; **44**: 7–26.
2 Seidman H, Mushinski MH & Geit SK *et al.* Probabilities of eventually developing or dying of cancer – United States, 1985. *Cancer* 1985; **35**: 36–56.
3 Carter HB & Coffey D. The prostate: an increasing medical problem. *Prostate* 1990; **16**: 39–48.
4 Brawer MK & Ellis WJ. Chemoprevention for prostate cancer. *Cancer* 1995; **75**: 1783–1789.
5 Jewett JJ. Significance of the palpable prostatic nodule. *JAMA* 1956; **160**: 838.

6 Thompson IM, Rounder JB, Teaque JL, Peak M & Spence CR. Impact of routine screening for adenocarcinoma of the prostate on stage distribution. *J Urol* 1987; **137**: 424–426.

7 Sika JV & Lindquist HD. Relationship of needle biopsy diagnosis of prostate to clinical signs of prostatic cancer: an evaluation of 300 cases. *J Urol* 1963; **89**: 737.

8 Gann PH, Hennekens CH & Stampfer MJ. A prospective evaluation of plasma PSA for detection of prostatic cancer. *JAMA* 1995; **273**: 289–294.

9 Ellis WJ, Chetner M, Preston S, Brawer MK. Diagnosis of prostatic carcinoma: the yield of serum PSA, DRE and TRUS. *J Urol* 1994; **152**: 1520–1525.

10 Cooner WH, Mosley RB, Rutherford CL Jr *et al*. Prostate cancer detection in a clinical urological practice by ultrasonography, digital rectal examination and prostate specific antigen. *J Urol* 1990; **143**: 1146–1152.

11 Lee F, Littrup PJ, Torp-Pederson ST, Mettlin C, McHugh TA & Gray JM. Prostate cancer: comparison of transrectal US and DRE for screening. *Radiology* 1988; **168**: 389–394.

12 Lee FR, Gray JM, McLeary RD *et al*. Prostatic evaluation by transrectal sonography: criteria for diagnosis of early carcinoma. *Radiology* 1986; **158**: 91–95.

13 Carter HB, Hamper UM, Sheth S, Sanders RC Epstein JI & Walsh PC. Evaluation of transrectal ultrasound in the early detection of prostate cancer. *J Urol* 1989; **142**: 1008–1010.

14 Partin AW, Carter HB, Chan DW *et al*. Prostate specific antigen in the staging of localized prostate cancer: influence of tumor differentiation, tumor volume and benign hyperplasia. *J Urol* 1990; **143**: 747–752.

15 Brawer MK & Nagle RB. Transrectal ultrasound guided prostate needle biopsy following negative digitally guided biopsy. *J Urol* 1989; **141**:278A.

16 Rifkin MD, Alexander AA, Pisarchick J & Matteucci T (1991). Palpable masses in the prostate: superior accuracy of ultrasound guided biopsy compared with accuracy of digitally guided biopsy. *Radiology* 1991; **179**: 41–42.

17 Hodge KK, McNeal JE, Terris MK & Stamey TA. Random systematic versus directed ultrasound-guided transrectal core biopsies of the prostate. *J Urol* 1989; **142**: 71.

18 Stamey TA & Kabalin JN. Prostate specific antigen in the diagnosis and treatment of adenocarcinoma of the prostate: I. Untreated patients. *J Urol* 1989; **141**: 1070–1075.

19 Oesterling J. Prostate-specific antigen: improving its ability to diagnose early prostate cancer. *JAMA* 1992; **267**: 2236–2238.

20 Brawer MK. PSA: a review. *Acta Oncol* 1991; **30**: 161–168.

21 Brawer MK. Laboratory studies for the detection of carcinoma of the prostate. *Urol Clin North Am* 1990; **17**(4): 759–68.

22 Partin AW & Oesterling JE. The clinical usefulness of prostate specific antigen: update 1994. *J Urol* 1994; **152**(5): 1358–1368.

23 Brawer MK, Rennels MA, Nagle RB, Schifman RA & Gaines J. Serum PSA and prostate pathology in men having simple prostatectomy. *Am J Clin Pathol* 1989; **92**: 760–764.

24 Brawer MK, Nagle RB, Pitts W, Freiha FS & Gamble SL. Keratin immunoreactivity as an aid to the diagnosis of persistent adenocarcinoma in irradiated human prostates. *Cancer* 1989; **63**: 454–460.

25 Bostwick DM & Brawer MK. PIN and early invasion in prostatic cancer. *Cancer* 1987; **59**: 788–794.

26 Bigler SA, Brown M, Deering RE & Brawer MK. Immunohistochemistry of type VII

collagen in human prostatic tissue. *J Urol* 1994; **151**(suppl): 277A.

27 Fuchs ME, Brawer MK, Rennels MA & Nagle RB. The relationship of basement membrane to histologic grade of human prostatic carcinoma. *Modern Pathol* 1989; **2**: 105–111.

28 Catalona WJ, Smith DS, Ratliff TL & Basler JW. Detection of organ-confined prostate cancer is increased through PSA-based screening. *JAMA* 1993; **270**: 948–954.

29 Brawer MK, Chetner MP, Beatie J, Buchner DM, Cessella RL & Lange PH. Screening for prostatic carcinoma with PSA. *J Urol* 1992; **147**: 841–845.

30 Catalona WJ, Richie JP, Ahmann FR *et al.* Comparison of DRE and serum PSA in the early detection of prostate cancer: results of a multicenter clinical trial of 6630 men. *J Urol* 1994; **151**: 1283–1290.

31 Brawer MK & Lange PH. PSA in the screening, staging and follow up of early-stage prostate cancer: a review of recent developments. *World J Urol* 1989; **7**: 7–11.

32 Brawer MK, Beattie J, Wener MH, Vessella RL, Preston SD & Lange PH. Screening for prostatic carcinoma with PSA. Results of the second year. *J Urol* 1993; **150**: 106–109.

33 Brawer MK, Beatie J & Wener MH. PSA as the initial test in prostate carcinoma screening: results of the third year. *J Urol* 1993; **149**(suppl): 299A.

34 Mettlin C, Jones G, Averette H, Gusberg SB & Murphy GP. Defining and updating the ACS guidelines for the cancer related check-up: prostate and endometrial cancer. *CA Cancer J Clin* 1993; **43**: 42–46.

35 Smith DS & Catalona WJ. The nature of prostate cancer detected through PSA based screening. *J Urol* 1994; **152**: 1732–1740.

36 Mettlin C, Murphy GP, Lee F *et al.* Characteristics of prostate cancers detected in a multimodality early detection program. *Cancer* 1994; **72**: 1701–1708.

37 Hammerer PG, McNeal JE & Stamey TA. Correlation between serum PSA levels and the volume of the individual glandular zones of the human prostate. *J Urol* 1995; **153**: 111–114.

38 Benson MC, Whang IS, Olsson CA, McMahon DJ & Cooner WH. The use of prostate-specific antigen density to enhance the predictive value of intermediate levels of serum prostate-specific antigen. *J Urol* 1992; **147**: 817–821.

39 Benson BC, Whang IS, Pantuck A *et al.* Prostate specific antigen density: a means of distinguishing benign prostatic hypertrophy and prostate cancer. *J Urol* 1992; **147**: 815–816.

40 Stamey TA, Yang N, Hay AR *et al.* Prostate-specific antigen as a serum marker for adenocarcinoma of the prostate. *N Engl J Med* 1987; **317**: 909–916.

41 Babaian RJ, Fritsche HA & Evans RB. PSA and prostate gland volume: correlation and clinical application. *J Clin Lab* 1990; **4**: 135–137.

42 Brawer MK, Aramburu EAG, Chen GL, Preston SD & Ellis WJ. The inability of PSA index to enhance the predictive value of PSA in the diagnosis of prostatic carcinoma. *J Urol* 1993; **150**: 369–373.

43 Bazinet M, Meshref AW, Trudel C *et al.* Prospective evaluation of prostate specific antigen density and systematic biopsies for early detection of prostatic carcinoma. *Urology* 1994; **43**: 44–51.

44 Rommel FM, Augusta VE, Breslin JA *et al.* The use of PSA and PSAD in the diagnosis of prostate cancer in a community based urology practice. *J Urol* 1994; **151**: 88–93.

45 Mettlin C, Littrup PJ, Kane RA *et al.* Relative sensitivity and specificity of serum PSA

level compared with age-referenced PSA, PSA density and PSA change. *Cancer* 1994; **74**: 1615–1620.

46 Oesterling JE, Jacobsen SJ, Chute CG *et al.* Serum PSA in a community-based population of healthy men. *JAMA* 1993; **270**: 860–864.

47 Dalkin BL, Ahmann FR & Kopp JB. PSA levels in men older than 50 years without clinical evidence of prostatic carcinoma. *J Urol* 1993; **150**: 1837–1839.

48 Catalona WJ, Hudson MA, Scardino PI *et al.* Selection of optimal PSA cutoffs for early detection of prostate cancer: receiver operating characteristic curves. *J Urol* 1994; **151**(suppl): 449A.

49 Petteway J & Brawer MK. Age specific vs. 4.0 ng/ml as a PSA cutoff in the screening population: impact on cancer detection. *J Urol* 1995; **153**: 465a.

50 Ellis WJ, Preston SD & Brawer MK. Diagnosis of prostatic carcinoma: the yield of serum PSA, digital rectal examination, and transrectal ultrasound. *J Urol* 1994; **151**(suppl): 404A.

51 Carter HB, Pearson JD & Metter EJ. Longitudinal evaluation of prostate-specific antigen levels in men with and without prostate disease. *JAMA* 1992; **267**: 2215–2220.

52 Carter HB & Pearson JD. PSA velocity for the diagnosis of early prostate cancer: a new concept. *Urol Clin North Am* 1993; **20**: 665.

53 Bernier P & Roehrborn CG. Predictive values of PSA rate of change in regards to the outcome of prostate biopsies in a longitudinally followed patient population. *J Urol* 1994; **151**(suppl) 293A.

54 Porter JR, Hayward R & Brawer MK. The significance of short-term PSA change in men undergoing ultrasound guided prostate biopsy. *J Urol* 1994; **151**(suppl): 293A.

55 Christensson A, Bjork J, Nilsson O *et al.* Serum prostate-specific antigen complexed to alpha 1-antichymotrypsin as an indicator of prostate cancer. *J Urol* 1993; **150**: 100–105.

56 Lilja H. Significance of different molecular forms of serum PSA. The free, non-complexed form of PSA versus that complexed to alpha-1-antichymotrypsin. *Urol Clin North Am* 1993; **20**: 681.

57 Stenman U, Leinonen J, Alfthan H, Rannikko S, Tuhkanen K & Althan O. A complex between PSA and α_1-antichymotrypsin is the major form of PSA in serum of patients with prostatic cancer: assay of the complex improves clinical sensitivity for cancer. *Cancer Res* 1991; **51**: 222.

58 Lilja H, Christensson A, Dahlen U *et al.* PSA in human serum occurs predominantly in complex with alpha-1 antichymotrypsin. *Clin Chem* 1991; **37**: 1618–1625.

59 Lilja H, Bjork T, Abrahamsson P *et al.* Improved separation between normals, BPH and carcinoma of the prostate by measuring free, complexed and total concentrations of PSA. *J Urol* 1994; **151**(suppl): 400A.

60 Stamey IA, Chen Z & Prestigiacomo A. Serum PSA binding alpha-1-antichymotrypsin: influence of cancer volume, location and therapeutic selection of resistant clones. *J Urol* 1994; **152**: 1510–1514.

61 Myrtle J, Kilmley P, Ivor L & Bruni J. Clinical utility of prostate specific antigen (PSA) in the management of prostate cancer. *Adv Cancer Diagn* 1986.

62 Chan DW, Bruzek DJ, Oesterling JE, Rock RC & Walsh PC. Prostate-specific antigen as a marker for prostatic cancer: a monoclonal and polyclonal immunoassay compared. *Clin Chem* 1987; **33**: 1916–1920.

63 Myrtle JF. More on 'hook effects' in immunometric assays for PSA. *Clin Chem* 1989; **35**: 2154.

64 Hortin GL, Bahnson RR, Daft M *et al*. Differences in values obtained with two assays of prostate-specific antigen. *J Urol* 1988; **139**: 762–765.

65 Vessella RJN & Lange PH. Clinical trial of an ultrasensitive prostate specific antigen (PSA) immunoassay. *Clin Chem* 1991; **37**: 1024.

66 Brawer MK, Wener MH, Daum PR & Close B. Method to method variation in assays for PSA. *J Urol* 1994; **151**(suppl): 450A.

67 Brawer MK, Daum P, Petteway JC & Wener MH. Assay variability in serum PSA determination. *Prostate* 1995; **27**: 1–6.

68 Graves HCB, Wehner N & Stamey TA. Comparison of a polyclonal and monoclonal immunoassay for PSA: need for an international antigen standard. *J Urol* 1990; **144**: 1516.

69 Murphy GP. The second Stanford conference on international standardization of PSA assays. *Cancer* 1995; **75**: 122–128.

70 Stamey TA. Second Stanford conference on international standardization of PSA immunoassays: September 1 and 2, 1994. *Urology* 1995; **45**: 173–184.

71 Feightner JW. The early detection and treatment of prostate cancer: the perspective of the Canadian task force on the periodic health examination. *J Urol* 1994; **152**: 1682–1684.

72 Gibbons RP, Correa RJ Jr, Brannen GE & Weissman RM. Total prostectomy for clinically localized prostatic cancer: long-term results. *J Urol* 1989; **131**: 564–566.

73 Hanks GE. External beam radiation treatment for prostate cancer: still the gold standard. *Oncology* 1992; **6**: 79.

74 Bagshaw MA, Kaplan ID & Cox RC. Radiation therapy for localized disease. *Cancer* 1993; **71**(suppl): 939.

75 Littrup PJ, Goodman AC & Mettlin CJ. The benefit and cost of prostate cancer early detection. *CA Cancer J Clin* 1993; **43**: 134–149.

76 Littrup PJ, Goodman AC, Mettlin CJ & Murphy GP. Cost analysis of prostate cancer screening: framework for discussion. *J Urol* 1994; **152**: 1873.

77 Chodak GW & Schoenberg HW. Progress and problems in screening for carcinoma of the prostate. *World J Surg* 1989; **13**: 60–64.

78 Faul P. Experience with the German annual preventive checkup examination. *Prostate Cancer* 1982; **3**: 57–68.

79 Gilbertsen VA. Cancer of the prostate gland: results of early diagnosis and therapy undertaken for cure of the disease. *JAMA* 1976; **215**: 81–84.

80 Jenson CB, Shahon DB & Wangensteen OH. Evaluation of annual examinations in the detection of cancer: special reference to cancer of the gastrointestinal tract, prostate, breast, and female reproductive tract. *JAMA* 1960; **174**: 1783–1788.

81 McWhorter WP, Hernandez AD, Meile AW *et al*. A screening study of prostate cancer in high risk families. *J Urol* 1992; **148**: 826–828.

82 Mueller EJ, Crain TW, Thompson IM *et al*. An evaluation of serial digital rectal examinations in screening for prostate cancer. *J Urol* 1988; **140**: 1445–1447.

83 Vihko P, Kontturi M, Lukkarinen O *et al*. Screening for carcinoma of the prostate: rectal examination, and enzymatic and radioimmunologic measurements of serum acid phosphatase compared. *Cancer* 1985; **56**: 173–177.

84 Waaler G, Ludvigsen TC, Runden TO *et al*. Digital rectal examination to screen for prostatic cancer. *Eur Urol* 1988; **15**: 34–36.

85 Devonec M, Chapeleon JY & Cathignol D. Comparison of the diagnostic value of

sonography and rectal examination in cancer of the prostate. *Eur Urol* 1988; **18**: 189–195.

86 Fritzsche PJ, Axford PO, Ching VC *et al*. Correlation of transrectal sonographic findings in patients with suspected and unsuspected prostatic disease. *J Urol* 1983; **30**: 272–274.

87 Hunter PT, Butler SA, Hodge GB *et al*. Detection of prostatic cancer using transretal ultrasound and sonographically guided biopsy in 1410 symptomatic. *J Endourol* 1989; **3**: 167.

88 Perrin P, Mouriquand P, Monsallier M *et al*. Irradiation of carcinoma of the prostate localized to the pelvis: analysis of tumor response and prognosis. *Int J Radiat Oncol Biol Phys* 1980; **6**: 555.

89 Ragde H, Bagley CM & Aldpae HC. Screening for prostatic cancer with high-resolution ultrasound. *J Endourol* 1989; **3**: 115.

90 Rifkin MD, Friedland GW & Shortliffe L. Prostatic evaluation by transrectal ultra-sonography: detection of carcinoma. *Radiology* 1986; **158**: 85–90.

91 Ercole CJ, Lange PH, Mathisen M, Chiou RV, Reddy PK & Vessela RL. Prostate specific antigen and prostatic phosphatase in the monitoring and staging of patients with prostatic cancer. *J Urol* 1987; **138**: 1181–1184.

92 Ferro MA, Barnes I, Roberts JBM & Smith PJB. Tumor markers in prostatic carci-noma. A comparison of prostate-specific antigen with acid phosphatase. *Br J Urol* 1987; **60**: 69–73.

93 Hudson MA, Bahnson RB & Catalona WJ. Clinical use of prostate specific antigen in patients with prostate cancer. *J Urol* 1989; **142**: 1011–1017.

94 Brawer MK & Lange PH, PSA. *Diag Clin Test* 1990; **28**: 16–21.

95 Babaian RJ & Camps JL. The role of PSA as part of the diagnostic triad and as a guide when to perform a biopsy. *Cancer* 1991; **68**: 2060–2063.

96 Catalona WJ, Smith DS, Ratcliff TL *et al*. Measurement of prostate-specific antigen in serum as a screening test for prostate cancer. *N Engl J Med* 1991; **324**: 1156–1161.

97 Cooner WH, Mosley BR & Rutherford CL Jr. Clinical application of transrectal ultrasonography and prostate specific antigen in the search for prostate cancer. *J Urol* 1988; **139**: 758–761.

98 Mettin C, Lee F, Drago & Murphy GP. The American Cancer Society National Prostate Cancer Detection Project: findings on the detection of early prostate cancer in 2425 men. *Cancer* 1991; **67**: 2949–2958.

99 Bazinet M. Personal communication, 1994.

100 Rommel FM. Personal communication, 1994.

7/Is There a Place for Transrectal Ultrasound in Diagnosis?

R. Clements

Introduction

Current programmes for the detection of prostate cancer are based on the diagnostic triad of the digital rectal examination (DRE), measurement of the serum prostate-specific antigen (PSA) and the appearances of the prostate on transrectal ultrasound (TRUS). Biopsy of the prostate is now most reliably performed as a TRUS-guided transrectal procedure as this improves the yield of prostate needle biopsy, but there is controversy about the ideal biopsy protocol. It is now clear that extensive cancer can be present with a normal PSA level, that even large-volume prostate cancer can remain impalpable on DRE, that not all hypoechoic areas are prostate cancer, that some cancers are isoechoic, and all this leads to confusion in the formulation of biopsy protocols for prostate cancer detection. The exact place of TRUS imaging within these complicated and controversial issues may be questioned.

The role of TRUS imaging in contemporary programmes to detect early prostate cancer can be understood by a consideration of the factors involved in the formulation of biopsy protocols for early prostate cancer. Protocols used since 1985 have concentrated on targeted biopsy of ultrasonically visible hypoechoic lesions in the peripheral zone of the prostate, but it is appreciated that this must also include biopsy of any palpable abnormality. This approach does not assess the transition zone satisfactorily, and it is now generally accepted that multiple systematic biopsies of palpably and ultrasonically normal prostate glands are an important supplement to biopsy protocols for patients with elevated PSA levels. But what is a 'normal' PSA level, and when is the PSA sufficiently abnormal to justify multiple systematic biopsy? In patients with a serum PSA over 10 ng/ml there is general agreement that multiple systematic biopsies should be performed but the need for such biopsies in patients with serum PSA levels between 4 and 9.9 ng/ml is controversial. The high detection rates reported in 1994 [1] from a multicentre screening programme using four-quadrant biopsies in addition to targeted biopsies of any palpable abnormality (but without particular reference to the TRUS appearances) in any patient with a serum PSA level over 4 ng/ml provides an argument for the much wider adoption of multiple biopsies in protocols for the diagnosis of early prostate cancer, but against this must be weighed the drawbacks of multiple systematic biopsies – the complications of the biopsy technique and the risk of diagnosis of foci of clinically insignificant cancer.

Safety of transrectal biopsy

The introduction of the spring-driven biopsy device in the late 1980s revolutionized the diagnosis of prostate cancer, and enabled extremely precise transrectal biopsy of focal ultrasonographic abnormalities of the prostate; multiple systematic biopsies of prostate glands with no focal ultrasonic or digital abnormality could also be easily undertaken. Historically, digitally guided prostate biopsy with a 14-gauge cutting needle had significant side-effects but ultrasound-guided biopsy with an 18-gauge needle and the automatic biopsy device has been associated with minimal side-effects. No preliminary anaesthetic or skin preparation is required for transrectal biopsy but this technique is usually performed under antibiotic cover. Complications of infection and haemorrhage may occur. Ultrasound-guided transrectal biopsy of the prostate should be performed under prophylactic antibiotic cover to minimize the chance of bacteraemia and prostatitis. The rate of infection is usually less than 1% but may approach 6% [2]. There are a variety of antibiotic regimens proposed for prostate biopsy. Current practice in our unit is the use of ofloxacin 400 mg twice daily for 3 days, giving the first dose half an hour before the biopsy. In a comparative trial of the use of intravenous gentamicin and oral ciprofloxacin [3] the incidence of bacteraemia and postbiopsy symptoms were less in patients given oral ciprofloxacin. Prostatic abscess development after biopsy may occur in diabetic patients, although in a report [2] no specific complications in 25 diabetic patients were noted; the only significant risk factor in this series was found in patients receiving steroid medication.

Significant haemorrhage is avoided by careful technique. Before needle insertion it is essential to check that the patient is not receiving therapy that may affect haemostasis, and anticoagulant medication and drugs such as acetylsalicylic acid and non-steroidal anti-inflammatory agents should be stopped days before the biopsy. Slight haematuria is often noted immediately after biopsy but significant haematuria is unusual with peripheral zone biopsies. Heavier haematuria may be noted if anterior transition zone biopsies have been taken. The slight haematuria may persist in 5–13% of patients for 2 days and haemospermia may be noted in about 9% [4]. Immediately after biopsy some bleeding from the rectal wall may be noticed and may persist in up to 2% of cases for 2 days [5]. Rectal wall bleeding may be more persistent with the multiple systematic biopsy approach.

The complication rate might generally be expected to increase as the number of biopsies sampled from a patient increases, particularly with the wider use of the multiple systematic biopsy approach. There are few reports in the literature on this issue, but when the number of samples taken increased from three to eight with the use of multiple systematic biopsies, the complication rate did not increase, although patients complained of increased discomfort [6].

Ultrasound-guided prostate biopsy is therefore a safe technique which patients find acceptable on an outpatient basis and it is this simplicity and patient acceptability, and the relatively low cost of the technique, that has led to its rapid and widespread adoption. On the basis of the report of Catalona and colleagues [1], the argument might be developed that all patients over 50 could be assessed for early prostate cancer by the taking of multiple systematic biopsies. This approach would expose large numbers of patients unnecessarily to the risks of prostate biopsy, and a more selective approach is needed. The problem is to define the criteria for any policy of selective prostate biopsy. Serum PSA level over 4 ng/ml is recognized by many as the threshold for active investigation but significant cancers occur in patients with PSA levels below 4 ng/ml. Should a PSA of 3 ng/ml, 2 ng/ml or 1 ng/ml be regarded as the threshold for investigation? Even with these thresholds, there will still be cancers detected purely by abnormalities of DRE and TRUS. Any selective biopsy protocol must therefore include these parameters in addition to a PSA threshold level.

Digital rectal examination and prostate cancer

DRE has been the traditional method to diagnose prostate cancer; nodules, asymmetry and/or focal induration may be palpated. Most cancers diagnosed by DRE are however too advanced for cure [7]. The positive biopsy rates for digitally guided transrectal or transperineal biopsies of palpably abnormal areas of the prostate have varied from 0.8% [8] to about 1.7% [7]. In a screening series reported in 1971, 5856 men were assessed with 28 407 routine DREs with a cancer detection rate of 1.3% [9]. Daniels *et al.* [10] studied 153 patients with tumours digitally localized to one prostate lobe with TRUS and bilateral biopsies, and 42% were found to have tumour in the clinically benign lobe as well as in the suspicious lobe.

Transrectal ultrasound and prostate cancer

The introduction of higher-frequency (i.e. around 7 MHz) transrectal transducers since 1985 has improved the spatial resolution of prostatic ultrasound and allowed considerable improvement in the imaging of internal prostate anatomy. Papers published before 1985 used lower-frequency ultrasound transducers (i.e. around 3.5 or 4 MHz) but modern transducers have enabled the ultrasonic criteria for prostate cancer to be revised with emphasis on the criteria for early cancer [11]. The commonest ultrasonic appearance of prostate cancer is a hypoechoic lesion in the peripheral zone (Fig. 7.1), but hyperechoic cancers can also rarely be found. Hypoechogenicity of the peripheral zone is a non-specific appearance for malignancy and biopsy of such peripheral zone lesions is necessary to establish the diagnosis.

About 40% of peripheral zone hypoechoic lesions are malignant, but the positive predictive value may be increased to 61% if the DRE of the corresponding area is abnormal [12]. The significance of peripheral zone hypoechoic areas in 83 patients with normal PSA levels – below 4 ng/ml – has been reported [13]. Sixteen men (19%) had cancer; 15 of 18 malignant lesions were over 1 cm in length, and in 47 patients there was correspondence between the digital and ultrasonographic findings. By contrast, only 3 of 36 patients with differences between the sonographic and digital findings had cancer.

Predictors of sonographic malignancy that can be used in the assessment of peripheral zone lesions in men with 'normal' PSA levels include lesion size,

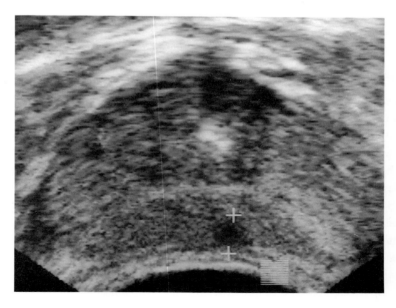

Fig. 7.1 Axial transrectal ultrasound scan with small hypoechoic cancer in the peripheral zone.

correspondence with digital abnormality and degree of hypoechogenicity [13]. Even with the improved resolution of modern transducers operating at about 7 MHz, many cancers are still isoechoic and this remains a major challenge to imaging of the prostate. Correlation of radical prostatectomy specimens with sonographic findings [14] showed that, whilst 75% of cancers were hypoechoic, 25% were isoechoic. It is a weakness of TRUS that early cancer may produce little change in echogenicity. It was hoped that the introduction of transducers capable of colour Doppler imaging might improve our ability to detect these isoechoic tumours but experience with colour Doppler in the prostate has been disappointing [15, 16] and has not made a major additional improvement to our ability to detect prostate cancer with ultrasound. The early results with colour Doppler imaging have suggested that this provides limited improvement over conventional grey-scale ultrasound in the differentiation of cancer from benign pathology. Rifkin *et al.* [15] diagnosed 132 cancers in 121 men in a series of 619 patients assessed with colour Doppler. Of the 132 cancers, 123 (93%) had corresponding grey-scale abnormalities and 114 (86%) demonstrated abnormal flow with colour Doppler imaging. Nine of the 132 cancers (7%) had no obviously identifiable grey-scale abnormality, but did have abnormal flow with colour Doppler. Similarly, Kelly *et al.* [16] found that colour Doppler imaging could improve the positive predictive value of TRUS but the improvement was insufficient to justify a major alteration to biopsy protocols.

Colour Doppler thus appears to offer relatively little over conventional grey-scale imaging in the assessment of the peripheral zone of the prostate but may be of some value in directing transition zone biopsies in large glands. Machines capable of transrectal colour Doppler imaging are usually more expensive, and the need for such higher-cost machines may be obviated by the use of the sonographically less demanding multiple biopsy approach which can detect many of these isoechoic tumours.

Hodge *et al.* [17] reported the use of multiple systematic biopsies, and this technique has been widely adopted subsequently as it is a sensitive means to detect prostatic cancer. The risk of diagnosing clinically insignificant non-palpable disease has been investigated mathematically [18], by performing multiple biopsies in clay models containing different volumes of coloured clay to denote tumour in the prostate. There was a direct correlation between volume of disease and the number of positive biopsies, but even in those models with only 2–5% disease, a single positive biopsy was obtained in 36% of attempts, suggesting that such low-volume disease can be detected by the multiple biopsy approach.

The claim that systematic biopsies risk diagnosing clinically insignificant prostate cancer has been investigated in a series of patients [19]. Defining clinically insignificant cancer as cancer less than 0.5 cm^3 in volume and using at least six biopsy samples per patient, they found that multiple systematic biopsies were positive for cancer in 442 of 816 patients, and 60 (14%) demonstrated only a minute focus of cancer (3 mm or less) in one of the six biopsy specimens. Twenty-seven of these patients with minute foci underwent radical prostatectomy, and 30% of the 27 patients had a cancer volume below 0.5 cm^3. The authors deduced that the risk of detecting insignificant cancer was 4% with six multiple systematic biopsies. They also found that by repeating the initial series of biopsies in patients with only one positive core out of six, they could decrease the risk of detecting insignificant cancer to 1.4%.

The multiple systematic biopsy approach introduced by Hodge *et al.* [17] involves taking six biopsy cores, three from each lobe at the base, mid-gland and apex of the prostate respectively, but taking four cores has also been advocated. Systematic four-quadrant biopsy in 580 men was reported by Spencer *et al.* [20]. Cancer was found by four-quadrant biopsy in 158 of 403 men with focal hypoechoic lesions, but only in 32 of 177 men (18%) with no hypoechoic lesion, and there was no significant change in Gleason score between the hypoechoic and isoechoic cancers. Multiple biopsies (four or six cores) have been most widely adopted to diagnose cancer in palpably and sonographically normal prostate glands with serum PSA levels over 10 ng/ml. Their role in patients with a PSA level below 10 ng/ml is more equivocal but the detection rate achieved by Catalona and colleagues [1] does demonstrate their potential value.

TRUS biopsy protocols have concentrated on an assessment of the peripheral zone of the prostate and relatively little attention has been given to the transition zone as grey-scale sonography has been inaccurate for assessment of the transition zone. Cancer originates in the peripheral zone in 68% of cases, but in the transition zone in 24%. Transition zone cancers have traditionally been diagnosed by transurethral resection of the prostate but are now often found by multiple systematic biopsies. Large organ-confined impalpable transition zone cancers, often associated with metastatic levels of PSA, do occur [21], and these cancers may be difficult to diagnose, as initial biopsies may be negative. Repeated systematic biopsies of the transition zone, including some relatively anterior cores, are needed for diagnosis of transition zone cancer.

Prostate-specific antigen levels and prostate cancer

The wide use of PSA since 1989 has caused a marked increase in the detection of prostate cancer since that time. PSA is covered in detail in Chapter 6, but its relevance to biopsy protocols needs to be considered in this chapter. PSA has been shown to be a useful initial test for prostate cancer but there are significant problems in using it as the primary modality for prostatic cancer detection, particularly as a large percentage of clinically significant cancers may have a serum PSA level below the 'normal' range. The prevalence and pathological extent of cancer in men with serum PSA levels between 2.9 and 4 ng/ml have been investigated [22] and cancer was found in 8 of 111 men (7.2%). All eight patients had organ-confined cancer; the digital examination was abnormal in two of the men, but all cases had abnormal sonographic findings.

Elevated levels of PSA occur in men with benign prostatic hypertrophy and other benign diseases and this lowers the specificity of PSA tests. Different approaches have been adopted to improve the effectiveness of PSA measurement. One approach is to relate the PSA to the ultrasound-measured gland volume (PSA density, predicted PSA). Another approach is to measure the rate of increase in PSA with time and this has been termed the PSA velocity or PSA change and it may be a sensitive indicator of malignancy in the prostate, and a third approach is to use higher values to define normal PSA levels in older age groups (age-related PSA).

Many patients with benign conditions of the prostate have a raised serum PSA level and a variety of approaches have been adopted to relate serum PSA level to prostate gland volume to achieve a more selective approach to prostatic biopsy. Brawer *et al.* [23] suggest that BPH rarely by itself causes elevation of the PSA level but that prostatitis, prostatic intraepithelial neoplasia (PIN) and occult carcinoma will explain most elevations. It is probable that BPH does cause some elevation of the PSA level and calculations related to ultrasound-measured prostate volume have been proposed based on Stamey and Kabalin's observations [24] that prostate cancer contributes a 10 times greater elevation in PSA per gram of prostate tissue than does benign prostatic hyperplasia. One such approach is the concept of predicted PSA. This was proposed by Lee and colleagues [25] from detailed analysis of 204 men who underwent TRUS and PSA prior to transurethral resection of the prostate. Using polyclonal PSA measurements and TRUS-measured prostate volume and a figure of 0.2 ng PSA/ml per gram of prostate tissue, the predicted PSA for the individual prostate was calculated, and by comparing this with the measured serum PSA, any 'excess' PSA unaccounted for in the gland volume alone could be calculated. It is the author's experience that predicted PSA aids TRUS by increasing the confidence to pursue aggressively subtle TRUS findings by biopsy.

Another approach is to use the quotient of serum PSA per prostate gland volume (PSA density, or PSA index). PSA density is obtained by dividing the serum PSA level by the volume of the entire prostate; Benson and colleagues [26] found that the mean PSA density for prostate cancer was 0.581 while that for benign prostatic hyperplasia was 0.044.

Longitudinal changes in PSA measurement with time (PSA change or PSA velocity) have also been evaluated as an index of suspicion for prostate cancer, with a suggestion that by monitoring this PSA change one may be able to differentiate 'fast-growing' malignancy from 'slow-growing' hyperplastic tissues.

Different PSA indices have been compared in a recent report using data from the American Cancer Society National Prostate Cancer Detection Project [27]. This study annually evaluates in a 5-year study a cohort of 2999 men with ages between 55 and 70 years with TRUS, DRE and PSA. Figures for specificity were deduced from 2011 patients with normal DRE and TRUS, and sensitivity from 171 men found to have cancer. A PSA change of 0.75 ng/ml per year was found to have the highest specificity (96%) and PSA density the lowest specificity (85%). PSA density had the highest sensitivity (75%) and PSA change the lowest sensitivity (55%), but these investigators concluded that none of these alternative PSA indices offered a particular advantage when compared with the 'normal' PSA concentration, defined as 4 ng/ml.

In the American Cancer Society National Prostate Cancer Detection Project [28], 2425 men were examined with 520 biopsies over a 3-year period and 88 cancers (17% of biopsies) were diagnosed. Ninety-three per cent of these cancers appeared to be tumours that were organ-confined. In 324 of these men (62%), the recommendation for biopsy was made solely on the TRUS findings; in 69 patients the biopsy recommendation was solely on DRE. In 116 patients (22%) DRE and TRUS were abnormal and in 11 patients (2%), in whom DRE and TRUS were normal, the biopsy was performed because of elevated PSA levels. TRUS was abnormal in 81% of men with cancer and the PSA levels and DRE were abnormal for 67% and 50% of cancers respectively.

The report by Catalona *et al.* [1] of a prospective multicentre trial of 6630 men aged over 50 assessed by DRE and PSA has produced important results. Four-quadrant biopsies were performed if the PSA level was greater than 4 ng/ml or if the DRE was suspicious, even if TRUS showed no suspicious hypoechoic areas. Cancer was found in 264 of 1167 biopsies. It was found that PSA detected more tumours than DRE and that the cancer detection rate was 3.2% for DRE, 4.6% for PSA and 5.8% for both modalities combined. Nearly 40% of cancers detected in this study were found in glands that were sonographically normal. The authors strongly recommend the use of four-quadrant biopsy if the serum PSA is greater than 4 ng/ml or if the DRE is suspicious.

In the above study suspicious sonographic findings were not used to determine whether to perform a biopsy. Many urologists and radiologists would currently only consider a biopsy in a patient with a serum PSA below 10 ng/ml if there were hypoechoic peripheral zone lesions on the scan or a palpable abnormality. On that basis, nearly 40% of the detected tumours in the above study would have been missed. The authors found that the positive predictive value was significantly greater for PSA over 4 ng/ml (32%) than for a suspicious DRE (21%), but that the addition of positive TRUS findings improved the positive predictive value in most (but not all) situations. Observations from the author's unit would support the importance of using both the serum PSA and the DRE findings as criteria for biopsy to detect early prostate cancer. In a recent unpublished UK programme to detect early prostate cancer in men aged between 55 and 70 years, 2078 men were assessed by DRE and PSA, and 508 men were further assessed by TRUS because of abnormal findings on the initial assessment. In 263 men, the serum PSA was over 4 ng/ml and in 316 men the DRE was suspicious. Sixty-one cancers were detected by biopsy of hypoechoic areas, palpable abnormalities, or by multiple systematic biopsies if the PSA was over 10 ng/ml. Of these 61 cancers, 14 were in men with a serum below 4 ng/ml and in 7 men the PSA was below 2 ng/ml, confirming the importance of including DRE in the biopsy protocol, irrespective of the serum PSA level.

Conclusions

It appears that a biopsy protocol based on the sampling of palpable abnormalities and multiple systematic sampling of the prostate in patients with an elevated PSA is supported by the literature as the current ideal biopsy protocol. Is TRUS imaging therefore unnecessary? In practice, imaging remains an important part of the biopsy process. Even with the multiple biopsy approach, the sampling tends not to be completely random but guided towards any suspicious hypoechoic areas that might be present, so that sampling is not blind. Higher-quality scanners can display more subtle alterations in texture (or focal areas of abnormal flow with colour Doppler) that the experienced sonologist will use to increase the accuracy of sampling and the cancer yield.

Does any other imaging modality offer advantage over TRUS for diagnosis of early prostate cancer? The prostate appears homogeneous on computed tomography (CT) scanning and CT therefore has no role in the diagnosis of early prostate cancer. The zonal anatomy of the prostate is demonstrated by magnetic resonance imaging (MRI), which is able to demonstrate peripheral zone cancer as areas of abnormal signal intensity (Fig. 7.2). The improved resolution of the prostate obtained with the endorectal MRI coil (Fig. 7.3) has

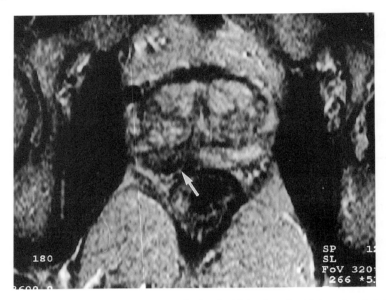

Fig. 7.2 Axial magnetic resonance image obtained with body coil with low-signal right peripheral zone cancer (arrow).

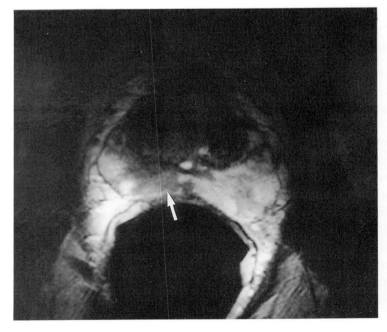

Fig. 7.3 Axial magnetic resonance image with endorectal coil with low-signal peripheral zone cancer (arrow).

enhanced visualization of the gland. However, MRI remains a technique for staging prostate cancer rather than initial diagnosis. The expense of this imaging system, together with the lengthy examination time, the relative scarcity of machines in some countries as well as the fact that some patients are unsuitable for MRI, means that primary diagnosis of early prostate cancer by MRI is not practical.

The simplicity of TRUS-guided biopsy means that TRUS will remain the imaging modality of choice for the diagnosis of prostate cancer into the first decade of the new millennium.

References

** 1 Catalona WJ, Richie JP, Ahmann FR *et al.* Comparison of digital rectal examination and serum prostate specific antigen in the early detection of prostate cancer: results of a multicenter clinical trial of 6630 men. *J Urol* 1994; **151**: 1283–1290.

2 Aus G, Hermansson CG, Hugosson J & Pedersen KV. Transrectal ultrasound examination of the prostate: complications and acceptance by patients. *Br J Urol* 1993; **71**: 457–459.

3 Roach MB, George WJ, Figueroa TE, Neal DE & McBride D. Ciprofloxacin versus gentamicin in prophylaxis against bacteremia in transrectal prostate needle biopsy. *Urology* 1991; **38**: 84–87.

4 Veneziano S, Pavlica P, Querze R, Nanni G, Lalanne MG & Vecchi F. Correlation between prostate-specific antigen and prostate volume, evaluated by transrectal ultrasonography: usefulness in diagnosis of prostate cancer. *Eur Urol* 1990; **18**: 112–116.

5 Puppo P, Perachino M, Ricciotti G, Vitali A, Arduino S & Di Ciolo L. Comparison between digital rectal examination, prostate-specific antigen and transrectal ultrasound in symptomatic patients. *Eur Urol* 1992; **21**(suppl): 87–91.

6 Dyke CH, Toi A & Sweet JM. Value of random US-guided transrectal prostate biopsy. *Radiology* 1990; **176**: 345–349.

7 Chodak GW, Keller P & Schoenberg HW. Assessment for screening for prostate cancer using digital rectal examination. *J Urol* 1989; **141**: 1136–1138.

8 Thompson IM, Ernst JJ, Gangai MP & Spence CR. Adenocarcinoma of the prostate: results of routine urological screening. *J Urol* 1984; **132**: 690–692.

9 Gilberson VA. Cancer of the prostate gland: results of early diagnosis and therapy undertaken for cure of the disease. *JAMA* 1971; **215**: 81–84.

10 Daniels GF, McNeal JE & Stamey TA. Predictive value of contralateral biopsies in unilaterally palpable prostate cancer. *J Urol* 1992; **147**: 870–874.

11 Griffiths GJ, Clements R, Jones DR, Roberts EE, Peeling WB & Evans KT. The ultrasound appearances of prostatic cancer with histologic correlation. *Clin Radiol* 1987; **38**: 219–227.

*12 Lee F, Torp-Pedersen S, Littrup PJ *et al.* Hypoechoic lesions of the prostate: clinical relevance of tumor size, digital rectal examination, and prostate-specific antigen. *Radiology* 1989; **170**: 29–32.

*Reference of special interest.
**Reference of outstanding merit

13 Spencer JA, Alexander AA, Gomella L, Matteucci T & Goldberg BB. Clinical and US findings in prostate cancer: patients with normal prostate-specific antigen levels. *Radiology* 1993; **189**: 389–393.

14 Dahnert WF, Hamper UM, Eggleston JC, Walsh PC & Sanders RC. Prostatic evaluation by transrectal sonography with histopathologic correlation: the echopenic appearance of early carcinoma. *Radiology* 1986; **158**: 97–102.

*15 Rifkin MD, Sudakoff GS & Alexander AA. Prostate: techniques, results, and potential applications of color Coppler US scanning. *Radiology* 1993; **186**: 509–513.

16 Kelly IMG, Lees WR & Rickards D. Prostate cancer and the role of color Doppler US. *Radiology* 1993; **189**: 153–156.

17 Hodge KK, McNeal JE, Terris MK & Stamey TA. Random systematic versus directed ultrasound guided transrectal core biopsies of the prostate. *J Urol* 1989; **142**: 71–75.

18 Stricker HJ, Ruddock LJ, Wan J & Belville WD. Detection of non-palpable prostate cancer. A mathematical and laboratory model. *Br J Urol* 1993; **71**: 43–46.

19 Terris MK, McNeal JE & Stamey TA. Detection of clinically significant prostate cancer by transrectal ultrasound-guided systematic biopsy. *J Urol* 1992; **148**: 829–832.

*20 Spencer JA, Alexander AA, Gomella L, Matteucci T & Goldberg BB. Ultrasound-guided four quadrant biopsy of the prostate: efficacy in the diagnosis of isoechoic cancer. *Clin Radiol* 1994; **49**: 711–714.

21 Stamey TA, Dietrick DD & Issa MM. Large, organ confined, impalpable transition zone prostate cancer: association with metastatic levels of prostate specific antigen. *J Urol* 1993; **149**: 510–525.

22 Colberg JW, Smith DS & Catalona WJ. Prevalence and pathological extent of prostate cancer in men with prostate specific antigen levels of 2.9 to 4.0 ng/ml. *J Urol* 1993; **149**: 507–509.

*23 Brawer MK, Rennels MA, Schiffman RA, Nagle RB & Gaines J. Serum prostate specific antigen and prostate pathology in men having simple prostatectomy. *Am J Clin Pathol* 1989; **92**: 760–764.

24 Stamey TA & Kabalin JN. Prostate specific antigen in the diagnosis and treatment of adenocarcinoma of the prostate. I. Untreated patients. *J Urol* 1989; **141**: 1070–1075.

25 Lee F, Littrup PJ, Loft-Christensen L *et al.* Predicted prostate specific antigen results using transrectal ultrasound gland volume. *Cancer* 1992; **70**: 211–220.

26 Benson MC, Whang IS, Pantuck A *et al.* Prostate specific antigen density: a means of distinguishing benign prostatic hyperplasia and prostate cancer. *J Urol* 1992; **147**: 815–816.

27 Mettlin C, Littrup PJ, Kane RA *et al.* and the Investigators of the American Cancer Society National Prostate Cancer Detection Project. Relative sensitivity and specificity of serum prostate specific antigen (PSA) level compared with age-references PSA, PSA density, and PSA change. *Cancer* 1994; **74: 1615–1620.

28 Babaian RJ, Mettlin C, Kane RA *et al.* and the Investigators of the American Cancer Society National Prostate Cancer Detection Project. The relationship of prostate-specific antigen to digital rectal examination and transrectal ultrasonography. *Cancer* 1992; **69**: 1195–1200.

8/The Limitations of Staging

D.A. Levy and M.I. Resnick

Introduction

In 1994, the American Cancer Society predicted that 200 000 newly diagnosed cases of prostate cancer would be recorded in the USA (a 20% increase over 1993), and 38 000 men would die as a result of the disease [1]. Furthermore, by the end of this decade a 37% increase in annual mortality is expected among those individuals diagnosed with prostate cancer [2]. The application of prostate-specific antigen (PSA) in the evaluation of patients deemed to be at risk for carcinoma of the prostate has had an impact on the dramatic increase in the incidence of prostate cancer over the past 5 years [2]. With the increasing number of newly diagnosed cases of prostate cancer there has been an immense effort to improve upon the accuracy of non-invasive staging modalities in an attempt to minimize the morbidity associated with the evaluation of these patients as well as to direct therapy more appropriately at those patients most likely to benefit from intervention.

Through continued research efforts, new data have been reported which have had an impact on the approach to patients diagnosed with prostate cancer. As these data continue to accumulate over the course of the next 5 years it seems likely that we will redefine which patients are most likely to benefit from aggressive interventional therapy, and hopefully during the next 15 years we will observe a positive impact on the natural course of the disease.

Traditional clinical staging techniques

Digital rectal examination

The limitations of traditional clinical staging modalities utilized in the direction of carcinoma of the prostate have been realized. Studies indicate that detection rates based solely upon the digital rectal examination (DRE) rarely exceed 1.7% [3, 4] and the accuracy of clinical staging based upon DRE alone is approximately 50% in men with a palpable lesion [4]. Furthermore, studies indicate that more than 70% of patients diagnosed by this modality will be upstaged at the time of pathological examination [5]. Additionally, DRE lacks specificity and studies have demonstrated false-negative rates as high as 36% for lesions believed to be suspicious based upon palpation alone [6]. In a recent large multicentre prostate cancer screening study in which 1060 men having a serum PSA greater than 4 ng/ml (Hybritech Tandem assay) or a suspicious DRE underwent transrectal ultrasound-guided quadrant biopsy of the prostate, only 11% (110) of the quadrants felt to be suspicious on DRE were actually positive on biopsy, which was not significantly different from the 9% of quadrants felt to be non-suspicious but which contained cancer [7]. Overall, 74% (308 of 418) of the quadrants containing cancer in this study were considered non-suspicious based on DRE alone. The positive predictive value for a suspicious DRE by quadrant was 11%.

While the DRE was a mainstay of prostate cancer detection in the past, recent studies have indicated conclusively that DRE lacks sensitivity and specificity and is not a reliable sole means of assessing a patient who is at risk for carcinoma of the prostate.

Transrectal ultrasonography

Ultrasonography was examined as an adjunct to DRE in an effort to improve upon detection rates as well as clinical staging of the disease. Initially, studies were carried out in an attempt to delineate a characteristic ultrasonographic appearance of prostate cancer, but the results were variable [8–10]. Recently, the accuracy of ultrasonography in detecting cancer was studied in 6630 men undergoing prostate cancer screening [7]. These data indicate that only 18% (153 of 855) of the sonographically suspicious quadrants actually had cancer, while 65% (282 of 435) of the quadrants considered to be non-suspicious based on ultrasonography were cancer-containing. Overall, of 251 patients with prostate cancer, 131 (52%) would have been missed if only the hypoechoic lesion was biopsied. These data are conclusive in that transrectal ultrasonography (TRUS) lacks the ability to differentiate between benign and malignant processes within the prostate gland, and is therefore not a reliable means of diagnosing carcinoma of the prostate. Furthermore, ultrasound cannot detect microscopic foci of tumour penetrating the prostatic capsule and therefore is not an accurate means of staging the disease. Indeed, in 1989, Rifkin *et al.* reported the accuracy of ultrasound in staging prostate cancer to be 58% (126 of 219 patients) with a specificity of 46 ± 5% and a sensitivity of 68% [11]. While initial investigations into the use of TRUS as a potential means of staging patients previously diagnosed with carcinoma of the prostate were promising, errors occurred primarily due to the presence of microscopic capsular invasion which cannot be detected by ultrasonography [11]. However, further studies into possible applications of ultrasonography indicate that it may be useful as an adjunctive means of evaluating a specific subgroup of patients with prostate cancer.

Recent investigations have indicated that TRUS may have merit in guiding seminal vesicle biopsies and thus aid in the preoperative staging of patients with prostate cancer [12]. In a study of 73 patients undergoing radical prostatectomy, preoperative TRUS-guided biopsies of seminal vesicle correctly diagnosed seminal vesicle involvement in 13 of 21 patients felt to have suspicious seminal vesicles based upon preoperative imaging studies [12]. These data support the use of preoperative TRUS-guided seminal vesicle biopsy in a select group of patients with carcinoma of the prostate.

Overall, the limitations of ultrasound are realized in the lack of sensitivity in differentiating benign from malignant lesions within the prostate gland with a high degree of certainty. Additionally, it is impossible to identify the extension of microscopic tumour foci into the capsule or beyond. While ultrasound has applicability to staging individuals with histologically proven carcinoma of the prostate, it is associated with considerable staging errors.

Computed tomography

Computed tomography (CT) is a popular imaging modality useful in assessing many different parts of the anatomy. Prior to the technological advancements in ultrasonography, CT scanning seemed to have relative merit in the evaluation of patients with prostate cancer. However, CT imaging lacks the sensitivity necessary to discern the internal architecture of the prostate gland [13], and due to the relative homogeneity of prostatic tissue, as well as the variable characteristics of carcinoma, CT scanning cannot differentiate neoplastic tissue from benign hyperplastic tissue. Furthermore, the utility of CT imaging in the evaluation of the anatomical capsule of the prostate and/or the seminal vesicles for the purposes of non-invasive staging has been disappointing [14–17]. Finally, CT scanning was evaluated for a possible role in the assessment of pelvic lymph nodes in patients with prostate cancer. The inability of CT to differentiate a suspicious lymph node (over 1.0 cm) from an abnormal lymph node (over 1.5 cm) as regards a benign inflammatory condition versus metastatic carcinoma renders CT a study of very limited value in the patient with prostate cancer.

CT has been applied to the assessment of the kidneys, adrenal glands and urinary bladder; however, its utility in the assessment of the patient with suspected of prostatic pathology is extremely limited. Considering the cost, sensitivity and specificity of CT scanning, there is little role for the routine use of CT scanning in the assessment of the patient with carcinoma of the prostate.

Magnetic resonance imaging

In the 1980s magnetic resonance imaging (MRI) became recognized as an accurate diagnostic modality for assessing various urological disorders, and provided significant improvements in the ability to image the internal architecture of the prostate [18, 19]. While studies utilizing MRI have indicated that both body surface and endorectal surface-coil MRI provide superior images of the zonal anatomy of the prostate compared to ultrasound, MRI cannot reliably differentiate benign from malignant lesions within the gland, nor can MRI accurately stage carcinoma when present [20, 21]. In a study of 28 patients with carcinoma of the prostate, Kahn *et al.* [20] reported that tumour was identified by MRI in 20 (70%) patients, and tumour volume was underestimated in 12 patients. While the accuracy of MRI in predicting extraglandular tumour was 82%, the sensitivity was only 37.5% and, furthermore, MRI identified only 10 of 19 patients with histologically proven benign hyperplasia. Similarly, in a recent report by Carter *et al.* [22], the sensitivity of MRI in the detection of non-palpable tumours within the prostate was only 58% while the specificity was 48%; however, it was 85% sensitive for non-palpable lesions. Finally, in a study of 22 patients with prostate cancer, endorectal coil MRI revealed an 82% accuracy rate in differentiating between stage B and C disease [23]. This study yielded an overall 16% increase in staging accuracy over that achievable with body-surface coil imaging. While sensitivity for detection of capsular invasion was 67% – a substantial improvement over the 44% sensitivity utilizing body coil imaging [24], – MRI remains a relatively inaccurate means of staging these individuals.

MRI has been applied to the detection of pelvic lymph node metastases in patients with prostate cancer, but MRI alone cannot differentiate an inflammatory node from a metastatic node based solely on image characteristics. Therefore, MRI lacks the necessary specificity to justify its use in the detection of pelvic lymph node metastases in patients with prostatic carcinoma.

While the majority of studies conducted on the prostate utilizing MRI have been carried out with body surface coils, perhaps there is a potential role for this non-invasive imaging modality in the staging of patients with previously diagnosed carcinoma of the prostate. Some centres are using this technology to confirm bony metastases on a routine basis. MRI is not sensitive or specific enough to be used as a routine diagnostic test and certainly the cost would also preclude this application. Additionally, there are insufficient data indicating the improved accuracy of MRI in the staging of locally advanced prostate cancer over TRUS. Further studies using the endorectal surface coils may provide the necessary information which will better define the role of MRI in the patient with prostate cancer.

New developments in staging

PSA was first discovered in seminal fluid by Hara *et al.* in 1971 [25]. Subsequently, extensive studies were carried out on PSA. Accurate serum half-lives were determined [26, 27], as well as proposed normal serum levels, and the role for this organ-specific protein in the monitoring of individuals with prostate cancer became evident. Numerous studies have been directed at further defining a potential role for PSA in the preoperative staging of patients with clinically localized adenocarcinoma of the prostate, but the shortcomings of PSA as an independent and accurate staging modality have become evident.

Lange *et al.* [28] critically reported that the positive and negative predictive values (78 and 61% respectively) for PSA to predict extracapsular disease were not sufficient to make this test useful as a sole means of non-invasively staging patients with carcinoma of the prostate. A study by Hudson and associates [29] demonstrated a significant overlap in serum PSA levels in men with varying stages of disease. Of patients with clinical stage A or B disease, 62% (64 of 103) had preoperative PSA values greater than 4 ng/ml, versus 72% (31 of 43) with clinical C or D lesions, and of 146 men evaluated in their series, 44% had PSA levels greater than 10 ng/ml, including 36% (37 of 103) with clinical A or B disease. When compared with pathological staging, the investigators found that preoperative PSA levels were inaccurate in predicting capsular penetration. There was a significant overlap of serum PSA levels among their study population regardless of clinical stage.

Overall, these data indicate that PSA alone is neither a sensitive nor an accurate indicator of clinical disease stage. To date there are no significant data to suggest that PSA alone is a reliable indicator of extracapsular disease, particularly at serum levels close to the normal range, nor can serum PSA levels reliably predict that disease is confined to the gland.

Efforts were subsequently directed at examining the use of PSA in conjunction with other basic tests used in the evaluation of patients with prostate cancer. Studies have indicated that, by combining the results of the preoperative serum PSA level, the presence of bilateral versus unilateral disease on biopsy and the Gleason score of the biopsy specimen, reasonably accurate predictions can be made as regards the likelihood of disease progression, lymph node involvement and capsular penetration [30–34].

In 1993, Walsh and colleagues reported on 185 individuals with clinical B disease followed for 5 years after radical prostatectomy [35]. Their findings indicate a significantly higher risk of disease progression with a mean Gleason score of 6.9 versus tumours with a mean Gleason score of 5.8 and the difference in Gleason score was significant at $P = 0.0001$. In this study only 13% of tumours with a Gleason score of < 7 showed evidence of disease progression compared to a 59% progression rate when the Gleason score was over 7 ($P < 0.0001$).

The presence of bilateral disease on transrectal needle biopsy of the prostate has been shown to be a clinically significant prognostic indicator of relative disease status. In a recently study of 57 patients with clinical B1 lesions who underwent radical prostatectomy, Daniels and colleagues reported that the presence of bilateral disease was associated with a 72% incidence of capsular penetration into periprostatic fat versus 28% for those individuals with unilateral disease on preoperative needle biopsy [34].

Furthermore, the combined utility of Gleason score, PSA and clinical stage was recently examined by Partin and colleages [30]. By performing a detailed multivariate analysis on 703 men with clinically localized prostate cancer, these investigators were able to develop nomograms and probability plots which more accurately predict the final pathological stage than any single variable. A combination of all three of these variables provided the most significant prediction. For example, based on these data, an individual with a PSA of 6 ng/ ml, a Gleason score of 4 and a clinical T2b lesion would have a 34% probability of capsular penetration, whereas an individual with a PSA of 6 ng/ml, Gleason score of 7 and a clinical T2b lesion would have a 68% probability of capsular penetration (Table 8.1). These data have proven to be quite useful in the preoperative planning for individuals diagnosed with prostate cancer, and with further evaluation, guidelines for candidacy for prostatectomy might be developed.

Summary

Over the past 3 years the incidence of prostate cancer in the American male population has increased from 133 000 in 1992 to over 200 000 in 1994. This dramatic increase can be attributed to several factors, including an overall increased awareness of the disease by the general population, widespread utilization of serum PSA determination by all health care providers, increasing numbers of patients undergoing prostate needle biopsies, and finally an ageing

Table 8.1 Nomogram for prediction of final pathological stage for prostate cancer based on the preoperative assessment of clinical stage, Gleason score and serum prostate-specific antigen (PSA). From Partin et al. [30] with permission.

PSA (ng/ml)	0.0–4.0						4.1–10						10.1–20						>20					
	Clinical stage						Clinical stage						Clinical stage						Clinical stage					
Score	Tla	Tlb	T2a	T2b	T2c	T3a	Tla	Tlb	T2a	T2b	T2c	T3a	Tla	Tlb	T2a	T2b	T2c	T3a	Tla	Tlb	T2a	T2b	T2c	T3a
Prediction of organ-confined disease																								
2–4	100	85	88	76	82	—	100	78	83	67	71	—	100	—	61	52	—	26	—	—	20	7	—	—
5	100	78	81	67	73	—	100	70	73	56	64	43	100	—	58	43	37	19	—	—	32	—	3	—
6	100	68	72	54	60	42	100	53	62	44	48	33	—	36	44	28	37	19	—	—	14	11	4	5
7	—	54	61	41	46	—	100	39	51	32	37	26	—	24	36	19	24	14	—	—	18	4	5	3
8–10	—	—	48	31	—	—	—	32	39	22	25	12	—	11	29	14	15	9	—	—	3	1	2	2
Prediction of established capsular penetration																								
2–4	0	15	14	26	17	—	0	22	19	34	27	—	0	—	40	49	—	—	—	—	80	94	—	—
5	0	22	20	34	26	—	0	29	28	45	34	58	0	49	43	58	61	75	—	—	68	—	97	—
6	0	30	29	46	38	59	0	45	38	56	49	68	—	62	56	73	59	82	—	—	86	90	96	95
7	—	43	39	59	50	—	0	58	49	68	59	75	—	73	64	81	73	86	—	—	80	96	95	98
8–10	—	—	50	68	—	—	—	64	59	77	71	87	—	87	70	86	82	92	—	—	97	99	97	98

Numbers represent probability (%). Dash represents lack of sufficient data to calculate probability.

141

population. With the recently reported age-specific PSA ranges [36] as well as the Food and Drug Administration approval of PSA use for early detection of prostate cancer, the incidence will inevitably continue to rise.

Historically, there has been little impact on the natural history of prostate cancer despite aggressive intervention. This perhaps can be attributed to the inability to select and treat those patients most likely to benefit from aggressive intervention. Currently, there are data to suggest that we can better predict which patients are more likely to have capsule-free disease, and therefore those most likely to be free of a biochemical as well as pathological recurrence during the extended postoperative period. Some centres are becoming much more selective based on patient age and serum PSA level with regard to who is a surgical candidate. Furthermore, lymph node dissections are not being performed on those individuals with a serum PSA < 10 ng/ml, unilateral disease and Gleason score of ⩽ 6. It is well-established that continence rates are superior in individuals who are younger (< 70 years old) and have lower Gleason scores (⩽ 7), and it seems likely that if more centres abide by these criteria there will be a significant impact upon the natural history of the disease and patients undergoing radical prostatectomy can expect better continence rates as well as disease-free survival.

References

* 1 Boring CC, Squires TS & Tong T. Cancer statistics, 1994. *Cancer* 1994; **44**: 7–19.
  2 Carter HB & Coffey D. The prostate: an increasing medical problem. *Prostate* 1990; **16**: 39–48.
  3 Chodak GW, Keller P & Schoenberg HW. Assessment of screening for prostate cancer using digital rectal examination. *J Urol* 1989; **141**: 1136–1138.
  4 Scardino PT. Early detection of prostate cancer. *Urol Clin North Am* 1989; **16**: 635–655.
* 5 The Veterans Administration Co-Operative Urologic Research Group. Treatment and survival of patients with cancer of the prostate. *Surg Gynecol Obstet* 1867; **124**: 1011.
  6 Wantanabe H, Igari D, Tanahashi Y, Harada K & Saitoh M. Transrectal ultrasonography of the prostate. *J Urol* 1975; **114**: 734–739.
  7 Flanigan RC, Catalona WJ, Richie *et al.* Accuracy of digital rectal examination and transrectal ultrasonography in localizing prostate cancer. *J Urol* 1994; **152**: 1506–1509.
  8 Rifkin MD, Frieland GW & Shortliffe L. Prostatic evaluation by transrectal endosonography: detection of carcinoma. *Radiology* 1986; **158**: 85–90.
* 9 Lee F, Gray JM, McLeary RD *et al.* Transrectal ultrasound in the diagnosis of prostate cancer: location, echogenicity, histopathology and staging. *Prostate* 1985; 7: 117–129.
  10 Dahnert W, Hamper UM, Eggleston JC, Walsh PC & Sanders RC. Prostatic evaluation by transrectal sonography with histopathologic correlation: the echopenic appearance of early carcinoma. *Radiology* 1986; **158**: 97–102.

* Reference of special interest.
** Reference of outstanding merit.

11 Rifkin MD, Zerhouni E, Gatsonis C *et al.* Comparison of magnetic resonance imaging and ultrasonography in staging early prostate cancer. *N Engl J Med* 1989; **323**: 621–626.

12 Terris MK, McNeal JE, Freiha FS & Stamey TA. Efficacy of transrectal ultrasound-guided seminal vesicle biopsies in the detection of seminal vesicle invasion by prostate cancer. *J Urol* 1993; **149**: 1035–1039.

13 Van Engleshoven JMA & Kreel L. Computed tomography of the prostate. *J Comput Assist Tomogr* 1979; **3**: 45.

14 Resnick MI. Noninvasive techniques in evaluating patients with carcinoma of the prostate. *Urology* 1981; **17**(suppl. 3): 25.

15 Denis L, Appel L, Broos J & Declerq G. Evaluation of prostatic cancer by transrectal ultrasonography and CT scan. *Acta Urol Belg* 1980; **48**: 71.

16 Peterson RW. Computed tomographic evaluation of alignancies of the bladder and prostate. *Comput Tomogr* 1977; **1**: 283.

17 Price JM & Davidson AJ. Computed tomography in the evaluation of the suspected carcinomatous prostate. *Urol Radiol* 1979; **1**: 39.

18 Kressel H. Magnetic resonance imaging. In: Pollack HM (ed.) *Clinical Urography.* Philadelphia: W.B. Saunders, 1990, pp. 433–455.

*19 Hricak H, Dooms GC, McNeal JE *et al.* MR imaging of the prostate gland: normal anatomy. *AJR* 1987; **148**: 51–58.

20 Kahn T, Burrig K, Schmitz-Drager B, Lewis JS, Furst G & Modder U. Prostatic carcinoma and benign prostatic hyperplasia: MR imaging with histopathologic correlation. *Radiology* 1989; **173**: 847–851.

21 Bryan PJ, Butler HE, Nelson AD *et al.* Magnetic resonance imaging of the prostate. *AJR* 1986; **146**: 543–548.

22 Carter HB, Bren RF, Tempany CM *et al.* Nonpalpable prostate cancer: detection with MR imaging. *Radiology* 1991; **178**: 523.

*23 Schnall MD, Imai Y, Tomaszewski J, Pollack HM, Lenkinsky RE & Kressel HY. Prostate cancer: local staging with endorectal surface coil MR imaging. *Radiology* 1991; **178**: 797–802.

24 Bezzi M, Kressel HY, Allen KS *et al.* Prostatic carcinoma: staging with MR imaging at 1.5T1. *Radiology* 1988; **169**: 339–346.

25 Hara M, Inorre T & Fukuyama T. Some physio-chemical characteristics of gamma-seminoprotein, an antigenic compound specific for human seminal plasma. *Jpn J Legal Med* 1971; **25**: 322.

26 Stamey TA, Yang N, Hay AR, McNeal JE, Freiha FS & Redwine E. Prostate specific antigen as a serum marker for adenocarcinoma of the prostate. *N Engl J Med* 1987; **317: 909–916.

27 Oesterling JE, Chan DW, Epstein JI *et al.* Prostate specific antigen in the preoperative and postoperative evaluation of localized prostate cancer treated with radical rostatectomy. *J Urol* 1988; **139**: 766–772.

*28 Lange PH, Ercole CJ, Lightner DJ, Fraley EE & Vessella R. The value of serum prostate specific antigen determinations before and after radical prostatectomy. *J Urol* 1989; **141**: 873–879.

29 Hudson MA, Bahnson RR & Catalona WJ. Clinical use of prostate specific antigen in patients with prostate cancer. *J Urol* 1989; **142**: 1011–1017.

*30 Partin AW, Yoo J, Carter HB *et al.* The use of prostate specific antigen, clinical stage and Gleason score to predict pathological stage in men with localized prostate cancer. *J Urol,* 1993; **150**: 110–114.

31 Partin AW, Carter HB, Chan DW *et al.* Prostate specific antigen in the staging of localized prostate cancer: influence of tumor differentiation, tumor volume and benign hyperplasia. *J Urol* 1990; **143**: 747–752.

32 Miller GJ & Cygan JM. Morphology of prostate cancer: the effects of multifocality on histological grade, tumor volume and capsule penetration. *J Urol* 1994; **152**: 1709–1713.

33 Epstein JI, Walsh PC & Brendler CB. Radical prostatectomy for impalpable prostatic cancer: the Johns Hopkins experience with tumors found on transurethral resection (stages T1A and T1B) and on needle biopsy (stage T1C). *J Urol* 1994; **152**: 1721–1729.

*34 Daniels GF, McNeal JE & Stameny TA. Predictive value of contralateral biopsies in unilaterally palpable prostate cancer. *J Urol* 1992; **147**: 870–874.

35 Epstein JI, Carmichael M, Partin AW & Walsh PC. Is tumor volume an independent predictor of progression following radical prostatectomy? A multivariate analysis of 185 clinical stage B adenocarcinomas of the prostate with 5 years followup. *J Urol* 1993; **149**: 1478–1481.

36 Oesterling JE, Jacobsen SJ, Chute CG *et al.* Serum prostatic-specific antigen in a community-based population of healthy men. Establishment of age-specific reference ranges. *JAMA* 1993; **270: 860–864.

9/Clinical Response – Can it be Predicted?

D.W.W. Newling

Introduction

When the large number of different treatments that have been introduced to treat prostate cancer are considered, the impact of these upon an understanding of the natural history of this disease can only be described as minimal. Apart from successes with radical prostatectomy or radiotherapy for some patients with localized prostate cancer, there are no other established curative treatments. However, it must be recognized that many of these patients did not need to be 'cured', as their disease posed no threat in their lifetime and there is little doubt that radical prostatectomy and radiotherapy have, in the past, been used somewhat indiscriminately. More recently, studies have been undertaken by careful analysis of prognostic factors present at the time of diagnosis to identify those patients with more aggressive disease for whom active therapy might be beneficial.

Palliative therapy of advanced prostate cancer probably improves survival time only marginally. It does, however, alleviate the symptoms of advanced disease and improves quality of life, if not its quantity. Patients diagnosed with advanced local or metastatic prostate cancer that cannot be cured exhibit prognostic factors that can indicate to their clinician the degree of urgency for starting treatment. In patients undergoing relapse after primary palliative therapy there are a number of important prognostic factors that can give an indication of anticipated survival and thus a possible time scale for further intervention.

When considering the prediction of clinical response to therapy for prostate cancer, prognostic factors in four different groups of patients need to be studied.

1 Those in whom prostate cancer is revealed incidental to an operation undertaken for supposedly benign disease.
2 Patients with obvious localized prostate cancer, with or without symptoms.
3 Patients with locally invasive prostate cancer or metastases.
4 Those in whom relapse occurs after response to initial palliative hormonal treatment.

Adverse prognostic factors in patients with incidental prostate cancer

Incidentally discovered prostate cancer (stage T1a, T1b, T1c/A1, A2) describes prostate cancers revealed incidentally by histological examination of tissue removed for clinically diagnosed benign disease. Schroder *et al.* [1] examined retrospectively 55 patients with incidentally discovered prostate cancers from a series of radical prostatectomy specimens. They examined the effect of several parameters on eventual outcome for patients in this study.

Histological/cytological features

The histological features included pleomorphism, the type of gland present in the tumour, the amount of tumour and stroma present. Cytological features were cell size, ratio of cytoplasm to nucleus, nuclear size and the presence or absence of nucleoli, vacuoles and mitosis.

Of the histological features, the amount of tumour present and gland differentiation were both of prognostic significance. Those patients described with 'medium' or 'much' tumour present (defined as 4–10 > 10 foci, or three or more microscopic fields × 100 magnification in the specimen) had a 35% chance of death from prostate cancer. No patients died if their tumours had been described as of 'small' volume. Glandular-type categories were based on Mostofi's classification [2], tumours with cribriform or solid glandular patterns were more dangerous than those with small, intermediate or large glands.

Examination of cytological parameters revealed that patients with large nuclear–cytoplasmic ratios appeared to have an increased chance of death from prostate cancer and mitoses also appeared to be disadvantageous.

Multifocal microscopic tumours (T1b; A2) in general carried a poorer prognosis than monofocal tumours, even if the tumour was palpable (T2; B1). Multifocality is associated with dedifferentiation and the prognostic potential of a tumour relates to its most dedifferentiated part [3].

Clinical parameters

Many patients with incidental prostate cancer are elderly and, if the tumour is of small volume with none of the adverse histological and cytological features mentioned above, it is unlikely that the cancer will influence the patient's survival. Certainly, if the anticipated survival of the patient is less than 15 years, it is most unlikely that treatment will ever be needed [4].

Prognostic factors in patients with cancer clinically localized to the prostate gland (T1–T4; B1, B2, C)

In a large retrospective study of 440 radical prostatectomy specimens, Schroder *et al.* [5] showed the following parameters to be prognostically significant.

Tumour volume

If described as 'much' or 'medium', the volume of a tumour had a significant impact on the likelihood of progression when compared with tumours described as 'small'. Large nuclei in individual cells were of significance indicating an adverse outlook. Marked nuclear anaplasia, and particularly grade, though more subjective, was of great significance. Those tumours which showed uniformly poor grade (i.e. G3 patterns) had a particularly poor and short prognosis with death from prostate cancer occurring in most patients. Thus, the important histological and cytological parameters identified in incidental carcinomas of the prostate have similar implications in tumours of larger volume. No single histological or cytological parameter could replace grading as a prognostic indicator. In addition, a number of other important prognostic factors could be identified in those tumours which were clinically detectable and locally advanced.

Gleason score

The use of Gleason's method of attributing a score to grade prostate cancer was a most important step forward towards an objective measurement of prognosis in prostate cancer [6]. In Gleason's method, the two most prominent grades of tumour were considered to be the most important prognostic factors with scoring between 2 and 10. For patients with clinically localized prostate cancer, a Gleason score greater than 6 carried a worse prognosis than a lower Gleason score. This scoring system is now widely used and has made it easier to compare studies of localized and advanced prostate cancer [7].

Local stage of tumour

Most patients with locally advanced prostate cancer (T3 or C) have tumours of larger volume than cancers which are confined to the prostate (T1, T2 or A1, A2, B1). There is little doubt from the literature that patients are more likely to die from prostate cancer if their cancers are locally advanced and not localized, regardless of the treatment they receive whether it is radical prostectomy or radiotherapy [7]. The impact of local stage on survival is not related to the stage itself but to the risk of undetected metastatic disease. For instance, with advancing local disease there is an increased risk of lymph node metastases [8] (Tables 9.1 and 9.2).

Table 9.1 Clinical stage and incidence of lymph node metastasis in 146 surgically staged patients with prostate cancer.

| Clinical stage | No. | Lymph node metastasis | |
		No.	%
A2	5	0	0
B1	3	0	0
B2	17	1	6
B3	50	21	42
C	71	40	56
Total	146	62	42

Table 9.2 Survival according to lymph node status.

Lymph nodes	No.	Alive without disease	Alive with disease
Negative	84	40 (48%)	10 (12%)
Positive	62	1 (2%)	9 (15%)

Locally advanced prostate cancers, especially when of high grade, have a greater tendency to spread through the prostatic capsule into seminal vesicles and other adjacent structures with early dissemination to pelvic lymph nodes and even distant metastases, even though these may not be detectable at the time of diagnosis. The role of neoadjuvant or adjuvant therapy for patients in these poor-prognosis groups to downsize T2 or even T3 prostate cancer is promising [9] but there is as yet no agreement about the best timing for adjuvant therapy.

Prostate-specific antigen

Prostate-specific antigen (PSA), when greater than 10 ng/ml in patients with clinically localized prostate cancer, is a significant adverse prognostic feature [10]. High PSA in such patients may indicate a large volume, penetration of the prostatic capsule or seminal vesicles locally, or pelvis lymph node spread. When the serum PSA is greater than 40 ng/ml, occult distant metastases may be present [11].

Prognostic factors in patients with locally advanced prostate cancer or metastatic disease

As in patients with early-stage prostate cancer, tumour volume present at initial diagnosis, whether local or metastatic, has a profound influence on prognosis. The prognostic factors identified by the European Organisation for Research and Treatment of Cancer (EORTC) Genito-Urinary (GU)-Group from ongoing analyses of all their studies on patients with metastatic prostate cancer showed that, with one exception, the type of palliative treatment prescribed has less influence on prognosis than the performance status of the patient, the level of alkaline phosphatase and haemoglobin (not shown by the EORTC), the stage and grade of tumour, the presence of symptomatic metastases in bone and of associated chronic disease.

Performance status

In an analysis of over 600 patients treated with antiandrogen therapy, de Voogt *et al.* [12] reported that performance status was the most influential factor that affected prognosis. Chodak *et al.* [13] confirmed these findings and also pointed out that patients with pain from metastases in bone which affected their performance status fared particularly badly.

Anaemia and serum levels of alkaline phosphatase

Several reports have indicated that the haemoglobin level at the time of diagnosis of metastatic prostate cancer is a significant factor for prediction of outcome [12, 14]. Usually, anaemia reflects malignant bone marrow involvement but it may also reflect haematuria or dietary deficiencies associated with a poor performance status. Elevated levels of alkaline phosphatase in the serum of men with metastatic prostate cancer are usually indicative of a high volume of skeletal metastatic deposits and are important harbingers of a poor chance of survival [12, 13]. However, for patients in whom serum alkaline phosphatase levels fall rapidly to normal ranges following endocrine treatment, the outlook is much brighter than for those in whom this does not occur [15].

Serum testosterone

Ishikawa *et al.* [16] and Chodak *et al.* [13] described independently that low serum testosterone levels at the time of diagnosis were associated with poor prognosis after treatment for metastatic prostate cancer. These observations confirmed earlier findings by Harper *et al.* [17] that the presence of low initial testosterone levels probably reflects prostate cancer capable of growth in a relatively androgen-deprived environment and is potentially hormone-independent with limited sensitivity to androgen withdrawal.

Stage and grade of prostate cancer

The EORTC GU-Group showed in over 1200 patients with metastatic prostate cancer that patients with advanced T-categories (T3, T4) have an appreciably worse outlook than those with tumours clinically localized to the prostate (T1, T2) [18]. Advanced local disease is more frequently of high grade and associated with pelvic lymph node spread.

As in localized prostate cancer, patients with high-grade tumours have a poorer prognosis than those with low-grade cancers. This is particularly true of patients with a pure G3 tumour, whose outlook is considerably worse than those with tumours of mixed pattern [19].

Metastatic factors

The presence of 15 or more skeletal metastases is a particularly poor prognostic sign [20], as is pain [13]. Soft-tissue metastases, especially in liver or distant lymph nodes, also carry a more sinister prognosis than skeletal metastases alone [21]. This is particularly true for patients in whom soft-tissue metastases continue to enlarge despite primary hormonal treatment.

Associated chronic disease

An interesting outcome of the analysis of prognostic factors carried out for the EORTC by de Voogt *et al.* [12] was the realization that chronic disease such as chronic obstructive airways disease, ischaemic heart disease or neurological disease was an adverse prognostic factor in men with advanced prostate cancer. This poses considerable problems since the presence of associated chronic disease can be hard to quantify so that it is impossible to assign patients to given treatments on the basis of such a prognostic variable. Nevertheless, it is a useful aid for clinicians when reviewing prognostic possibilities in individual cases.

Influence of treatment on prognosis

Androgen ablation remains the most important palliative therapy for prostate cancer. There appears to be little difference between medical and surgical orchidectomy, steroidal antiandrogen monotherapy, non-steroidal anti-androgen monotherapy, oestrogen therapy, treatment with combined chemohormonal agents, e.g. Estracyt® (apart from poorly differentiated tumours), or maximal androgen blockade (luteinizing hormone releasing hormone therapy or surgical castration combined with a non-steroidal antiandrogen). Any differences in the outcome of treatment are of less prognostic consequence than the prognostic factors already described, especially performance status, anaemia, serum, alkaline phosphatase and stage of the primary tumour. However, for patients with small-volume metastatic prostate cancer, maximal androgen blockade has been shown to confer some benefit over castration alone as time to progression increased and there was improved overall and cancer-specific survival time [22]. Nevertheless, a recent meta-analysis has not shown this difference to be significant in 22 different studies comparing standard androgen ablation with maximal androgen blockade [23]. Therefore, on the issue of maximal androgen ablation, all that can be said with some certainty is that it would appear to have a useful role to treat a closely defined group of men with small-volume metastatic prostate cancer, but the majority of patients presenting with metastatic disease do not come within this category.

Prognosis in hormone relapse

Newling *et al.* [24] have defined prognostic factors in relation to different types of disease progression when relapse occurred after maximal androgen blockade (Table 9.3). The most common indication of hormone escape was an increase in the serum PSA and from that time survival was about 1 year. When disease progression was manifested by a demonstrable increase of skeletal metastases, survival was less than 1 year. Weight loss, deterioration of performance status, increased anaemia and the appearance of soft-tissue metastases indicated an increasingly limited outlook which was not affected favourably by chemotherapeutic or other secondary treatments.

It is likely that, following a rise of serum PSA after hormonal therapy and before clinical symptoms of relapse become evident, there could be a window of opportunity to administer agents (when they become available) to treat hormone-insensitive prostate cancer since at that time most patients would be asymptomatic and in good condition so that a real survival benefit could be expected.

Table 9.3 Prognostic importance of progression.

Type of progression	% Progress survival*	Median risk†	Relative progression‡	Median
Prostate-specific antigen	45	52	1.93	24 months
Bone	40	41	1.39	30 months
Pain	37	32	2.51	34 months
Performance status	32	24	2.57	‡
Acid phosphatase	24	43	1.62	‡
Haemoglobin	18	22	2.40	‡
Alkaline phosphatase	17	35	1.79	‡
Urological symptoms	9	48	1.51	‡
Weight	6	12	4.26	‡
Lung	4	11	2.04	‡
Regional lymph nodes	3	28	1.61	‡
Liver	2	10	5.42	‡
Distant lymph nodes	2	33	1.15	‡

* Median survival after progression in weeks.
† Relative risk of death in patients progressing.
‡ Not yet attained.

New prognostic factors

DNA content and ploidy

Nearly 40 years ago, Atkin and Richards [25] reported that the characteristic biological feature of malignant cells is the presence of aneuploidy. Cytogenic studies are difficult in solid tumours because of the lack of consistent high-quality metaphase preparations and therefore measurement of DNA content by flow-cytometry may provide independent information about prognosis [26].

Green *et al.* [27] showed that in prostate tumours of small volume, there is early evidence of aneuploidy which suggests that this is an early event in the development of prostate neoplasia. It has also been shown that aneuploidy is an individual prognostic factor of importance [26, 28]. If a cut-off point of 1.40 is used in place of the more usual value of 1.05, aneuploidy becomes a highly significant individual prognostic factor. Ekman *et al.* [29] have shown that DNA aneuploid tumours are more androgen receptor-negative than diploid prostatic tumours.

However, the importance of ploidy as an overall prognostic factor in all stages of prostate cancer appears to be less significant than local tumour extension, grade of tumour and the presence or absence of lymph node metastases.

Oncogenes and tumour suppressor genes

The results of studies of oncogene activity in prostate carcinoma have been conflicting. The ERB-B2 oncogene [30] is strongly expressed in benign prostatic hyperplasia (BPH) but has also been found in a small number of patients with very aggressive prostate cancers. This oncogene is highly homologous with the receptor for epidermal growth factor (EGF). However, when compared with less aggressive prostate cancer, there is not sufficient evidence to consider ERB-B2 as an important individual prognostic factor.

The *ras* oncogene [31] has been found in a number of poorly differentiated prostate cancers but the inconsistent expression of its product, the P21 protein, has led to doubts about its clinical significance. It is most commonly expressed, however, in metastatic sites of prostate cancer and a P21 protein can usually be identified. There is, therefore, the possibility that this oncogene could prove to be a useful indicator of metastatic potential.

The tumour suppressor gene, p53 [32] has been shown to be present in its mutated form in a significant number of poorly differentiated metastatic prostate cancers. It appears that tumours with a high expression of mutated p53 are most frequently poorly differentiated, have a high metastatic potential and are associated with a high risk of death from prostate cancer.

The retinoblastoma suppressor gene RBI [33] appears to be implicated in the genesis of prostate cancer. The DU145 prostatic carcinoma cell line contains an abnormal RBI suppressor gene; this gene is responsible for preventing the cell from entering the G1 phase from G0 and thus, if it mutates, will allow more rapid proliferation of malignant cells.

Growth factors

The identification of the importance of EGF and transforming growth factor-α (TGF-α) in the proliferation of prostate cancer in the LNCaP prostatic cancer cell line has led to a search for these products in human prostate cancers and even in the serum of patients with advanced disease. There is little doubt that these growth factors are two of many that are involved with the final common path of hormonal control of prostate cancer and, when identified in histological sections or in serum of patients, appear to be related to a poor prognosis [34].

Other growth factors such as transforming growth factor-β (TGF-β) seem to have a role in preventing cell proliferation and can be demonstrated in higher concentrations in histological sections of well-differentiated tumours with a better clinical prognosis [35].

Cellular proliferation markers

Counting mitoses is a relatively rough-and-ready method of assessment of cellular proliferation. Techniques that measure accumulation of radioactive-labelled thymidine or bromodeoxyuridine show that in carcinomas uptake may be 30 times greater than in normal tissue of BPH [36]. A good correlation has been found between the ^{3}H thymidine labelling index and the measurement of the S-phase fraction by flow-cytometry. These parameters are higher in aneuploid than in diploid tumours and are associated with rapid progression of disease. Of particular interest is the observation that measurement of these factors appears to delineate a group of patients with localized disease but with a high potential for metastases.

Ki-67 is an antibody that recognizes poorly characterized nuclear antigen expressed in proliferating cells, in contrast to cells in the G0 phase of the cell cycle. High Ki-67 staining in tumour tissue from prostate cancer patients treated with endocrine therapy has been shown to be associated with a short time to progression [37].

Proliferating cell nuclear antigen (PCNA) is a useful marker of cell proliferation in many different malignancies. PCNA expression is difficult to measure and has only recently been shown to have a loose association with poor prognosis after examination of needle biopsies of patients with prostate cancer [38].

Conclusion

Analysis of prognostic factors present at the time of diagnosis of prostate cancer can help to identify some patients with localized tumour who may deserve early, aggressive therapy, as well as other patients with more advanced disease who could respond well to palliative hormonal treatment. After failure of attempted curative treatments and subsequent hormonal therapy, the pattern of progression of prostate cancer is an important prognostic factor relating to prediction of survival. It has to be recognized that there has been little advance during the past 50 years in understanding and changing the natural history of prostate cancer, which is now the most commonly diagnosed cancer of men. It is, therefore, necessary to continue searching for new prognostic factors at both cellular and molecular level to plan treatments more precisely in relation to the biology of prostate cancer of individual patients with the ultimate objective of controlling the rising death toll from this disease.

References

1 Schroder FH, Blom JHM, Hop WCJ & Mostofi FK. Incidental carcinoma of the prostate treated by total prostatectomy in the prognostic impact of microscopic tumor extension and grade. *World J Urol* 1983; **1**: 15–23.

2 Mostofi FK. Problems of grading carcinoma of the prostate. *Semin Oncology* 1976; **3**: 161–169.

3 Elder JS, Gibbons RP & Brennan GE. Efficacy of radical prostatectomy for stage A2 carcinoma of the prostate. *Cancer* 1985; **56**: 2051–2054.

4 Epstein JH, Ekkelstein JC, Paul G & Walsh PC. Prognosis of untreated stage A1 prostatic carcinoma. A study of 94 cases with an extended follow-up. *J Urol* 1986; **136**: 837–838.

5 Schroder FH, Blom JHM, Hop WCJ & Mostofi FK. Grading of prostatic cancer. An analysis of the prognostic significance of single characteristics. *Prostate* 1985; **6**: 81–100.

6 Gleeson DF. Histological grading and clinical staging of prostate cancer. In: *Urologic Pathology of the Prostate*, Tannenbaum M, ed. Philadelphia: Lea & Febiger; 1977, pp. 171–197.

7 Fowler JA & Mills SE. Operable prostatic carcinoma, correlation among clinical stage, pathological, Gleason histological score and early disease free survival. *J Urol* 1985; **133**: 49–52.

** 8 Freiha FS. Carcinoma of the prostate – non metastatic disease. In: *Combination Therapy in Urological Malignance*, Smith PH, Ed. Berlin: Springer-Verlag, 1989, pp. 119–141.

9 Sassini AM & Schulman CC. Neoadjuvant hormonal deprivation before radical prostatectomy. *Eur J Urol* 1993; **24**(suppl. 2): 46–50.

10 Oesterling JA, Chan DW, Epstein JJ *et al.* PSA in preoperative and postoperative of localised prostate cancer treated with radical prostatectomy. *J Urol* 1988; **139**: 766–772.

11 Brawer MK. PSA – a review. *Acta Oncol* 1991; **30**: 161–168.

*12 de Voogt HJ, Smith PH, Pavone-Macaluso M *et al.* and members of the EORTC GU-group. Cardiovascular side effects of diethylstilbestrol, CPA, medroxyprogesterone acetate and estramustine phosphate used for the treatment of advanced prostatic caner: results from EORTC trials 30761 and 30762. *J Urol* 1986; **135**: 303–307.

13 Chodak GW, Vogelzang J, Caplan RJ, Soloway M & Smith JA. Independent prognostic factors in patients with metastatic (stage D2) prostate cancer. *JAMA* 1991; **265**: 618–621.

14 Mulders PFA, Dijkman GA, Fernandez de Moral P, Theeuwes AGU & Debruyne FMJ. Analysis of prognostic factors in disseminated prostatic cancer. *Cancer* 1990; **65**: 2758–2761.

15 Cooper EH & Armatage TG. Tumor markers in monitoring the treatment of advanced prostate cancer. *Prog Biol Clin Res* 1990; **59**: 65–72.

16 Ishikawa S, Soloway MS, Van der Zwaag R & Todd B. Prognostic factors in survival free of progression after androgen deprivation therapy for treatment of prostatic cancer. *J Urol* 1989; **141**: 1139–1142.

17 Harper ME, Peeling WB, Cowley T *et al.* Plasma steroid and protein hormone concentrations in patients with prostatic carcinoma before and during oestrogen therapy. *Acta Endocrinol* 1976; **81**: 409–429.

18 Newling DWW. European Trials and the management of prostate cancer. *Semin Surg Oncol* 1995; **11**: 65–71.

* Reference of special interest.
** Reference of outstanding merit.

19 Gallee MPW, Ten Kate FJW, Mulder PGH, Blom JHM & van der Heul RO. Histological grading of prostatectomy specimens. Comparison of prognostic accuracy of five grading systems. *Br J Urol* 1990; **65**: 368–375.

20 Ernst DS, Hanson J & Venner PM. Analysis of prognostic factors in men with metastatic prostate cancer. *J Urol* 1991; **146**: 372–376.

21 Prout GR, Heaney JA, Griffing PP, Daly J & Shipley WU. Nodal involvement as a prognostic indicator in patients with prostatic carcinoma. *J Urol* 1980; **124**: 226–231.

22 Denis L, Whelan P, Carneiro de Moura JL *et al.* Goserelin acetate and flutamide vs bilateral orchiectomy. A phase III EORTC trial (30853). *Urology* 1993; **42**: 119–130.

23 Dalesio O, Peto R & Schröder F for the Prostate Cancer Trialists Collaborative Group. Maximum androgen blockade in advanced prostate cancer – an overview of 22 trials with 3289 deaths in 5710 patients. *Lancet* 1995; **346**: 265–269.

24 Newling DWW, Fossa SD, Tunn UW, Kurth KH, De Pauw M & Sylvester R. Mitomycin V vs Estramustine in the treatment of hormone resistant metastatic prostate cancer: the final analysis of the EORTC GU group prospective randomized phaase III study (30865). *J Urol* 1993; **150**: 1840–1844.

25 Atkins NB & Richards BM. DNA in human tumors as measured by microspectrophometry of Feulgen stain: a comparison of tumors rising at different sites. *Br J Cancer* 1956; **10**: 229–241.

26 Visakorpi T, Kallioniemi OP, Koivula T & Isola J. New prognostic factors in prostatic carcinoma. *Eur Urol* 1993; **24: 438–449.

27 Green DR, Taylor SR, Whelan TM & Scardino PT. DNA aneuploidy by image analysis of individual foci of prostate cancer. A preliminary report. *Cancer Res* 1991; **5**: 4084–4089.

28 Visakorpi T. Preliperation activity determined by DNA flowcytometry and proliperating cell nuclei antigen (PCNA). Immunohistochemistry as a prognostic factor in prostatic carcinoma. *J Pathol* 1992; **168**: 7–13.

29 Ekman P, Svennerus K, Zetterberg A & Gustafson JÅ. Cytophometric DNA analyses and steroid receptor content in human prostatic carcinoma. *Scand J Urol Nephrol* 1981; (suppl. 60): 85–88.

30 Waxman J & Sikora K. *The Molecular Biology of Cancer.* Oxford: Blackwell Scientific Publications 1989; pp. 41–43.

31 Barbacid M. RAS genes. *Ann Rev Biochem* 1987; **56**: 779–827.

32 Rubin SJ, Hallahan DE, Ashman CR *et al.* Two prostate carcinoma cell lines demonstrate abnormalities in tumor suppressor genes. *J Surg Oncol* 1991; **46**: 31–36.

33 Goodrich DW, Wang NP, Qian YW, Lee EYHP & Lee WH. The retinoblastoma gene product regulates progression through the G phase of the cell cycle. *Cell* 1991; **67**: 293–302.

34 Mellon K, Thompson S, Charlton RG *et al.* p53, c-erbB-2 and the epidermal growth factor receptor in the benign and malignant prostate. *J Urol* 1992; **147**: 496–499.

35 Wilding G, Valverius E, Knabbe C & O'Elman EP. Role of transforming growth factor β in human prostate cancer cell growth. *Prostate* 1989; **15**: 1–12.

36 Meyer JS, Sufrin G & Martin SA. Proliferative activity of benign human prostate, prostatic adenocarcinoma and seminal vesicle evaluated by thymidine labelling. *J Urol* 1982; **128**: 1353–1356.

37 Gallee MPW, Visser-De Jong E, Ten Kate FJW, Schröder FH & Van der Kwast TH.

Monoclonal antibody Ki-67 defined growth fraction in benign prostatic hyperplasia and prostatic cancer. *J Urol* 1989; **142**: 1342–1346.

38 Yu CCW, Hall PA, Fletcher CDM *et al*. Haemangiopericytomas: the prognostic value of immunohistochemical staining with a monoclonal antibody to proliferating cell nuclear antigen (PCNA). *Histopathology* 1991; **12**: 29–33.

Part 3
Initial Treatment Policies

10/Organ-Confined Prostate Cancer – Is Surgery the Only Option?

R.L. Byrne and D.E. Neal

Introduction

The best treatment strategy for men with organ-confined (T1–2, N0 M0) prostate cancer remains controversial. The main reason is that appropriate randomized controlled trials have not been performed to compare radical prostatectomy, radiotherapy and conservative treatment. Until such trials take place management will remain a matter of informed clinical opinion rather than clinical science. In the absence of an active screening programme in the UK, only a third of newly diagnosed patients with prostate cancer have clinically localized tumours. Treatment options for this group of men include radical prostatectomy, external beam radiotherapy, brachytherapy, hormonal manipulation and deferred treatment or 'watchful waiting'. More recent treatments include cryosurgery, hyperthermia and laser therapy. Heightened public awareness about prostatic disease and the advent of screening will lead to an increase in the proportion of organ-confined prostate cancers.

What is the risk of a conservative approach for organ-confined (T1/2 N0 M0) cancers?

Expectant treatment policy

Expectant treatment of localized prostate cancer is a real alternative because some men have low rates of progression and current data do not clearly demonstrate superior survival following radiotherapy or radical prostatectomy. In the Veterans Administration Cooperative Urological Research Group (VACURG) of men with localized prostate cancer (stage T1 and T2), the death rate attributable to prostate cancer was only 3–6% (follow-up 6.8–13.5 years) [1]. In a further VACURG prospective study [2], 111 men with T1 and T2 prostate cancer were randomized to watchful waiting or radical prostatectomy. After 15 years of follow-up there was no difference in overall survival between the two groups. However, the authors pointed out that the sample size was too small to detect accurately a large difference in survival.

George [3] undertook a prospective study of conservative therapy for 363 rather elderly men with histologically proven, bone scan-negative, localized prostate cancers. Actuarial survival rates (excluding non-cancer deaths) at 5 and 7 years were 80 and 75% respectively. However, 84% of men exhibited local progression. Similar results were reported by Johansson *et al.* [4]. In this study, 223 patients with localized prostate cancer were followed up with a watchful waiting policy. The observed 5-year survival rate was 68.8%, but more than 80% of deaths were due to causes other than cancer and the corrected 5-year survival was 92.8%. In the Johansson study, many men with high-grade tumours were excluded from conservative treatment and given radiotherapy. In both the George and Johansson studies many men were elderly with tumours that had been diagnosed incidentally after prostatectomy. This is a problem because more than 10 years' follow-up is needed to demonstrate the true impact of prostate cancer on survival.

Survival

It has been claimed that survival of men with untreated T1 tumours is similar to that of an age-matched control population [5], which is not surprising because autopsy studies have shown that 20% of 60-year-old men have microscopic foci of prostate cancer [6]. Adolfsson and colleagues [7] followed up 122 patients with well or moderately differentiated T1 or T2 tumours: the risk of death from prostate cancer was 1% after 5 years and 16% after 10 years in men not dying from other causes. The authors concluded that the risk of dying from intercurrent disease was higher than the risk of dying from prostate cancer. However, none of these patients had a poorly differentiated tumour.

These suggestions that watchful waiting is a good treatment for some men with localized tumours have been supported by Waason and colleagues [8]. These authors carried out a structured literature review of studies of men managed by radical prostatectomy, irradiation or watchful waiting published in the preceding 25 years. No convincing evidence was found for the superiority of one treatment over another in survival rates. In view of this finding and that both surgical and radiotherapeutic options are associated with varying degrees of morbidity, Waason *et al.* suggested that watchful waiting was superior because of the lack of complications. However, differences in cancer-related death rates in non-randomized studies can result purely from case selection if elderly men with low life expectancy and small, low-grade incidentally found tumours are treated by watchful waiting and if men with more advanced high-grade tumours are offered radiotherapy. Clearly, if men undergoing radical prostatectomy are found to have lymph node metastases during surgery and are then excluded from prostectomy, better survival rates will be found after surgery.

Treatment strategies

Decision analysis modelling three treatment strategies for localized prostate cancer (radical prostatectomy, external-beam radiation therapy and watchful waiting with delayed hormone therapy if metastatic disease developed) has been carried out [9]. Data were obtained from a literature review and analysis of Medicare claims. It was reported that for patients with well-differentiated tumours, treatment appears to offer little benefit over watchful waiting in terms of quality-adjusted life expectancy. Curative treatment of men with well-differentiated prostatic cancers resulted in a survival benefit of less than 6 months and may have actually diminished quality of life for some patients. In particular, this report stated that men over the age of 75 years would be best managed by watchful waiting.

It is clear that men with localized prostate cancer do not form a homogeneous group. Not only are there differences of outcome between T1 and T2 tumours, but also there are differences related to histological grade. Chodak *et al.* [10] performed an analysis of 828 case records from six non-randomized studies published since 1985 of men with localized tumours treated conservatively by means of observation or delayed hormone therapy, but not by radical surgery or irradiation. Ten years after diagnosis, disease-specific survival was recorded as 87% for men with grade 1 or 2 tumours and 34% for those with grade 3 tumours. This led the authors to conclude that initial conservative management would be suitable for some men with grade 1 or 2 clinically localized prostate cancer. Jewett [11] concluded that, although most T1 tumours are latent in the true sense or have a low biological potential, there is still a group, probably those with a higher clinical grade or those that are diffuse, that tend to progress and require additional therapy.

Disease progression

Of concern is that progression to distant metastases has been shown to occur in 16% of patients with untreated T1a tumours [12]. This often happens without detectable change in the primary lesion. However, others [13] have quoted normal 15-year life expectancies for those with low-grade T1 lesions and a normal 10-year, but diminished 15-year, life expectancy for men with high-grade lesions. Expectant management of patients with T2 tumours has resulted in 5-, 10- and 15-year survival rates of 71, 58 and 28% respectively [14]. As with T1 lesions, histological grade for T2 tumours has been shown to be a predictor of both prostate cancer death and disease progression [4]. Thus there are subsets of men, partly defined by histological grade, within each stage who are associated with a poor outcome. It is hoped that newer molecular biological studies will enable better prognostic markers to be defined.

Understaging of localized prostate cancer is common. In a study by Zincke *et al.* [15], 148 men with T1 and T2 tumours underwent radical prostatectomy, and pathological examination showed that 63% had organ-confined disease. The difficulty of detecting capsular invasion or minor degrees of extension through the apex or base of the gland is not surprising given the limitations of present-day imaging.

There is little doubt that low-grade incidentally defined prostate cancers (T1a) have a low rate of progression – at least up to 5 years after diagnosis. There is a definite role for conservative treatment in this group of men. Caution with this approach must be exercised in younger men with life expectancies of greater than 10 years because of the increased rate of progression after time. On the other hand, the rate of progression of T1b tumours is much greater [16], being in the order of 32% at 4 years.

High-quality data on death rates from prostate cancer in larger series of T2a and T2b tumours treated conservatively are not available, but it is likely that after 10 years death rates from cancer are in the order of 15–30% and that overall progression rates are in the order of 40–50%. Hence, there is a definite role for watchful waiting in this group if men have a life expectancy of less than 10 years at diagnosis. Whether radical prostatectomy should be offered is dependent not only on long-term survival rates, but also on morbidity after operation.

Radical prostatectomy

Radical perineal prostatectomy was first described and popularized by Hugh Young in 1905. The radical retropubic prostatectomy was introduced by Millin in 1947 and more recently the anatomical nerve-sparing prostatectomy has been described by Walsh *et al.* [17]. Both perineal and retropubic radical prostatectomies are still widely practised and each procedure has its advocates. The main disadvantage of the perineal approach is the need for a further procedure, either by means of laparotomy or laparoscopy, to allow assessment of the pelvic lymph nodes. Studies have shown no significant differences between the two approaches in terms of operative time, incidence of positive surgical margins and in-hospital or long-term complication rates [18]. However, there was a significantly greater estimated blood loss and transfusion rate for patients undergoing retropubic prostatectomy.

Radical prostatectomy remains the modality of choice for many urologists to treat men with organ-confined prostate cancer. It has to be stressed, however, that this preference is not based on hard scientific data. One randomized trial [19] of 97 patients with clinically localized prostate cancer compared radical prostatectomy with radiotherapy. All patients had normal serum levels of prostatic acid phosphatase, and bone scans, and no pelvic node involvement was indicated by staging pelvic lymphadenectomy. With time to first evidence of treatment failure used as the end-point for determination of treatment efficacy, radical prostatectomy was shown to be more effective than megavoltage radiation in establishing local disease control. No recent long-term data are available from this study and the numbers would have precluded the detection of even quite large differences in outcome.

Several observational studies have however been reported. Belt and Schroder [20] followed 464 patients for up to 20 years after total perineal prostatectomy. Of patients who had disease histologically confined within the capsule, only 7.6% died of prostate cancer. Similar results were reported by Gibbons *et al.* [21] who followed 52 patients who had undergone total perineal prostatectomy for a minimum of 15 years, none of whom received adjuvant therapy. Seventeen per cent had recurrence and 10% died of prostate cancer. The actual overall survival rate at 15 years was 64%, the actuarial survival was 67% and the cause-specific survival was 90%. Gibbons *et al.* concluded that if long-term survival, free from disease, is the most important outcome for men with clinically localized disease then total prostatectomy would be the treatment of choice. It was stated that the life expectancy of these patients was similar to that of the general male population of the same age in the same region during the same interval. However, essentially the same outcome can be achieved at 10 years, with conservative management of men with grade 1 or grade 2 localized prostate cancer [10]. In a literature review the disease-specific survival at 10 years was found to be 93% compared with 83% for deferred treatment and 74% for external radiation therapy [22]. These figures are subject to bias, however, because of different criteria used in selection of treatment.

In reports of operative series, the majority undergo preoperative lymphadenectomy, those with positive nodes are excluded from surgery and hence often go into a different follow-up group and may not be reported in studies of surgical treatment. The proportion of patients with a clinically localized prostate cancer found to have positive lymph nodes is between 4 and 28% [23, 24]. As men who undergo radiotherapy do not have formal assessment of lymph node status, then it is likely that a proportion of patients will have lymph node spread. Given that it is probable that surgeons would refer for radiotherapy patients with less favourable tumours, the lymph node-positive rate will be at least 25%. This would obviously create bias when comparing different treatment groups and needs to be considered when reviewing results of different treatment strategies.

Morbidity and mortality

An important consideration when deciding to undertake radical prostatectomy is the cost to the patient in terms of mortality and morbidity. Until recently, radical prostatectomy was followed by impotence in nearly all patients and by incontinence in up to 20%. However, the introduction of nerve-sparing technique by Walsh [17] has improved outcome. Steiner *et al.* [25] evaluated the effects of the anatomical radical prostatectomy in the first 593 consecutive patients to undergo this procedure in the same centre as Walsh. Complete urinary control was achieved in 92% of patients and mild stress incontinence was present in the remaining 8%. Six per cent wore one or fewer pads per day and only 2 patients (0.3%) required an artificial sphincter. None of the patients in this series was totally incontinent. The same group also published results regarding postoperative sexual function [26]. This was evaluated in 600 consecutive men who were 34–72 years old. Sixty-eight per cent of those who were potent preoperatively were potent after operation; sexual function was preserved in 91% of men less than 50 years old, 75% of men 50–60 years old and 25% of men 70 years old or older.

Although this technique provides vastly improved results for postoperative impotence and urinary continence, it has been questioned whether this occurs at the price of adequate tumour excision. Stamey *et al.* [27] reported that 83–90% of tumours that extend beyond the prostatic capsule do so in the area of the neurovascular bundles. However, Eggleston and Walsh [28] showed no evidence of compromise with the nerve-sparing operation. In the results published by Walsh *et al.* [29] of anatomical radical prostatectomy for 955 men with clinically localized prostate cancer, 10-year actuarial analysis demonstrated a 7% likelihood of distant metastases and local recurrence rates of 4%. Thus it does not appear that such a procedure when undertaken by an experienced operator compromises cancer cure compared with a standard approach. Walsh points out that the neurovascular bundles should be sacrificed if there is suspicion of local invasion.

Other considerations are the morbidity and mortality associated with this procedure in an elderly population. The 30-day mortality is in the order of 0.3%, even in series which report outcome from many different centres. Morbidity includes cardiopulmonary complications in 4% of men aged 65–69 years and 7.4% of men aged 75–79 years [30], with an incidence of pulmonary embolism of 0.6% [31]. Rectal injuries can usually be recognized during surgery and repaired as appropriate; more serious rectal injuries occur infrequently, with fewer than 1% of patients requiring a colostomy. The rate of vesical neck contracture has been reported as between 4.7 and 8.7% [31].

Does surgery cure prostate cancer?

The aim of radical prostatectomy is cancer cure. Paulson and colleagues [23] reported on the results of 441 patients with T1 or T2 disease who had normal preoperative bone scans and no evidence of nodal extension, as judged by staging pelvic lymphadenectomy. Histological examination of the surgical specimens found that 28% of tumours had disease extending to the margins of the specimen and 17% had disease extending beyond the prostate but confined to the specimen. Failure rate was defined on the grounds of increases in serum acid phosphatase or on grounds of metastatic disease or on the basis of local recurrence detected by digital rectal examination (DRE) and confirmed by biopsy. For the 55% who had organ-confined disease there was a 12% failure rate at 10 years; for men with specimen-confined disease, the failure rate at 10 years was 30% and for men who were margin-positive, the failure rate was 60%. Thus cancer cure cannot be guaranteed even in those with no preoperative evidence of tumour extension beyond the prostate and histological evidence of complete resection.

There does appear to be a role for radical prostatectomy in the management of localized prostate cancer and a life expectancy of more than 10 years. However, even with histological evidence of complete tumour excision, there is still no guarantee of cure. Although the major complications of incontinence and erectile impotence still occur, the incidence has been significantly reduced by newer techniques.

Radiotherapy

The techniques of radiotherapy utilized in the treatment of localized prostate cancer include external-beam radiotherapy, interstitial radioisotope implantation or a combination of both. External-beam radiotherapy for the treatment of prostate cancer was pioneered by Bagshaw in the early 1950s. The interest in radiotherapy developed when it was realized that hormone manipulation was unable to provide anything other than palliation for prostate cancer. In addition, the high rates of incontinence and impotence associated with radical surgery at that time made the development of an alternative, with lower morbidity and mortality, an attractive proposition. Although external-beam radiotherapy appeared to have benefit, there were problems with major bowel and bladder complications, which occurred in 10–12% [32]. This was probably because of the need to administer high doses for a significant effect on the tumour to occur. There is evidence that gastrointestinal and urinary complications have gradually become less frequent and less severe as a result of improvements in radiation techniques. Because of the damaging effects of external-beam radiotherapy on other tissues, brachytherapy for prostate cancer was developed; its advantages include delivery of high local doses with limited injury to adjacent organs. The need for surgery to place the radioactive seeds provides an opportunity to perform pelvic lymphadenectomy simultaneously and thus provide more accurate staging information. More recently, brachytherapy, delivered using ultrasound control, without the need for operation, has become increasingly popular.

External-beam radiotherapy

The only randomized clinical trial comparing radical surgery with megavoltage radiation therapy [19] showed surgery to be more effective than radiotherapy in establishing disease control. Such results were challenged by Bagshaw *et al.* [33] who reported that survival 15 years following radiotherapy for T1 tumours did not deviate significantly from an age-matched peer group. For patients with T2 tumours, survival after 15 years was 5% less than an age-matched group of men. As pointed out by Bagshaw and colleagues, these excellent results were despite the absence of knowledge of lymph node status and capsular penetration. Similar results were reported by others [34].

Can external-beam radiotherapy cure prostate cancer?

To determine the ability of radiotherapy to achieve cure it is necessary to look at disease progression and deaths following treatment. El-Galley *et al.* [35] reviewed 191 patients who underwent external-beam radiotherapy for localized disease between 1982 and 1991; 52% had T1 or T2 disease. Five-year survival rates were 77% for T1 disease, 70% for T2 disease and 50% for T3 disease. Long-term local control was 80, 65 and 22% for patients with T1, T2 and T3 disease respectively. The development of metastases was also related to stage: 20% in T1 disease, 40% in T2 disease and 80% in T3 disease. These results implied that radiotherapy was less effective than surgery in providing local control and long-term cure or that a proportion of patients were understaged and radiotherapy was more effective than might be indicated; or it may be that neither treatment was better than conservative treatment. This dilemma emphasizes the real need for large-scale long-term randomized studies.

The importance of accurate staging when assessing results is illustrated in the study by Lee and Sause [36] who carried out staging lymphadenectomy before external-beam radiotherapy. For 20 patients with localized disease who were node-negative, the 15-year actuarial survival, cause-specific survival and local control rates were 40, 75 and 92% respectively. The 5-year survival for this group was 85% overall, but with 100% cause-specific survival and 100% local control at 5 years. Similar results have been reported by Bagshaw *et al.* [33] and Hanks [34].

Postirradiation prostatic biopsies have been used to determine the local failure rate of external-beam radiotherapy. Forman *et al.* [37] found that 15% of patients with T1 or T2 disease had a positive biopsy 2 years after the completion of radiotherapy treatment. In the study by Schellhammer *et al.* [38] the incidence of negative biopsy 18 months or more after therapy was 65%. There was no difference in the biopsy results for those treated by external-beam radiotherapy or brachytherapy, but a positive biopsy was associated with a poor outcome. However, Leach and colleagues [39] found that a positive biopsy following irradiation did not predict disease-free survival, overall survival or death from prostatic cancer in patients followed for 10 years.

Thus the ability of external-beam radiotherapy to control and possibly cure prostate cancer in the long term remains uncertain. Certainly, short-term results (5 years) approach those of radical surgery or watchful waiting. Mortality is rare with any of the radiotherapy techniques (< 1%). El-Galley *et al.* [35] reported that, although 36% of patients had late bowel complications, none were severe and none required surgical intervention; only 4% developed severe late radiation toxicity affecting the bladder. Leach *et al.* [39] reported minor and major complication rates of 25 and 3% respectively; major complications were confined to men who received 7000 rad. The incidence of erectile dysfunction following external-beam radiotherapy varies from 14 to 46% [40]. However, Goldstein *et al.* [41] reported sexual dysfunction in 79% of patients treated with external-beam radiotherapy.

Brachytherapy

The technique of brachytherapy for prostate cancer was developed by Carlton and Hudgins in 1965. The rationale was that the equivalent of 7000–7500 rad could be administered with fewer complications than occurred with the same dosage of external-beam irradiation. However, the procedure still required surgery. In order to exclude the need for a surgical procedure, ultrasound-guided brachytherapy using iodine-125 seed implantation was introduced by Holm *et al.* in the early 1980s [42]. Priestly and Beyer [43] reported on 157 men who underwent transperineal ultrasound-guided radioactive seed implantation for localized prostate cancer between 1988 and 1991. The main postoperative complication was difficulty with urination and transurethral resection of the prostate was commonly required 6–8 weeks prior to the procedure. Mild dysuria and haematuria postprocedure were common, although only 1 patient had urinary retention. The incidence of impotence was less than 10% and there were no deaths and no significant bowel complications. There was a 90% reduction in tumour size at 9 months, as indicated by DRE and transrectal ultrasound. The advantage reported by the authors of this paper is that it is a procedure that is relatively easy to perform, taking less than 1 h, and patients can go home the same day without a catheter *in situ*. They recommend it as an alternative for patients who are unfit for radical surgery, but for whom curative treatment is indicated.

Kaye *et al.* [44] reported that 28% of patients developed irritative or obstructive symptoms following iodine-125 implantation for localized prostate cancer, but only 7% had severe symptoms. These men underwent seed implantation by a percutaneous approach. Superficial urethral necrosis with haematuria occurred in 3%; this developed 2–3 years following implantation and was treated by transurethral resection of the prostate. Of patients who had good sexual function before treatment, 81% maintained good erections at 8–12 months of follow-up. Clinical progression-free survival was 51% for those with tumours less than 2 cm on DRE and Gleason score of less than 7, although the mean follow-up was only 26 months. The long-term results of brachytherapy are yet to be assessed.

Recommended treatment for T1–2 N0 M0 prostate cancer

Even in patients with T1 or T2a disease who have normal prostate-specific antigen, bone scans and lymph nodes, the results of radical prostatectomy show that 10-year survival rates are in the order of about 90% with local recurrence rates of 5–8%. In the absence of appropriate randomized controlled trials, it is not possible to offer definitive guidance about treatment protocols. Clearly, in such circumstances, the provision of up-to-date information to men and allowing them to play an important role in decision-making are vital.

Men with a less than 10-year life expectancy

Most urologists would not offer radical treatment to men with a less than 10-year survival and would offer watchful waiting with delayed hormonal therapy.

T1a tumours

These small, low-grade tumours can be carefully observed with sequential prostate-specific antigen measurement and DRE.

T1b tumours

These tumours are often of high grade and have a high incidence of lymph node metastasis. Progression rates at 5–10 years are significant and in men with a good life expectancy treatment may range from conservative treatment and delayed hormonal treatment, radiotherapy or radical prostatectomy.

T2a, T2b tumours

These are the ideal tumours to be considered for radical prostatectomy because of the lower rate of lymph node metastasis and the high rate of organ-confined disease. Despite this observation, men should be given the choice between such surgery, radiotherapy and watchful waiting with delayed hormonal therapy.

References

** 1 Byar DP, Corle DK and VACURG. VACURG randomised trial of prostatectomy for stage I and II prostate cancer. *Urology* 1981; **17**(suppl): 7–11.

2 Graverson HP, Nielson KT, Gasser TC, Corle DK & Madsen PO. Radical prostatectomy versus expectant primary treatment in stages I and II prostate cancer. *Urology* 1990; **36**: 493–498.

3 George NJR. Natural history of localised prostatic cancer managed by conservative therapy alone. *Lancet* 1988; **i**: 494–497.

** 4 Johansson J-E, Adami H-O, Anderson S-O, Bergstrom R, Krusemo UB & Kraaz W. Natural history of localised prostatic cancer. *Lancet* 1989; **i**: 799–803.

** 5 Byar DP. VACURG studies on prostatic cancer and its treatment. In: *Urologic Pathology*. New York: Lea & Febiger, 1977, pp. 241–267.

* 6 Breslow N, Chan CW, Dhom G *et al.* Latent carcinoma of the prostate at autopsy in seven areas. *Int J Cancer* 1977; **20**: 680–688.

7 Adolfsson J, Carstensen T & Lowhagen T. Deferred treatment in localised prostate cancer. *Br J Urol* 1992; **69**: 183–187.

8 Waason JH, Cushman CC, Bruskewitz RC, Littenberg B, Mulley AG & Wennberg JE. A structured literature review of treatment for localised prostate cancer. Prostate disease patient outcome research team. *Arch Family Med* 1993; **2**: 487–493.

9 Fleming C, Waason JH, Albertson PC, Barry MJ & Wennberg JE. A decision analysis of

* Reference of special interest.
** Reference of outstanding merit.

alternative treatment strategies for clinically localised prostate cancer. *JAMA* 1993; **269**: 2650–2658.

*10 Chodak GW, Thisted RA, Gerber GS *et al.* Results of conservative management of clinically localized prostate cancer. *N Engl J Med* 1994; **330**: 242–248.

11 Jewett HJ. The present status of radical prostatectomy for stages A and B prostatic cancer. *Urol Clin North Am* 1975; **2**: 105–124.

12 Epstein JI, Paul G, Eggleston JC & Walsh PC. Prognosis of untreated stage A1 prostatic carcinoma: a study of 94 cases with extended follow-up. *J Urol* 1986; **136**: 837–839.

13 Hanash KA, Utz D & Cook EN. Carcinoma of the prostate: a 15 year follow-up. *J Urol* 1972; **107**: 450–453.

14 Barnes R, Hirst A & Rosenquist R. Early carcinoma of the prostate, comparison of stages A and B. *J Urol* 1976; **115**: 404–405.

15 Zincke H, Blute ML, Fallen MJ & Farrow GM. Radical prostatectomy for stage A adenocarcinoma of the prostate: staging errors and their implications for treatment recommendations and disease outcome. *J Urol* 1991; **146: 1053–1058.

*16 Cantrell BB, DeKlerk DP, Eggleston JC, Boitnott JK & Walsh PC. Pathological factors that influence prognosis in stage A prostatic cancer: the influence of extent versus grade. *J Urol* 1981; **125**: 516–520.

17 Walsh PC, Lepor H & Eggleston JC. Radical prostatectomy with preservation of sexual function. Anatomical and pathological considerations. *Prostate* 1983; **4: 473–485.

18 Frazier HA, Robertson JE & Paulson DF. Radical prostatectomy: the pros and cons of the perineal versus retropubic approach. *J Urol* 1992; **147**: 888–890.

19 Paulson DF, Lin GH, Hinshaw W & Stephani S. Radical surgery versus radiotherapy for adenocarcinoma of the prostate. *J Urol* 1982; **128: 502–504.

20 Belt E & Schroder FH. Total perineal prostatectomy for carcinoma of the prostate. *J Urol* 1972; **107**: 91–96.

*21 Gibbons RP, Correa RJ, Brannen GE & Weissman RM. Total prostatectomy for clinically prostatic cancer: long term results. *J Urol* 1989; **141**: 564–566.

*22 Adolfsson J, Steineck G & Whitmore WF. Recent results of management of palpable clinically localized prostate cancer. *Cancer* 1993; **72**: 310–322.

23 Paulson DF, Moul JW & Walther PJ. Radical prostatectomy for clinical stage T1–2 N0 M0 prostatic adenocarcinoma: long-term results. *J Urol* 1990; **144**: 1180–1184.

24 Middleton RG & Smith JA Jr. Radical prostatectomy for stage B2 prostatic cancer. *J Urol* 1982; **127**: 702–703.

25 Steiner MS, Morton RA & Walsh PC. Impact of anatomical radical prostatectomy on urinary continence. *J Urol* 1991; **145**: 512–515.

26 Quinlan DM, Epstein JI, Carter BS & Walsh PC. Sexual function following radical prostatectomy: influence of preservation of neurovascular bundles. *J Urol* 1991; **145**: 998–1002.

27 Stamey TA, McNeal JE, Freiha FS & Redwine E. Morphometric and clinical studies on 68 consecutive radical prostatectomies. *J Urol* 1988; **139**: 1235–1241.

28 Eggleston JC & Walsh PC. Radical prostatectomy with preservation of sexual function: pathological findings in the first 100 cases. *J Urol* 1985; **134**: 1146–1148.

29 Walsh PC, Partin AW & Epstein JI. Cancer control and quality of life following anatomical radical retropubic prostatectomy: results at 10 years. *J Urol* 1994; **152: 1831–1836.

30 Lu-Yao GL, McLerram D, Waason J & Wennberg JE. An assessment of radical pros-

tatectomy. Time trends, geographic variation and outcome. *JAMA* 1993; **269**: 2633–2636.

31 Zincke H, Oesterling JE, Blute ML, Bergstalh EJ, Myers RP & Barrett DM. Longterm (15 years) results after radical prostatectomy for clinically localized (stage T2C or lower) prostate cancer. *J Urol* 1994; **152: 1850–1857.

32 Bagshaw MA, Ray GR, Pistenma DA, Castellino RA & Meares EM Jr. External beam radiation therapy of primary carcinoma of the prostate. *Cancer* 1975; **36**: 723–728.

33 Bagshaw MA, Cox RS & Ramback JE. Radiation therapy for localised prostate cancer. *Urol Clin North Am* 1990; **17: 787–802.

34 Hanks GE. External beam radiation therapy for prostate cancer clinically confined to the gland. *Urology* 1989; **33**(suppl.): 21–26.

35 El-Galley RES, Howard GCW, Hawkyard S *et al.* Radical radiotherapy for localized adenocarcinoma of the prostate. A report of 191 cases. *Br J Urol* 1995; **75**: 38–43.

36 Lee JR & Sause WT. Surgically staged patients with prostatic carcinoma treated with definitive radiotherapy: fifteen-year results. *Urology* 1994; **43**: 640–644.

37 Forman JD, Oppenheim T, Liu H, Montie J, McLaughlin PW & Porter AT. Frequency of residual neoplasm in the prostate following three-dimensional conformal radiotherapy. *Prostate* 1993; **23**: 235–243.

38 Schellhammer PF, El-Mahdi AM, Higgins EM, Schultheiss TE, Ladaga LE & Babb TJ. Prostate biopsy after definitive treatment by interstitial 125 iodine implant or external beam radiation therapy. *J Urol* 1987; **137**: 897–901.

39 Leach GE, Cooper JF, Kagan AR, Synder R & Forsythe A. Radiotherapy for prostatic carcinoma: post-irradiation prostatic biopsy and recurrence patterns with long term followup. *J Urol* 1982; **128**: 505–509.

40 Zinreich ES, Derogatis LR, Herpst J, Auvil G, Piantadosi S & Order SE. Pre and post treatment evaluation of sexual function in patients with adenocarcinoma of the prostate. *Int J Rad Oncol Biol Phys* 1990; **19**: 1001–1004.

41 Goldstein I, Feldman M & Deckers PJ. Radiation associate impotence: a clinical study of its mechanism. *JAMA* 1984; **251**: 903–910.

*42 Holm HH, Juul N, Pedersen JF, Hansen H & Stroyer I. Transperineal 125 iodine seed implantation in prostate cancer guided by transrectal ultrasound. *J Urol* 1993; **103**: 283–628.

43 Priestly JB & Beyer DC. Guided brachytherapy for treatment of confined prostate cancer. *Urology* 1992; **40**: 27–32.

44 Kaye KW, Olson DJ & Payne JT. Detailed preliminary analysis of ^{125}I implantation for localized prostate cancer using percutaneous approach. *J Urol* 1995; **153**: 1020–1025.

11/Organ-Confined Prostate Cancers – Which are Dangerous?

G.D. Steinberg, C.W. Rinker-Schaeffer and C.B. Brendler

Introduction

There has been an extraordinary increase in the incidence of prostate cancer in the USA (60% from 1990 to 1993), and the incidence continues to rise. In addition, the number of radical prostatectomies performed in the USA has increased almost fivefold from 1987 to 1992. This increase in the number of radical prostatectomies is also true for men in their seventh decade of life. Olsson and Goluboff predict that, because of changing methods of detection of prostate cancer in the USA, approximately 52% of newly diagnosed patients will be treated with radical prostatectomy [1].

Because of the poor prognosis for men with locally advanced and metastatic prostate cancer, efforts to control this disease have focused on aggressive screening to detect the cancer while still organ-confined and potentially curable. A potential complication of such screening is the high prevalence of 'histological' cancers that pose little health risk. For example, autopsy studies indicate that 30% of men 50–60 years old and 50% of those 70–80 years old have histological prostatic cancers which did not produce symptoms during their lifetime. Additional studies have demonstrated that this high age-related prevalence of histological prostatic cancer is observed throughout the world's male population [2]. In contrast, the prevalence of clinically manifest prostatic cancer varies by more than 15-fold between the high incidence rate in Americans versus the low incidence rate in Japanese, although their average life spans are equal. These results suggest that many histologically detected, asymptomatic prostate cancers may never become life-threatening during the life time of the host [3]. The majority of these lesions may not produce clinical symptoms because they have not undergone all of the genetic changes necessary for malignant progression (i.e. have not acquired metastatic ability).

It is estimated that screening may identify up to 10 million men with prostate cancer; however, only about 900 000 would die of their cancer if left untreated [4]. At this time it is not possible to identify which histologically localized cancers will complete malignant progression and, therefore, require aggressive therapy as opposed to those which are truly indolent, possibly best treated conservatively. Clinically useful markers for substaging individual tumours and predicting the clinical course of disease are being studied by various investigators. True progress will not be made until delineation of the cellular and molecular pathways of metastatic progression is identified.

Pathological features of prostate cancer

The problem presented by prostatic cancer is that currently it is difficult to predict the clinical course of the disease for individuals. Approximately 50% of men with prostatic cancer have clinically advanced (i.e. non-organ-confined) disease at the time of initial diagnosis. One-third of the remaining 50% of men with clinically localized disease actually have more advanced disease found pathologically [5]. In some men prostatic cancer metastasizes rapidly, while other men survive untreated for many years with localized disease that does not progress clinically [6]. If organ-confined, prostatic cancer can be cured by surgery alone (i.e. radical prostatectomy) [7]. Unfortunately, if diagnosed when non-organ-confined, prostatic cancer is a fatal disease for which at present there is no curative treatment [8, 9]. Because of the poor prognosis for men with metastatic prostatic cancer, aggressive screening programmes have been suggested for men starting at the age of 50 in order to permit early detection of prostate cancer while organ-confined and therefore potentially curable. However, the questions remain as to whether we are overtreating some men with prostate cancer, and, if so, can we identify those patients who need aggressive treatment and those who do not.

Significance of tumour grade

Currently prostate cancer is detected by an abnormal digital rectal examination (DRE) and/or an elevated serum prostate-specific antigen (PSA). Transrectal ultrasound (TRUS)-guided biopsies provide histological material for examination. The histological grade of the primary prostatic cancer lesion is evaluated using the Gleason grading system [10]. In this system, grading is based upon the degree of glandular differentiation and growth pattern of the tumour as it relates to the prostatic stoma. The pattern may vary from well-differentiated (grade 1) to poorly differentiated (grade 5). This system takes into account tumour heterogeneity by scoring both the primary and secondary tumour growth patterns. For example, if the majority of the tumour is moderately differentiated (grade 3) and the secondary growth pattern is poorly differentiated (grade 4), the combined score would be a Gleason grade of 7. This system is predictive of biological potential for tumours with either very low (i.e. < 5) or very high (i.e. 8–10) combined scores; however, it is of limited use for tumours with intermediate (5–7) scores. This limitation is of particular importance since most tumours (76%) are in this intermediate category [11].

In addition, predicting the biological potential of prostatic cancer based upon histology of the needle biopsy alone is problematic. In several studies comparing needle biopsies with subsequent radical prostatectomies, 20–58% of the needle biopsy specimens were diagnosed as well-differentiated with substantially fewer of the radical prostatectomies showing well-differentiated tumour [12, 13]. This is due to a tendency to undergrade limited amounts of intermediate-grade tumour on needle biopsy, the presence of higher-grade tumour present elsewhere in the prostate and the presence of higher-grade tumour within the same tumour. Using restrictive criteria for low Gleason grading, Epstein and Steinberg [14] reported that 47% of radical prosta-tectomy specimens had higher-grade tumour present. Thus, because of diffi-culty in identifying Gleason score from preoperative needle biopsies, it is uncertain that conservative therapy should be recommended, even for patients with very-low-grade cancer on needle biopsy. In addition, Epstein *et al.* [15] reported on 153 radical prostatectomy specimens removed for non-palpable prostate cancer. Nine per cent of the prostates contained tumour foci that were predominantly Gleason pattern 4 or 5 and measured 1 cm^3 or less. Therefore, prostate cancer can be high-grade early in its course, and patients followed conservatively should undergo widespread needle sampling of the prostate to enhance detection of multifocal high-grade disease.

Ohori *et al.* [16] reported that patients with a Gleason score of 7 or greater had a higher cancer progression rate when treated with radical prostatectomy than patients with Gleason score less then 7. However, $85 \pm 18\%$ of patients with high-grade organ-confined prostate had no evidence of progression at 5 years and did as well as patients with low-grade disease. Partin *et al.* [17] reported the clinical outcome of 72 men with Gleason scores 8–10 on needle biopsy and clinically localized disease. Sixty-three men underwent radical prostectomy, while 32% had positive pelvic lymph nodes, of whom nine did not undergo radical prostatectomy. The actuarial likelihood of having an undetectable PSA at 5 years was 45% for men with specimen-confined disease. Thus, the Gleason score does not necessarily predict biological aggressiveness in all patients with localized prostate cancer. Moreover, radical prostatectomy is potentially curative in some men with high-grade organ-confined prostate cancer.

Walsh and colleagues from Johns Hopkins recently presented 10 years of experience with anatomical radical retropubic prostatectomy [18]. The actuarial likelihood of an elevated serum PSA increased with higher pathological stage and Gleason score. The 10-year likelihood of freedom from PSA relapse was 85% for men with organ-confined disease, 82% with focal capsular penetration, 54% with established capsular penetration and Gleason score less than 7, 42% with established capsular penetration and Gleason score 7 or greater, and 43% with seminal vesicle involvement. Thus, radical prostatectomy appears to cure most men with localized disease. However, it is still unclear which patients with apparently unfavourable pathology would benefit from adjuvant therapy.

Clinical stage T1c prostate cancer

The widespread use of serum PSA and TRUS to screen for prostate cancer has resulted in the earlier detection of tumours, many of which are non-palpable (T1c) by DRE. The biological significance of these tumours is uncertain; the question arises whether these early detection techniques are diagnosing histologic or 'latent' prostate cancers of low biological potential.

The clinical and pathological characteristics of non-palpable prostate cancers identified with PSA screening have recently been reported in several studies. Incidental prostate cancers detected at the time of cystoprostatectomy have a mean tumour volume of only 0.04 cm^3, 78% are less than 0.5 cm^3, and 87% are organ-confined [19]. In contrast, T1c prostate cancers are about 50 times larger and generally more extensive. Oesterling *et al.* [20] reported on 208 patients treated with radical prostatectomy. Only 53% of the patients had organ-confined prostate cancer (11% less than 0.5 cm^3 of tumour), 34% positive surgical margins, 9% seminal vesicle invasion and 3% positive pelvic lymph nodes. Humphrey and Catalona reported on 53 men undergoing radical prostatectomy for stage T1c prostate cancer [21]. Only 19% of these tumours were less than 0.5 cm^3, 43% demonstrated extracapsular extension and/or positive surgical margins and only 8% of tumours were Gleason score 2–4. Epstein *et al.* reported on 157 stage T1c prostate cancer patients treated with radical prostatectomy [22]. Only 51% of the patients had organ-confined prostate cancer (26% less than 0.5 cm^3 of tumour), 34% had extensive extracapsular extension, 17% positive surgical margins, 6% seminal vesicle invasion and 4% positive pelvic lymph nodes. Thus, most of stage T1c prostate cancers appear to be clinically significant tumours.

Epstein *et al.* also examined multiple preoperative clinical and pathological parameters in an attempt to identify patients with insignificant tumours who might be considered for conservative therapy. Patients were accurately predicted to have minimal tumours (tumour volume less than 0.5 cm^3) by having a PSA density less than 0.1, no Gleason grade 4 or 5 tumour on needle biopsy, fewer than three positive biopsy cores, and less than 50% involvement of any single biopsy core.

However, these findings in non-palpable prostate cancer still do not completely address the question of which patients with favourable pathology need treatment and which ones do not. To answer this question will require an understanding of the molecular and genetic changes associated with prostatic cancer growth and progression.

Intracellular markers of prostate cancer progression

Cellular changes, or markers, which are associated with the neoplastic transition from locally invasive prostatic cancer to metastatic disease have been identified by a number of laboratories. In some cases these changes seem to be involved in multiple steps in the progression of prostatic cancer (e.g. cellular pleomorphism/genetic instability) while others seem to occur at specific points along the progression pathway (e.g. changes in nuclear shape, increased angiogenesis) [23]. While the role that each of these factors plays in the progression of prostatic cancer remains uncertain, a temporal relationship of cellular events is being established.

DNA ploidy

A well-established principle of tumour biology is that tumours progress to more aberrant phenotypes with time. In human prostate cancers, the least malignant cells initially have a diploid DNA content [24]. Flow-cytometric analysis of the DNA content per cell has demonstrated that fewer than 10% of histologically detected, low-volume (i.e. stage T1a) human prostatic cancers are aneuploid, in comparison to about 40% of higher-volume cancers [25, 26]. These findings are clinically relevant since patients with aneuploid tumours have a shorter time to progression and decreased survival as compared to patients with diploid tumours [27–30]. Repeated fine-needle aspiration biopsies of untreated patients with localized prostatic cancer demonstrated that 25% of these patients progressed towards increased aneuploidy during 24 months or more of surveillance. Moreover, this progression in DNA aneuploidy has also been correlated with progression towards less well-differentiated histological phenotypes (i.e. higher histological grades of cancer) [31]. Montgomery *et al.* [29] found ploidy to be the best independent predictor of prognosis in organ-confined prostate cancer. Gleason grade enhanced prognostication when added to ploidy. Carmichael *et al.* [32] reported that DNA ploidy analysis was able to predict disease recurrence in patients with well to moderately differentiated (Gleason score less than 7) clinical stage T2 prostate cancer treated with radical prostatectomy. DNA ploidy analysis was of no additional predictive value in men with high-grade tumours. In this study tumour volume was also predictive of progression in patients with well to moderately differentiated tumours. However, in a multivariate analysis of tumour volume, Gleason score and ploidy, ploidy was not an independent predictor of prognosis.

Cytogenetic changes

In addition to changes in ploidy during metastatic progression, cytogenetic aberrations have been observed in human prostatic cancer tissue. Brothman *et al.* found that cells from localized prostatic cancer did not exhibit consistent chromosomal changes [33]. In contrast, Atkin and Baker demonstrated that prostatic cancer cells from metastatic cancer patients had a consistent deletion in the q arm of chromosome 10 in the region of 10q23–qter [34]. Deletions in 10q23 have also been observed in presently available human prostatic cancer cell lines. These results suggest that structural alterations, specifically 10q23 deletions, are associated with the progression of prostatic cancer to a more malignant phenotype. Thus, malignant progression of human prostatic cancer is associated with the development of aneuploidy and non-random cytogenetic changes.

Nuclear morphometry

The inaccuracies and poor reproducibility of grading systems for prostate cancer have led many investigators to search for more objective and quantitative methods for grading prostate cancer. Morphometry has permitted a more careful quantification of these nuclear characteristics. Diamond *et al.* [35, 36] were the first to employ a simple nuclear shape factor (nuclear roundness) to describe the shape of cancerous nuclear in patients with stage B1 and B2 (Whitmore–Jewett staging) prostate cancer. In these studies the outcome for these patients was accurately predicted. Since then, several investigators have used this method to predict prognosis for patients with various stages of prostate cancer [37–41]. More recently, a multivariate analysis of the variance of nuclear roundness, clinical stage, Gleason score and the patient's age have been used to predict the disease-free survival among a group of 100 men treated by radical prostatectomy [42]. Recent advances in computer and image analysis technologies have made this quantitative modality available for routine analysis of patient samples in clinical practice. This information may aid in

Chapter 11

stratifying patients into high-risk and low-risk groups for testing adjuvant therapies for prostate cancer.

Nuclear matrix proteins in prostate cancer

The nuclear matrix consists of the insoluble structural framework of the nucleus. Nuclear matrix protein patterns analysed with two-dimensional gel electrophoresis were found to be cell-type-specific in human cultured breast carcinoma cell lines [43]. Subsequently, it was demonstrated that nuclear matrix protein patterns have tissue specificity in rat sex-accessory tissues and characteristic differences in a series of rat prostate cancer cell lines and tumours [44]. Additional studies have demonstrated that there are differences in the nuclear matrix protein patterns between normal prostate, benign prostatic hyperplasia (BPH) and prostate cancer in fresh human tissue collected from 21 men undergoing surgery for either clinically localized prostate cancer or BPH [45]. Fourteen different nuclear matrix protein changes that are specific for BPH and prostate cancer were identified. One nuclear matrix protein, PC-1, was identified in all prostate cancer specimens (14 of 14) but not in any normal prostate (0 of 13) or BPH (0 of 14) specimens. Thus, PC-1 may be a candidate nuclear matrix marker for prostate cancer [45].

Cellular motility

Until recently, methods did not exist for study of the dynamic biological properties of *living* cancer cells. Time-lapse videomicroscopy of living cancer cells has revealed that some cancer cells exhibit dynamic forms of cell motility. Time-lapse studies of cancer cells using the Dunning R3327 system of rat prostatic adenocarcinomas demonstrated various distinct types of cell motility, including cell membrane ruffling, pseudopodal extension, undulation and cell translation [46]. Time-lapse films were made and visually graded using isolated cells taken from seven (four low metastatic and three highly metastatic) Dunning variants. Marked differences were found between cells taken from the highly metastatic cell lines and those from the low metastatic lines. The identification of different types of cell motility may aid the study of individual live cancer cells and help to identify patients with aggressive tumours.

Extracellular markers of prostate cancer progression

Extracellular matrix interactions

The interactions between prostatic cancer cells and the extracellular matrix (ECM) must be considered in any models of prostatic cancer invasion and metastasis. The involvement of the basement membrane and extracellular as both a barrier and store for growth and angiogenesis factors has been well-established [47]. In order for prostatic cancer cells to metastasize they must be able to degrade the basement membrane, traverse the ECM, adhere to a distant site and establish a blood supply (i.e. induce tumour angiogenesis). Functionally it has been demonstrated that initiation of this process requires the secretion of proteolytic enzymes, increased cellular motility, altered cell substrate interactions and induction of tumour angiogenesis.

Metalloproteinase activity

The degradation of the basement membrane by type IV collagenases and other proteases has been suggested to be the first step in invasion and metastasis. In particular, the role of 72 kDa type IV collagenase has been the subject of extensive study. Stearns and Wang have found increased collagenase expression in malignant human prostatic cancer tissue as compared to benign controls [48]. Specifically, they found that the levels of 72 kDa collagenase RNA and protein were undetectable in benign prostatic tissue but were consistently high in prostatic cancer tissue (Gleason grades 1–8), suggesting a role for 72 kDa collagenase expression in the transition from benign to invasive phenotypes. Further evidence for the role of matrix metalloproteinases in the development of prostatic adenocarcinoma is provided by the work of Pajouh *et al.* [49]. In addition to increased levels of 72 kDa collagenase, they also found increased expression of the matrix metalloproteinase matrilysin. These data support a model in which increased metalloproteinase expression is involved in initiating prostatic cancer invasion. This may be a useful marker to test in future clinical trials to assess biological aggressiveness.

Cell adhesion molecules

Besides extracellular matrix interaction, tumour intercellular interactions are also critical for the metastatic process. For example, recent studies have indicated a role for E-cadherin, a calcium-dependent cellular adhesion molecule (CAM), in invasion and metastasis [50]. E-cadherin is a large protein molecule that spans the cell membrane and, in effect, connects the intracellular cytoskeleton to similar molecules extending from neighbouring cells. It has been shown that when E-cadherin is expressed in some cancer cells, its structure is disorganized, thus perturbing the attachment to the internal cellular skeleton. This perturbation may be due to a dysfunctional catenin protein, the molecule that links E-cadherin to the cytoskeletal actin. In recent studies of human prostatic cancer specimens, E-cadherin was found at normal levels in moderately differentiated tumours but was diminished or absent in poorly differentiated, higher-stage tumours and in positive lymph nodes [51]. In those samples which had decreased or undetectable levels of E-cadherin, there was an inverse correlation between the level of E-cadherin and invasion. These results suggest that a reduction in E-cadherin protein expression may be an important determinant in the acquisition of metastatic ability in prostatic cancer.

Angiogenesis

There is a large body of evidence that the ability of cancer to grow and metastasize is critically dependent upon the induction of tumour angiogenesis (i.e. development of new blood vessels). Recent studies have demonstrated that the intensity of angiogenesis within an individual tumour can predict metastatic potential in malignant melanoma, breast cancer, non-small cell lung cancer and prostatic cancer. Bigler *et al.* demonstrated a critical role for angiogenesis in prostate cancer [52]. These authors reported a significantly increased density of microvessels within invasive, clinically detected, human prostatic cancer relative to normal prostatic stroma. In addition, they found a significant difference in vascularity even in poorly differentiated, clinically detected human prostatic cancers between those that metastasized and those that were organ-confined. Recently, Weidner *et al.* have also reported that increasing microvessel density (i.e. degree of angiogenesis) is correlated with the acquisition of metastatic ability by human prostatic cancers [53].

The observation that poorly differentiated prostatic carcinomas which metastasized had a significantly higher mean microvessel density (greater tumour angiogenesis) than similar tumours that did not metastasize suggests that poorly differentiated histology is not sufficient for metastases to occur. A concomitant alteration to a highly angiogenic phenotype appears to be as important as development of a poorly differentiated morphology in the acquisition of metastatic ability. Studies are presently under way at various centres to see if microvessel density can be a clinically significant marker of biological aggressiveness in prostate cancer.

Molecular markers of prostate cancer progression

The role of oncogene expression

Genes controlling cellular proliferation

The progression of normal cells to a fully malignant phenotype involves initiation, promotion and progression. The molecular mechanisms for these events generally involve or are associated with the activation or overexpression of one or more oncogenes. Molecular analysis of both primary and metastatic human prostatic cancer tissues obtained from patients with clinically detected disease has demonstrated that none of the *ras* family of oncogenes (i.e. H, K or N) is commonly mutated [54]. In contrast, Viola *et al.* have reported that enhanced expression of the H-*ras* p21 protein is associated with increasing histological grade (i.e. loss of histological differentiation) in human prostatic cancer [55]. Sumiya *et al.* likewise reported a direct correlation between loss of histological differentiation and *ras* p21 protein expression [56]. These results suggest that enhanced expression, not mutation, of p21 *ras* protein is involved in the progression of prostatic cancer in both human and rat tumours. Thus, overexpression of H-*ras* p21 appears to be not an early event in the initiation of prostatic carcinogenesis but is involved in the progressional stage due to enhancement of genetic instability of the cancer cells.

Genes controlling cellular death

The oncogene *bcl*-2 has been found to be involved in the inhibition of apoptosis or programmed cell death. The role of *bcl*-2 in the development and progression of carcinoma of the prostate has been examined by McDonnell *et al.* [57]. Using immunohistochemical techniques, they found that *bcl*-2 is not usually expressed in androgen-dependent prostatic cancer cells, whereas it was expressed in androgen-independent prostatic cancer cells. These findings suggest that expression of *bcl*-2 protein in carcinomas of the prostate is associated with the transition to androgen independence. The expression of this oncogene may be useful in future adjuvant chemotherapy trials for metastatic prostate cancer.

The role of tumour suppressor genes

Acquisition of metastatic ability by prostatic cancer cells represents the most lethal aspect of prostatic cancer progression. It is now clear that malignant progression involves not only gains in critical transforming functions but also requires the loss of regulatory functions which normally suppress tumor-igenesis and metastasis. The first chromosomal alterations observed to be associated with cancer cells were cytogenetic changes, such as the addition, deletion or translocation of large portions of chromosomes. More recently, it has become possible to identify smaller, submicroscopic chromosomal dele-tions and mutations. The loss of heterozygosity (LOH) of markers on various chromosomes suggests the presence of a tumour suppressor gene at that site. The involvement of such suppressor genes is supported by the correlation of chromosomal deletions with prostatic cancer progression. Specifically, dele-tions on chromosomes 13, 17 and 18 may affect the expression of the known tumour suppressor genes Rb, p53 and DCC respectively, and may alter the expression of tumour suppressor functions [58]. Recently Bova *et al.* reported evidence which strongly indicates the presence of a tumour suppressor gene on chromosome 8, specifically in the region of 8p22 [59]. Using eight poly-morphic markers for 8p they found that 32 of 51 (63%) of the informative tumours showed loss of at least one locus. The most frequently deleted region was observed at chromosome 8p22–8p21.2. This study confirms previous findings of frequent loss of 8p loci in human prostate cancer. Furthermore, it defines the most likely region for tumour suppressor genes on 8p to a 14 cM area around the MSR locus at 8p22. These results demonstrated the highest rates of LOH observed for any chromosome involved with prostate cancer progression, and may therefore represent an early event in prostatic carcino-genesis.

Recent studies support a role for p53 in the suppression of human prostatic cancer progression [60]. Accumulation of mutant p53 has been found in histologically poorly differentiated and metastatic prostatic cancers [61]. Such accumulation was not detected in hormone-dependent lesions. These results support a role for p53 mutation in the progression from hormone-dependent to hormone-independent and metastatic tumours. Immunocytochemical data indicate the prostatic cancer cells expressing the wild-type p53 gene are growth-arrested. These results suggest a functional role for p53 gene in sup-pressing prostatic tumorigenesis.

Alterations in the retinoblastoma (Rb) gene product may also be important in prostate cancer tumorigenesis. Allelic loss of chromosome 13q (i.e. the location of the Rb gene) has been detected in approximately 25% of localized human prostate cancers [62]. In addition, decreased levels of Rb protein have been observed in approximately 50% of surgical specimens obtained from metastatic sites of human prostatic cancers.

The putative tumour suppressor gene DCC, which is located on chromosome 18q, was identified by its frequent deletion in human colorectal cancer. The role of reduced DCC expression and/or LOH in prostatic cancer is presently under investigation. In patient samples, 12 of 14 prostate cancers (86%) showed reduced expression of DCC and 5 of 11 informative cases (45%) showed LOH of the DCC locus [63]. This would indicate that down-regulation of the DCC gene, by either reduced expression or LOH at the DCC locus, is a common feature of prostatic cancer While these data indicate a correlation between LOH of the DCC locus and prostatic cancer, a functional role for DCC in the initiation or progression of prostatic cancer has not yet been identified.

Thus, immunohistocytochemical analysis of human prostate cancer specimens for p53, Rb, DCC and other tumour suppressor genes may aid in predicting the prognosis of men with prostate cancer. However, these genetic changes may occur relatively late in prostatic carcinogenesis. Patients with potentially curable organ-confined prostate cancer may have earlier genetic alterations, not yet identified, that increase the likelihood for further genetic alterations and biological aggressiveness.

The role of metastatic suppressor genes

Currently an intensive effort to identify chromosomal regions and genes involved in metastasis suppression is underway. Initially, these studies consisted of fusing non-metastatic and highly metastatic Dunning rat prostatic cancer cells. The hypothesis was that if the loss or inactivation of metastasis suppressor genes is involved in malignant progression, then the somatic cell hybrids from such a fusion would be non-metastatic since chromosomes from the non-metastatic parental cell would supply the lost suppressor gene functions. From these experiments Ichikawa *et al.* found that the tumorigenicity and *in vivo* growth rates of the hybrid clones, which contained a full complement of parental chromosomes, were not affected at all [64]. In contrast, none of the animals bearing hybrid tumours developed distant metastases. When these non-metastatic primary tumours were passaged *in vivo*, animals occasionally developed distant metastases. Cytogenetic analysis of eight of these metastatic revertants had a consistent loss of a copy of normal rat chromosome 2. This study demonstrates that prostatic cancer metastasis is associated with the loss of specific chromosomes which do not affect the growth rate or tumorigenicity, only metastatic ability. The location of homologous metastasis suppressor genes is currently being mapped [65].

In an attempt to identify other genes involved in the suppression of prostatic cancer metastasis, a panel of cells which contain defined portions of human chromosomes has been constructed. The general construction scheme employs microcell-mediated chromosome transfer specifically to transfer individual human chromosomes to the recipient cells of interest. Using this method, specific human chromosomes have been introduced into highly metastatic rat prostatic cancer and breast cancer cell lines. The effects of human chromosomes on the tumorigenic and metastatic potential of the aforementioned lines are being tested. By comparing the results in each of these systems, both general and specific mediators of metastasis will be identified. Studies using these cells as recipients for human chromosomes have identified metastasis suppressor activities on human chromosomes 8 [66], 11 [67] and 17 [68]. Spontaneous deletion of portions of human chromosome 11 in some of these clones demonstrates that the minimal portion of this chromosome capable of suppressing prostatic cancer metastasis involves a region between 11p11.2 and 13 and does not include the Wilms tumour-1 locus. In contrast, transfer of human chromosome 11 into highly metastatic, oestrogen-independent rat mammary cancer cells has no effect on the tumour growth rate or metastatic ability. This indicates that the metastatic suppressor genes in human chromosome 11p11.2–13 is prostate cancer-specific [69]. Using these methods a gene (KAI-1) has been identified [70]. The KAI-1 gene maps to 11p11.2–p13, is strongly expressed in normal human prostatic tissues and is down-regulated in metastatic human prostate cancer cell lines. The ability of KAI-1 to function as a metastasis suppressor *in vivo* was tested and these studies demonstrated that KAI-1 expression suppressed metastasis to the same extent as the 11p11.2–p13 region.

By studying a combination of these microcell-mediated chromosome transfer hybrid cell panels, it should be possible to construct a molecular map of chromosomes specifically involved in prostatic cancer metastasis, and to use this information for positional cloning of genes involved in this process. These results demonstrate that there are genetic alterations which are uniquely required for the acquisition of metastatic ability of tumorigenic prostatic cancer cells. Furthermore, these findings support a model in which tumorigenicity and metastatic ability are distinct properties of cancer cells requiring both common and unique genetic alternations. Currently it is not known whether the activities encoded by these chromosomes represent separate 'brakes' for metastasis, or if they possibly function in the same biochemical pathways. The identification of these putative prostate cancer metastasis suppressor genes may aid in predicting prognosis and identifying those patients with prostate cancer who may need aggressive treatment or more conservative therapy.

Conclusions

There has been a recent emphasis on early detection and screening of men for prostate cancer. Enhanced screening has already resulted in a significant increase in the number of histologically localized prostate cancers detected each year. This increases the long-standing clinical problem of determining which of these patients should be followed conservatively and which should undergo immediate therapy. If immediate therapy is given, it must be determined which of these patients should be given adjuvant therapy in addition to definitive local treatment. Cellular and molecular markers for malignant progression, especially the transition to metastatic ability, must be identified to allow the development of an accurate substaging method for prostatic cancers so that therapy can be individualized for each patient. Since mass screening could identify 10 million American men with prostate cancer, and the lifetime probability of dying from prostatic cancer is only about 2.9%, only approximately 7% of men with histological prostatic cancer eventually die due to the progression of their disease. This raises the critical issue as to the optimal therapy for the remaining 93% (i.e. approximately 9 300 000) of men with potential diagnosable histological prostatic cancer. The magnitude of this figure illustrates clearly the urgent need for a clear understanding of the cellular and molecular events involved in the progression of prostatic cancer.

References

1 Olsson CA & Goluboff ET. Detection and treatment of prostate cancer: perspective of the urologist. *J Urol* 1994; **152**: 1695–1699.
2 Carter HB, Piantadosi S & Isaacs JT. Clinical evidence for and implications of the multistep development of prostate cancer. *J Urol* 1990; **143**: 742–746.
3 Thompson IM & Chodak GW. The natural history of adenocarcinoma of the prostate. *J Cell Biochem* 1992; **16H**: 20–25.
4 Scardino PT, Weaver R & Hudson MA. Early detection of prostate cancer. *Hum Pathol* 1992; **23**: 211–222.
5 Carter HB & Coffey DS. Prostate cancer: the magnitude of the problem in the United States. In *A Multidisciplinary Analysis of Controversies in the Management of Prostate cancer*, Coffey DS, Resnick MI, Dorr FA, Karr JP, eds. New York: Plenum Press, 1988, pp. 1–9.
6 Johannson JE, Adami HO, Anderson SO, Bergstrom R, Krusemo UB & Kraaz W. Natural history of localized prostatic cancer. *Lancet* 1989; **ii**: 799–803.
7 Walsh PC & Jewett HJ. Radical surgery for prostatic cancer. *Cancer* 1980; **45**: 1906–1911.

* Reference of special interest.
** Reference of outstanding merit.

8 Raghaven D. Non-hormone chemotherapy for prostate cancer: principles of treatment and application to the testing of new drugs. *Semin Oncol* 1988; **15**: 371–389.

9 Crawford ED, Eisenberger MA, McLeod DC *et al*. A controlled trial of leuprolide with and without flutamide in prostatic cancer. *N Engl J Med* 1989; **321**: 419–424.

10 Gleason DF. Classification of prostatic carcinomas. *Cancer Chemother Rep* 1966; **50** 125–128.

11 Gleason DF, Mellinger GT and the Veterans Administrative Cooperative Urological Research Group. Prediction of prognosis for prostatic adenocarcinoma by combined histological grading and clinical staging. *J Urol* 1974; **111**: 58–64.

12 Garnett JE, Oyasu R & Grayhack JT. The accuracy of diagnostic biopsy specimens in predicting tumour grades by Gleason's classification of radical prostatectomy specimens. *J Urol* 1984; **131**: 690–694.

13 Mills SE & Fowler JE. Gleason histologic grading of prostatic carcinoma: correlations between biopsy and prostatectomy specimens. *Cancer* 1986; **57**: 346–349.

*14 Epstein JI & Steinberg GD. The significance of low-grade prostate cancer on needle biopsy. *Cancer* 1990; **66**: 1927–1932.

*15 Epstein JI, Carmichael M, Partin AW & Walsh PC. Small high grade adenocarcinoma of the prostate in radical prostatectomy specimens performed for nonpalpable disease: pathogenetic and clinical implications. *J Urol* 1994; **151**: 1587–1592.

16 Ohori M, Goad JR, Wheeler TM, Eastham JA, Thompson TC & Scardino PT. Can radical prostatectomy alter the progression of poorly differentiated prostate cancer? *J Urol* 1994; **152**: 1843–1849.

17 Partin AW, Lee BR, Carmichael M, Walsh PC & Epstein JI. Radical prostatectomy for high grade disease; a reevaluation 1994. *J Urol* 1994; **151**: 1583–1586.

18 Walsh PC, Partin AW & Epstein JI. Cancer control and quality of life following anatomical retropubic prostatectomy: results at 10 years. *J Urol* 1994; **152**: 1831–1836.

19 Kabalin JN, McNeal JE, Price HM, Freiha FS & Stamey TA. Unsuspected adenocarcinoma of the prostate in patients undergoing cystoprostatectomy for other causes: incidence, histology and morphometric observations. *J Urol* 1989; **141**: 1091–1094.

20 Oesterling JE, Suman VJ, Zincke H & Bostwick DG. PSA-detected (clinical stage Tlc or B0) prostate cancer; pathologically significant tumors. *Urol Clin North Am* 1993; **20**: 687–693.

21 Humphrey PA & Catalona WJ. Clinical and pathological characteristics of non-palpable prostate cancers. *J Urol* 1995 (in press).

22 Epstein JI, Walsh PC, Carmichael M & Brendler CB. Pathologic and clinical findings to predict tumor extent of nonpalpable (stage Tlc) prostate cancer. *JAMA* 1994; **271: 368–374.

23 Rinker-Schaeffer CW, Partin AW, Isaacs WB, Coffey DS & Isaacs JT. Molecular and cellular changes associated with the acquisition of metastatic ability by prostate cancer cells. *Prostate* 1994; **25**: 249–265.

24 Frankfort OS, Chin JL, Englander LS, Greco WR, Pontes JE & Rustum YM. Relationship between DNA ploidy, glandular differentiation, and tumor spread in human prostate cancer. *Cancer Res* 1985; **45**: 1418–1423.

25 McIntire TL, Murphy WM, Coon JS *et al*. The prognostic value of DNA ploidy combined with histologic substaging for incidental carcinoma of the prostate gland. *Am J Clin Pathol* 1988; **89**: 370–373.

26 Miller GJ. Prostate cancer: DNA ploidy, volume and other prognostic factors. In:

Comprehensive Textbook of Genitourinary Oncology, Vogelzang NJ, Scardino PT, Shipley WV & Coffey DS, eds. Baltimore, MD: Williams & Wilkins, 1995 (in press).

27 Winkler HZ, Rainwater LM, Myers RP *et al*. Stage D1 prostatic adenocarcinoma: significance of nuclear DNA ploidy patterns studied by flow cytometry. *Mayo Clin Proc* 1988; **63**: 103–112.

28 Nativ O, Winkler HZ, Raz Y *et al*. Stage C prostatic adenocarcinoma: flow cytometric nuclear DNA ploidy analysis. *Mayo Clin Proc* 1989; **64**: 911–919.

29 Montgomery BT, Nativ O, Blute ML *et al*. Stage B prostatic adenocarcinoma: flow cytometric nuclear DNA ploidy analysis. *Arch Surg* 1990; **125**: 327–331.

30 Adolfsson J, Ronstrom L, Hedlund P-O, Lowhagen T, Cartensen J & Tribukait B. The prognostic value of modal deoxyribonucleic acid in low grade, low stage untreated prostatic cancer. *J Urol* 1990; **144**: 1404–1407.

31 Adolfsson J & Tribukait B. Evaluation of tumor progression by repeated fine needle biopsies in prostatic adenocarcinoma: modal deoxyribonucleic acid value and cytological differentiation. *J Urol* 1990; **144**: 1408–1410.

*32 Carmichael MJ, Veltri RW, Partin AW, Miller MC, Walsh PC & Epstein JI. Deoxyribonucleic acid ploidy analysis as a predictor of recurrence following radical prostatectomy for stage T2 disease. *J Urol* 1995; **153**: 1015–1019.

33 Brothman AR, Peehl, DM, Patel AM & McNeal JE. Frequency and pattern of karyotype abnormalities in human prostate cancer. *Cancer Res* 1990; **50**: 3795–3803.

34 Atkin NB & Baker MC. Chromosome study of five cancers of the prostate. *Hum Genet* 1985; **70**: 359–364.

35 Diamond DA, Berry SJ, Umbricht C, Jewett HJ & Coffey DS. Computerized image analysis of nuclear shape as a prognostic factor for prostatic cancer. *Prostate* 1982; **3**: 321–332.

36 Diamond DA, Berry SJ, Jewett HJ, Eggleston JC & Coffey DS. A new method to assess metastatic potential of human prostate cancer: relative nuclear roundness. *J Urol* 1982; **128**: 729–734.

37 Paulson DF, Stone AR, Walther PJ, Tucker JA & Cox EB. Radical prostatectomy: anatomical predictors of success or failure. *J Urol* 1986; **136**: 1041–1046.

38 Clark TD, Askin FB & Bagnell CF. Nuclear roundness factor: a quantitative approach to grading in prostatic carcinoma, reliability of needle biopsy tissue, and the effect of tumor stage on usefulness. *Prostate* 1987; **10**: 199–206.

39 Mohler JL, Partin AW, Isaacs WI & Coffey DS. Time lapse videomicroscopic identification of Dunning R3327 adenocarcinoma and normal rat prostate cells. *J Urol* 1987; **137**: 544–547.

40 Miller GJ & Shikes JL. Nuclear roundness as a predictor of response to hormonal therapy of patients with stage D2 prostatic carcinoma. In: *Prognostic Cytometry and Cytopathology of Prostate Cancer*, Karr JP, Coffey DS & Gardner W, eds. New York: Elsevier Science, 1988, pp. 349–354.

41 Partin AW, Walsh AC, Pitcock RV, Mohler JL, Epstein JI & Coffey DS. A comparison of nuclear morphometry and Gleason grade as a predictor of prognosis in stage A2 prostate cancer: a critical analysis. *J Urol* 1989; **142**: 1254–1258.

42 Partin AW, Steinberg GD, Pitcock RV *et al*. Use of nuclear morphometry. Gleason histologic scoring, clinical stage and age to predict disease free survival among patients with prostate cancer. *Cancer* 1991; **70**: 161–168.

43 Fey EG & Penman S. Nuclear matrix proteins reflect cell type of origin in cultured human cells. *Proc Natl Acad Sci USA* 1988; **85**: 121–125.

44 Getzenberg RH, Pienta KJ, Huang YW & Coffey DS. Identification of nuclear matrix proteins in the cancer and normal rate prostate. *Cancer Res* 1991; **51**: 6514–6520.

*45 Partin AW, Getzenberg RH, Carmichael MJ *et al*. Nuclear matrix proteins in benign prostate hyperplasia and prostate cancer. *Cancer Res* 1993; **53**: 744–746.

46 Mohler JL, Partin AW, Isaacs WI & Coffey DS. Time lapse videomicroscopic identification of Dunning R3327 adenocarcinoma and normal rat prostate cells. *J Urol* 1987; **137**: 544–547.

47 Liotta LA, Steeg PS & Stetler-Stevenson WG. Cancer angiogenesis and metastasis: an imbalance of positive and negative regulation. *Cell* 1991; **64**: 327–336.

48 Stearns ME & Wang M. Type IV collagenase (Mr 72 000) expression in human prostate: benign and malignant tissue. *Cancer Res* 1993; **53**: 878–883.

49 Pajouh NS, Nagle RB, Breatnnack R, Finch JS, Brawer MK & Bowden GT. Expression of metalloproteinase genes in human prostate cancer. *J Cancer Res Clin Oncol* 1991; **117**: 144–150.

*50 Frixen UH, Behrens J, Sachs M *et al*. E-cadherin-mediated cell–cell adhesion prevents invasiveness of human carcinoma cells. *J Cell Biol* 1991; **112**: 173–185.

*51 Umbas R, Schalken JA, Aalders TW *et al*. Expression of the cellular adhesion molecule E-cadherin is reduced or absent in high-grade prostatic cancer. *Cancer Res* 1992; **52**: 5104–5109.

52 Bigler SA, Brawer MK & Deering RE. Neovascularization in carcinoma of the prostate: a quantitative morphometric study. *Modern Pathol* 1990; **5**: 50a.

53 Weidner N, Carroll PR, Flas J, Blumenfeld W & Folkman J. Tumor angiogenesis correlates with metastasis in invasive prostate cancer. *Am J Pathol* 1993; **143**: 401–409.

*54 Carter BS, Epstein JI & Isaacs WB. *ras* gene mutations in human prostate cancer. *Cancer Res* 1990; **50** 6830–6832.

55 Viola M, Fromowitz F, Oravez *et al*. Expression of *ras* oncogene p21 in prostate cancer. *N Engl J Med* 1986; **314**: 133–137.

56 Sumiya H, Masai M, Akimoto S, Yatani R & Schimazi J. Histochemical examination of the expression of *ras* p21 protein and R-1881-binding protein in human prostatic cancers. *Eur J Cancer* 1990; **26**: 786–789.

57 McDonnell TJ, Troncoso P, Brisbay SM *et al*. Expression of protooncogene *bcl-2* in the prostate and its association with emergence of androgen-independent prostate cancer. *Cancer Res* 1992; **52**: 6940–6944.

*58 Isaacs WB & Carter BS. Genetic changes associated with prostate cancer in humans. *Cancer Surv* 1991; **11**: 15–24.

59 Bova GS, Carter BS, Bussemakers MJG *et al*. Homozygous deletion and frequent loss of chromosome 8p22 loci in human prostate cancer. *Cancer Res* 1993; **53: 3869–3873.

60 Isaacs WB, Carter BS & Ewing CM. Wild-type p53 suppresses growth of human prostatic cancer cells containing mutant p53 alleles. *Cancer Res* 1991; **51**: 4716–4720.

61 Navone N, Troncoso P, Pisters LL, Palmer JL, von Eshenbach AC & Conte CJ. P53 protein accumulation in the progression of human prostate carcinoma. *SBUR abstracts*, 1993.

62 Carter BS, Ewing CM, Ward WS *et al*. Allelic loss of chromosomes 16q and 10q in human prostate cancer. *Proc Natl Acad Sci* 1990; **87**: 8751–8755.

63 Gao X, Honn KV, Grignon D, Sakr W & Chen YQ. Frequent loss of expression and loss of heterozygosity of the putative tumor suppressor gene DCC in prostatic carcinomas. *Cancer Res* 1993; **53**: 2723–2727.

*64 Ichikawa T, Ichikawa Y & Isaacs JT. Genetic factors and suppression of metastatic ability of prostatic cancer. *Cancer Res* 1991; **51**: 3788–3792.

65 Smith RC & Rinker-Schaeffer CW. Molecular genetics and cell biology of genitourinary cancers. In: *Comprehensive Textbook of Genitourinary Oncology*, Vogelzang NJ, Scardino PT, Shipey WV & Coffey DS, eds. Baltimore, M D: Williams & Wilkins, 1995, (in press).

66 Ichikawa T, Nihei N, Suzuki H *et al*. Suppression of metastasis rat prostatic cancer by introducing human chromosome 8. *Cancer Res* 1994; **54**: 2299–2302.

67 Ichikawa T, Ichikawa Y, Dong JT *et al*. Localization of metastasis suppressor gene(s) for prostatic cancer to the short arm of chromosome 11. *Cancer Res* 1992; **52**: 3486–3490.

68 Rinker-Schaeffer CW, Hawkins AL, Ru N *et al*. Differential suppression of mammary and prostate cancer metastasis by human chromosomes 17 and 11. *Cancer Res* 1994; **54**: 6249–6256

69 Ichikawa T, Ichikawa Y, Dong JT *et al*. Localization of metastasis suppressor gene(s) for prostatic cancer to the short arm of chromosome 11. *Cancer Res* 1992; **52**: 3486–3490.

70 Dong JT, Lamb PW, Rinker-Schaeffer CW *et al*. *KAI 1*, a metastasis suppressor gene for prostate cancer on human chromosome IIp II.2. *Science* 1995; **268: 884–886.

12/When should Pelvic Lymphadenectomy Precede Treatment?

W.G. Bowsher

Introduction

During the past decade there has been a rekindling of interest in pelvic lymphadenectomy for prostate cancer. It is easy to attribute this to the development of laparoscopic techniques but the interest has also been stimulated by a more aggressive attitude towards the treatment of local disease in selected patients. With the rapid development of laparoscopic surgery, better understanding of prostate-specific antigen (PSA) and new imaging techniques, the precise indications for lymphadenectomy can seem unclear. At a recent round-table discussion at the Société Internationale d'Urologie, it was concluded that the role of lymph node dissection and prostatectomy is basically staging. There was no claim on the part of the report that therapeutic benefit resulted from lymphadenectomy. The decreasing incidence of positive nodes in association with total prostatectomy was noted. It was felt that this probably related to better case election before surgery and a better understanding of the impact of high-grade tumours [1]. It is apparent that this method of staging should be regularly compared with the alternatives. Currently, the technique does have a role.

Open surgery

A lower midline or Pfannenstiel incision is made. Through an extraperitoneal approach, the nodes in the obturator triangle can be palpated and dissected out. This triangle is defined between the medial edge of the external iliac vein, the obturator nerve and the pelvic side wall. Lymphatics are sealed during the dissection by the judicious use of pen-and-scissor diathermy along with the application of clips. One of the best descriptions of the technique was by Peters [2] (see also Chapter 13).

Laparoscopic surgery

There has been increasing interest recently in laparoscopic surgery. The technique of laparoscopic lymphadenectomy is relatively new and worthy of elaboration. Patients can be admitted as day-cases or for an overnight stay. Informed consent is obtained for both laparoscopic pelvic node dissection and laparotomy. Blood is grouped and saved. Antithrombotic stockings are prescribed.

Under general anaesthesia, place the patient in the lithotomy position on Lloyd Davies stirrups with each arm beside the trunk. Hyperextend the pelvis by placing a rolled blanket under the buttocks with 10° of Trendelenburg tilt. Prepare the abdomen and drape to allow access to both iliac fossae. The surgeon stands on the side undergoing surgery, with a camera operator opposite and the assistant between the patient's legs. A 14 F urethral catheter is placed in the bladder and left on free drainage. A Veress needle is inserted through a subumbilical incision and a pneumoperitoneum produced and maintained at 14 mmHg. An 11 mm trocar is inserted through this incision and the telescope is inserted into the peritoneal cavity to visualize the crucial landmarks on the television monitors. Where necessary, the Trendelenburg tilt is increased to displace the bowel from the pelvis.

Place two 10 mm ports in the right iliac fossa under camera vision and use with 5 mm adaptors as working channels. Blunt grasping forceps are used to pick up the peritoneum midway between the medial umbilical ligament and the pulsation of the external iliac artery. A peritoneal incision is then made between these two structures using hook diathermy and the peritoneal window extended using blunt dissection with two pairs of grasping forceps. The vas deferens is identified at the base of the wound, lifted with the hook diathermy, coagulated and divided. The medial aspect of the external iliac vein is then exposed by teasing the adjacent fat with two pairs of blunt grasping forceps. Lymph nodes in the area between the medial aspect of the external iliac vein, the pelvic side wall and over the obturator nerve are then cleared using blunt grasping forceps, hook diathermy and diathermy scissors. These are withdrawn piecemeal through the most convenient 10 mm port after removing the 5 mm adaptor or, when necessary, the endoscope is moved to one of the 10 mm ports and the nodes extracted through the 11 mm port in 11 mm cup forceps. Bleeding small vessels are secured using either coagulating diathermy or clips after they are clearly seen with the help of a suction irrigation device (irrigating with 1000 units heparin/litre of Hartmann's solution). The 10 mm ports are then removed and the associated wounds closed with nylon. The procedure is then repeated on the left, retracing the sigmoid colon, where necessary, in blunt grasping forceps. At the end of each operation, haemostasis is carefully checked using irrigation and aspiration of the operative fields. After desufflation of the abdomen, the wounds are closed with nylon. All nodes are sent for paraffin section.

When nodes appear to be infiltrated by carcinoma, an individual node biopsy is performed: a node is dissected free using blunt dissection with grasping forceps and sharp dissection with diathermy scissors, removed in 11 mm cup forceps through the 11 mm port and sent for frozen section. When this proves positive, the dissection goes no further.

If persistent bleeding cannot be controlled during the operation, a laparotomy has to be carried out, haemostasis obtained and the procedure completed by open operation. With experience, the operating time compares favourably with the open operation.

Advantages of pelvic lymphadenectomy

Lymph node dissection is the most accurate method available for assessing pelvic lymph node involvement with carcinoma of the prostate. Both computed tomography (CT) and magnetic resonance imaging (MRI) are unlikely to detect tumour in normal-sized nodes [3]. Pedal lymphography is less accurate than node dissection [4] and prostatic lymphoscintigraphy lacks the precision and clarity required for disease staging [5].

It is obviously appropriate to include a staging lymphadenectomy when the decision has already been made to proceed to radical retropubic prostatectomy. Knowledge of such nodal disease may be sufficient evidence to institute early hormonal therapy [6, 7].

In PT3 tumours with established capsular penetration, one-third have positive nodes. It appears that with a small focus of capsular penetration, PT3 tumours have a difference in outcome depending on nodal status [1]. Careful histological examination of pelvic lymph nodes may avoid inappropriate local therapy for carcinoma of the prostate [8]. Therefore, lymphadenectomy may be appropriate as a staging prognostic tool in such patients with focal capsular penetration. There is evidence that once this disease has spread to pelvic nodes, distant metastases can be expected within 2–3 years [9].

In the past, pelvic node dissection for carcinoma of the prostate has been criticized owing to the risk of lymphocoele, suprapubic and genital oedema as well as thromboembolic disease. The technique for laparoscopic node dissection described in this review includes some modifications that are important in this respect. The incidence of lymphoedema is greatly reduced by leaving the deep inguinal nodes and those along the lateral border of the external iliac artery, and the risk of venous thrombosis is reduced by avoiding manipulation of the pelvic veins [10]. Furthermore, the incidence of lymphocoele is likely to be reduced by a transperitoneal approach.

The use of laparoscopic pelvic lymph node dissection has several implications. The surgical assault on the patient is lessened, resulting in a comfortable and speedy return to normal activity. The operation is possible without making great demands on hospital bed occupancy. As a result, node dissection is more appealing as an investigation and staging procedure. If nodal status is known, a fairer comparison of treatments is possible: for example, a more accurate audit of the results of radical prostatectomy versus radiotherapy for localized carcinoma of the prostate. Some enthusiasts argue that laparoscopic pelvic lymph node dissection followed by perineal prostatectomy could be less morbid in some hands than retropubic lymph node dissection plus prostatectomy at the same time. Whether this will be proven to be true is as yet unknown.

Disadvantages of pelvic lymphadenectomy

There is a risk of overutilizing the technique if insufficient notice is taken of imaging and PSA results. With increased experience of this surgery and appropriate preoperative imaging, the diagnosis of positive nodes may be very rare. In a recently published series of 409 patients subjected to pelvic lymph node dissection at the time of radical prostatectomy, only 15 (3.7%) had positive nodes [11]. This raises questions about the routine use of frozen section of nodes during this procedure.

There is a major controversy concerning laparoscopic ablative procedures for potentially curable cancers in view of the potential but unproved risk of tumour dissemination and inadequate resection. An enhanced risk of dissemination and seedling implantation may reflect only a theoretical concern since there is no hard evidence for increased dissemination of tumours by laparoscopy but this potential phenomenon cannot be ignored and it merits detailed investigation by clinical and experimental studies. There is a very long list of possible factors which may enhance the spread of cancer during laparoscopic surgery: the hormonal effects of a positive-pressure pneumoperitoneum, the increased handling and exfoliation of malignant cells, the dissemination of exfoliated cells by carbon dioxide convection, reduced portal perfusion and possible oppression of the hepatic reticuloepithelial function, the vasodilatory effect of carbon dioxide, the enhanced growth and implantation of exfoliated tumour cells by the carbon dioxide–air mix, the production of toxic compounds by smoke generated by high-frequency electrosurgery in a closed environment and, finally, the creation of multiple raw wounds with a fibrin seal which may produce immunoprotection for exfoliated implanted cells [12].

Summary of indications for pelvic lymphadenectomy

1 If a patient is taken to the operating theatre for radical retropubic prostatectomy.

2 If radical prostatectomy or radiotherapy is being considered but preliminary staging investigations are equivocal.

3 Prior to radical perineal prostatectomy, a laparoscopic lymphadenectomy should be considered.

The future

It is likely that, during the next decade, prostate cancer will be diagnosed with increased frequency. This will be a reflection of the possible increased incidence of the disease as well as more sophisticated methods of diagnosis. Furthermore, there may also be an association with increased audit and research of the role of screening for prostate cancer [13]. Until urological surgeons have access to more sophisticated tumour markers, there will still be areas of doubt about the precise staging of the disease in particular patients and lymph node dissection, either open or laparoscopic, will retain a role in important clinical decision-making.

References

1 Donoghue JP. The role of lymph node dissection in urologic cancer surgery: summary of discussion and conclusions. *SIU Newlett* April 1995, p. 23.

2 Peters J. Open pelvic lymph node dissection. In *Technical Aspects of Prostate Cancer Treatment: The Present and the Future.* Oxford: Clinical Communications, 1994, pp. 6, 7.

* 3 Chadwick DJ, Cobby M, Goddard P *et al.* Comparison of transrectal ultrasound and magnetic resonance imaging in the staging of prostate cancer. *Br J Urol* 1991; **67**: 616–621.

4 O'Donoghue EPN, Shridar P, Sherwood T *et al.* Lymphography and pelvic lymphadenectomy in carcinoma of the prostate, 1976; **48**: 689–696.

5 Stone AR, Merrick MV & Chisholm CD. Prostatic lymphoscintigraphy. *Br J Urol* 1979; **51**: 556–560.

6 Pollen JJ. Endocrine treatment for prostatic cancer. *Urology* 1983; **21**: 555–558.

** 7 van Aubel OGJM, Hoekstra WJ & Schroder FH. Early orchidectomy for patients with stage D1 prostatic carcinoma. *J Urol* 1985; **134**: 292.

** 8 McDowell GC, Johnson JW, Tenney D *et al.* Pelvic lymphadenectomy for staging clinically localized prostate cancer. *Urology* 1990; **35**: 476–482.

9 Catalona WJ & Kelly DR. Accuracy of frozen section detection of lymph node metastases in prostatic carcinoma. *J Urol* 1983; **127**: 460.

* Reference of special interest.
** Reference of outstanding merit.

*10 Lytton B. Early prostatic cancer. In *The Prostate*, Blandy JP & Lyddon B, eds. London: Butterworth, 1986, p. 166.

11 Levran Z, Gonzalez JA, Diokno SZH *et al*. Are pelvic computed tomography, bone scanning and pelvic lymphadenectomy necessary in the staging of prostatic cancer? *Br J Urol* 1995; **75** 778–781.

12 Cuschieri A. Laparoscopic management of cancer patients. *J R Coll Surg Edin* 1995; **40**: 1–9.

13 Hall R. Radical prostatectomy and prostate cancer screening. The need for national audit and research. *Ann R Coll Surg Engl* 1994; **76**: 367–372.

13/Keeping Out of Trouble with Radical Prostatectomy

J. Peters

Introduction

Radical prostatectomy has been described for over 80 years but did not gain popularity to any large extent until around 15 years ago.

Walsh and Donker [1] first described the anatomy of the neurovascular bundles as they course beside the prostate and urethra.

Having addressed one of the major causes of impotence following radical prostatectomy, the procedure had a resurgence of interest. Since then, further definition of the pelvic anatomy and, in particular, the musculature of the urethra and periurethral tissues have been more widely understood [2].

The key to the operation is now an improved understanding of the tissue planes, the anatomy of the dorsal venous complex and the position of the neurovascular bundles.

Patients now accept radical prostatectomy more readily as with modern techniques there is a chance of potency postoperatively from the procedure with much less morbidity as well as an opportunity of cure from prostate cancer.

Further modifications of the technique to decrease the changes of bladder-neck contracture have been put forward by Walsh with his mucosal eversion at the bladder neck [3]. All these factors have made radical retropubic prostatectomy much less threatening to the surgeon. It has also led to a much lower incidence of impotence and incontinence. For a superb description of the operation and its anatomy, I do not believe one can go past Walsh's description of radical retropubic prostatectomy in the current edition of *Campbell's Urology* [3]. This chapter looks at how one stays out of trouble during the procedure or gets out of difficulty if problems arise.

Preoperative preparation

Part of the reason why radical prostatectomy has gained a poor reputation is the high incidence of positive surgical margins, seminal vesical involvement of capsular penetration in the pathology specimens as a result of understaging preoperatively.

Accur..te preoperative staging of the disease is critical and if there is any hint that the tumour is close to seminal vesicles or to the capsule, it would be wise to regard the disease as extraprostatic and consider radiotherapy rather than surgery.

If the patient has had a previous transurethral resection of the prostate, the operation is generally delayed for approximately 8 weeks. In those patients who have had a transrectal ultrasound-guided needle biopsy of the prostate there may be periprostatic induration and fibrosis and those patients are easier to operate on after a delay of a few weeks.

All my patients for radical prostatectomy have 3 units of autologous blood donation and are under 70 years of age. They are admitted to hospital 24–36 h preoperatively and are given 2 litres of Go-litely® bowel preparation. The positioning of the patient on the operating table is very important and I use the supine position with a rolled towel directly under the buttocks. This elevates the pelvis and makes operative access to the depths of the pelvis much easier. It is important that the towel is not placed underneath the lumbar spine, as this does not help elevation and thus exposure within the pelvis.

Epidural anaesthesia is used for the procedure and is continued for 2–3 days postoperatively to give the patient adequate pain relief and allow for early mobilization.

Surgical technique

A lower midline incision is used from the symphysis pubis to 2 cm above the umbilicus. The linea alba is incised and the retropubic space entered. The transversalis fascia is separated bluntly from the undersurface of the rectus muscle. It is important to avoid bleeding from the inferior epigastric vessels. The transversalis fascia can also be sharply incised vertically just left of the midline at the level of the umbilicus and continuing superiorly. This will release more of the transversalis fascia, allowing it to fall posteriorly and thus allow more room to operate in the pelvis.

Pelvic lymphadenectomy

A modified pelvic lymphadenectomy is performed. It is important to realize that the lymphatic tissue is surrounded by a fascial envelope. This fascial envelope runs from the external iliac vein to just above the obturator nerve and vessels.

The first manoeuvre in lymphadenectomy is to get into the plane over the midpoint of the external iliac vein and with a sucker to dissect directly underneath the vein to the musculature of the lateral wall of the pelvis. Use a right-angle directly above the obturator nerve and vessels so that the lymph node package is free in its mid-extent. This then leaves a tube of lymph node tissue which is attached inferiorly, where it can be clipped and divided. I do not divide the aberrant obturator vessels as these may be important in the maintenance of potency postoperatively. This then leaves the lymph node package attached at its superior extent. With a sucker, the dissection can be carried superiorly and it is worth noting that the lymph node package itself divides around the obturator nerve. There is thus a medial and lateral attachment that can be separately clipped and divided. It is not necessary to divide the vas. If one carefully dissects out the lymph node package in its fascia, bleeding is seldom a problem and the specimen can be removed as one. All grossly abnormal lymph nodes outside this area should also be sent for frozen section. Once the frozen section has been returned negative for malignancy, the prostatectomy itself can proceed.

The endopelvic fascia and mobilization of prostate

The visceral and parietal layers of the endopelvic fascia join just lateral to the prostate. One should carefully use a sucker to remove any of the flimsy fat overlying this layer and identify the point of incision in it. This should be just lateral to the prostate and I find it best to use a scalpel to open the fascia only and no deeper. An incision too medial will result in bleeding from the veins over the capsule of the prostate and thus obscure vision. An incision too lateral will get into the fibres of the levator ani. In the correct plane, it will be very easy to place a finger through the hole in the endopelvic fascia and fully mobilize down to the apex of the prostate (Fig. 13.1). It is not recommended to use scissors for this manoeuvre as they may pierce more deeply than a scalpel and result in inadvertent and unnecessary bleeding from the lateral venous plexus of the prostate. Once this manoeuvre has been performed, one can then turn attention to the dorsal venous complex.

Division of puboprostatic and dorsal venous complex

This is generally where the operation is somewhat threatening. After incision of the endopelvic fascia, there is a wide band of tissue over the distal surface of the prostate and the puboprostatic ligaments. With the use of a sucker and forceps, the fat both medial and lateral to the puboprostatic ligaments can be gently teased out. The superficial dorsal vein is tied with 0 chromic and divided. This then generally exposes the puboprostatic ligaments but there is also a

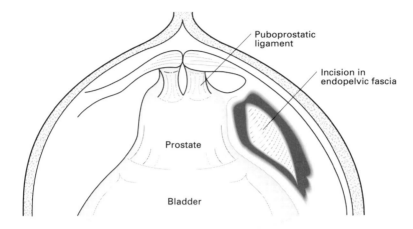

Fig. 13.1 Incision in the endopelvic fascia allowing blunt finger dissection down beside the prostate.

fibrous band of tissue lateral to these. This is the anterior extent of the pelvic fascia and usually contains vessels which run from the lateral surface of the prostate to the levator ani. These have been referred to as the lateral veins of Kelly [4]. There is generally a little triangle of tissue between this condensation of fascia and the puboprostatic ligament on each side (Fig. 13.2). Using a

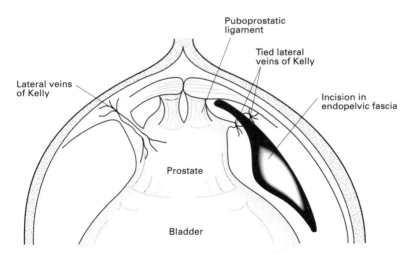

Fig. 13.2 The lateral veins of Kelly and accompanying overlying fascia can be divided and ligated to narrow the dorsal vein complex.

right-angle forceps, dissection between these two structures is completed and the lateral veins of Kelly can be divided and ligated with an 0 chromic tie. Once this is done on both sides the dorsal venous complex will become more readily apparent and will in fact be narrower than initially thought and thus easier to manage.

The puboprostatic ligaments are divided with a scalpel at their junction with the symphysis pubis but every care should be taken not to cut too deeply. Scratch the surface of the puboprostatics and once it is apparent that most of the division has been done, use a finger to depress and thus break the more deeply placed fibres. This protects the dorsal venous complex below this, as any dissection with scissors or any deeper dissection with a knife can result in bleeding which can be difficult to control. Having divided the puboprostatics one can then use the index finger on both hands to identify the urethra with its 20 French Foley catheter *in situ*. The dorsal venous complex is then felt to be quite narrow but is about 2–3 cm deep (Fig. 13.3). With blunt dissection using the index finger of both hands, the plane between the dorsal venous complex

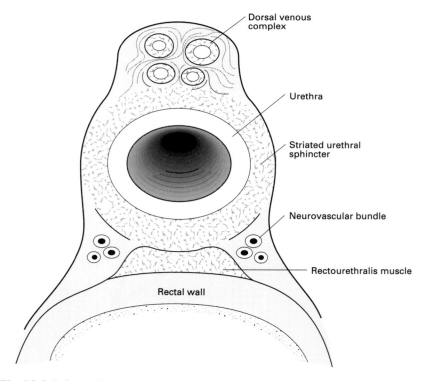

Fig. 13.3 Relationship of urethra to surrounding structures. The dorsal vein complex is quite deep.

and the anterior surface of the urethra can be felt. A right-angled forceps is passed to pick up a ligature of chromic catgut with which to tie the dorsal venous complex. It is important to ensure that this is on the anterior surface of the urethra, otherwise troublesome bleeding may occur (Fig. 13.4). At this point, pass a right-angled forceps just above this tie and divide the dorsal venous complex with scissors or diathermy. It is very important at this stage not to get into the anterior surface of the prostate. Once the complex has been divided, there may be some back-bleeding from the surface of the prostate, which is quite easy to deal with.

Sometimes the tie on the dorsal venous complex slips off, in which case the venous bleeding can be easily controlled with a 2–0 chromic suture on a Thompson–Walker (Bozeman) needle holder (Fig. 13.5). This needle holder is invaluable as it gives excellent access to the pelvis and is far superior to straight needle holders because its angled shaft eliminates the difficulty of placing a needle underneath the symphysis pubis. When underrunning the

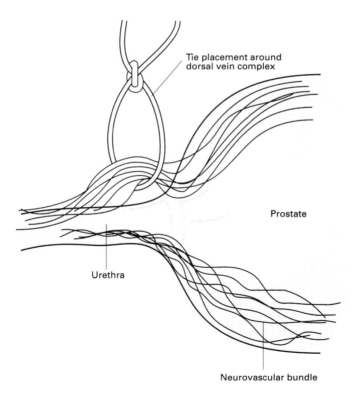

Tie placement around
dorsal vein complex

Prostate

Urethra

Neurovascular bundle

Fig. 13.4 The tie placement should be deep enough so as to tie off all of the dorsal vein complex. Stay far enough away from the capsule of the prostate.

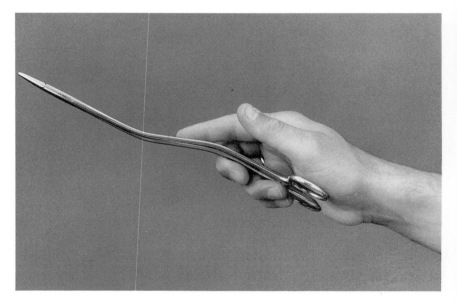

Fig. 13.5 The Thompson–Walker (or Bozemann) needle holder allows easy access to the pelvic floor for suture placement.

dorsal venous complex with a 2–0 chromic, it is important to start on one side, tie the suture and then run it horizontally across to the other side. Do not attempt to bunch the whole of the complex with a single suture as this invariably leads to tearing and more bleeding. The prostatourethral junction should now be well seen and visualization should be excellent.

Urethral division

You are now looking at the prostatourethral junction, which can be clearly seen. Just laterally and posteriorly are the neurovascular bundles. Use a right-angle forceps to enter the plane directly behind the urethra so as to separate this from the neurovascular bundles laterally and the posterior aspect of the striated urethral sphincter and rectourethralis posteriorly (Fig. 13.6). The next step is to incise the anterior aspect of the prostatourethral junction with scissors and identify the urethral catheter. Here place a 2–0 chromic suture on the anterior surface of the urethra and take a little piece of the dorsal venous complex and striated urethral sphincter anterior to it (Fig. 13.7). This is used for later identification of the urethral margin and as the anterior suture in the urethrovesical anastomosis. The suture is brought out through the wound and

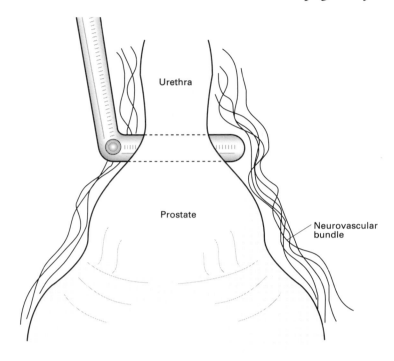

Fig. 13.6 Placement of right-angled clamp behind the urethra to separate the neurovascular bundles from the line of urethral transection.

clipped. The urethral catheter is then pulled out through this opening, clamped, divided and used for traction.

This exposes the posterior aspect of the urethra, with striated external sphincter together with Denonvilliers fascia and rectourethralis below it. A right-angled forceps is passed behind the urethra, which is divided. This then leaves tissue of the striated external sphincter, rectourethralis and Denonvilliers fascia under which a right-angled forceps is placed. This tissue is then sharply divided so that the plane between Denonvilliers fascia and the rectum is exposed. This manoeuvre can be quite difficult after a needle biopsy and it is here that one must be very careful not to enter the rectum. If you are in the correct plane, you will be able to place a finger between the rectum and the Denonvilliers fascia and dissect bluntly and very easily up the posterior surface of the prostate.

If this dissection is difficult then you are not in the correct plane and will usually be working too superficially. Blunt finger dissection is preferable to

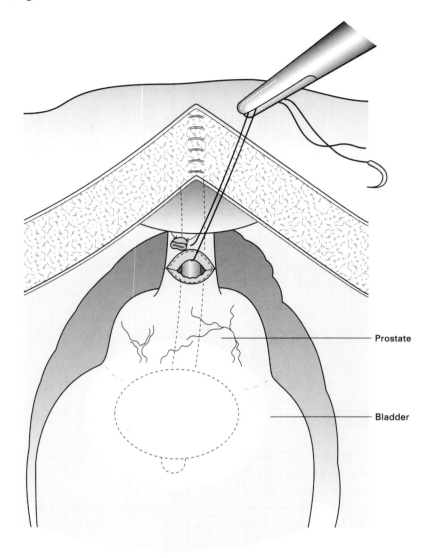

Fig. 13.7 The anterior aspect of the urethra is opened. The catheter is seen and a urethral marker suture of 2–0 chromic placed at 12 o'clock.

perform this manoeuvre rather than sharp dissection although Walsh points out that it may lead to traction on the neurovascular bundle and thus injure the nerves. It should then be possible to feel up to the superior border of the prostate and laterally the lateral pedicles of the prostate, beneath which the neurovascular bundle should be apparent. The lateral pelvic fascia is a flimsy band laterally which can be divided sharply and then the lateral pedicles of the prostate can be clipped or tied above the neurovascular bundle on each side. Care must be taken not to produce a traction injury on the neurovascular bundle when doing this. Mobilization of the prostate and division of its lateral pedicles can then be continued up superiorly. Close to the bladder neck these pedicles can be thick and it is probably better to divide these so that the lateral border of the seminal vesicle is easily identified on each side. The neurovascular bundle runs very close to the seminal vesicle on each side, particularly on its superior aspect. Care is therefore essential when tying and dividing the pedicles in this area.

At this stage of the operation, the prostate is free inferiorly and the seminal vesicles and ampulla of the vas can be attended to (Fig. 13.8). It is easiest to do this from below, before division of the bladder neck. To identify the seminal vesicles and ampulla of the vas on each side, it is necessary to incise back through Denonvilliers fascia. It is very easy to identify the vesicles on each side

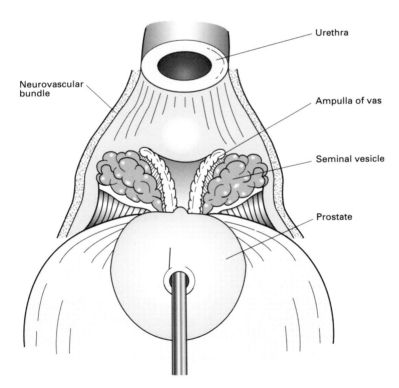

Fig. 13.8 The prostate has been fully mobilized, showing the ampulla of the vas and seminal vesicle on each side.

but the ampullae of the vas tend to be deeper in the dissection, i.e. slightly ventral to the plane of the vesicles. Use scissors to dissect the midline to identify one ampulla of vas. It is easier to use a right-angled forceps and bisect the ampulla free of the vesicle so it can then be clamped, divided and ligated with 0 chromic. The other ampulla can then be located, clamped, divided and ligated similarly. With further dissection, the correct plane behind the seminal vesicles can be entered but it is important not to get too far away from the surface of the vesicle itself, as this will make dissection quite difficult. For this, use scissors to get right on to the plane of the vesicle and then grasp it with a Babcock clamp. Using a sucker, the vesicle can be mobilized in its entirety.

The ampulla of the vas generally has a dense fascial connection to the seminal vesicle and if this is divided sharply the vesicle will free up quite easily. This leaves the base of the seminal vesicle, which can be clamped, ligated with an 0 chromic and divided. Once both vesicles and vasal ampullae have been mobilized and divided, you can turn your attention to the bladder neck.

Division of bladder neck

I use a diathermy to divide the junction of prostate and bladder anteriorly. It is important to make certain that the line of incision is away from the prostate and not cutting into it at this point. Once the balloon on the catheter has been seen, it can be removed, the balloon deflated, a clamp placed and the catheter used as a traction device. A gauze swab is placed in the bladder and a small Deaver retractor in the bladder neck enables both ureteric orifices to be identified. If the anaesthetist has been giving the patient plenty of fluids, there will be a good efflux of urine from each orifice, which will be clearly seen to lie well away from the bladder neck. With a combination of diathermy and ties, it is possible to continue around the bladder neck and stay well away from the ureteric orifices. This will generally leave some more of the lateral pedicles on each side which can either be divided with cautery or tied with 0 chromic catgut. When dividing the posterior aspect of the bladder neck, use a diathermy to mucosa and then place dissecting scissors in the midline and punch through posteriorly so only lateral tissue remains to be divided. This clarifies identification of the lateral pedicles so that ligation of the remaining tissue is much easier, especially if the vasa and seminal vesicles have been previously divided from behind.

Once the prostate has been removed use the index and middle finger of the right hand to mobilize bluntly under the bladder neck (Fig. 13.9). This gives more mobility to the bladder base and makes it easier for the bladder to come down and sit in the pelvis with little, if any, tension during the anastomosis.

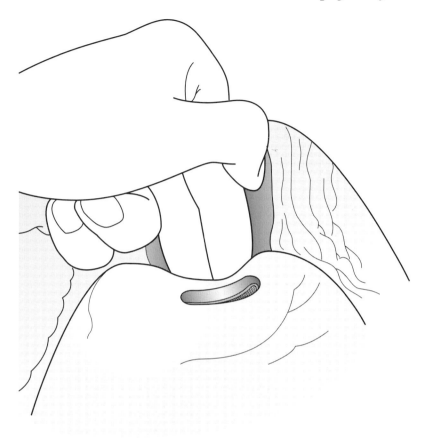

Fig. 13.9 Gentle finger dissection posteriorly allows for greater mobility of the bladder base and less tension of the anastomosis.

The specimen is now removed and the pelvis can be inspected for any bleeding. It may be necessary to use 2–0 chromic suture to stop little vessels bleeding from the lateral pedicles. It is also important to look very carefully at the site of ligation of the seminal vesicles and ampullae of the vas, as frequently there may be a little bleeder that needs either diathermy or clipping. You should now have a very good haemostasis.

Preparation of the bladder neck

There will now be a very good view of the ureteric orifices and the bladder can be prepared for the anastomosis. Walsh [3] has described mucosal eversion of the bladder neck with interrupted sutures of 4–0 chromic after racket-handle closure of the bladder neck has been performed (Fig. 13.10). It may be easier to use a continuous running suture of 4–0 chromic catgut. This is a sero-muscular to mucosal suture which is run from outside in from the 3 o'clock to 9 o'clock position posteriorly on the bladder neck and prolapses the mucosa well out, like a bottom lip (Fig. 13.11). If this suture is run from inside out, there will generally be some tearing and the mucosa will not prolapse out easily. After this has been done, inspect the ureteric orifices. They are usually well away from the proposed site of the anastomosis and are thus safe. I then carry out a racket-handle closure of the bladder neck with a running 2–0

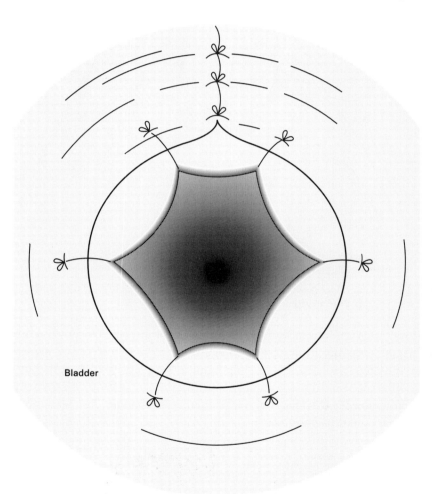

Fig. 13.10 Interrupted 4–0 chromic mucosal eversion sutures. Note that not all of the mucosa prolapses out.

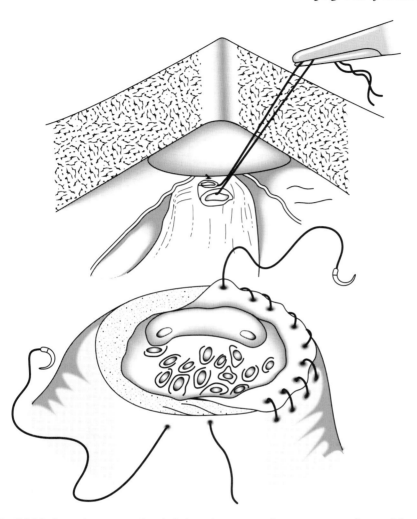

Fig. 13.11 A continuous running 4–0 chromic suture prolapses mucosa well out of the anastomosis.

chromic suture placed anteriorly so that the vesicourethral anastomosis is to be constructed on the posterior aspect of the bladder neck, that is, that area of the bladder closest to the ureteric orifices (Fig. 13.12). This gives better access to the pelvis and results in less tension at the anastomosis. Close the bladder neck down to approximately 1 cm.

211

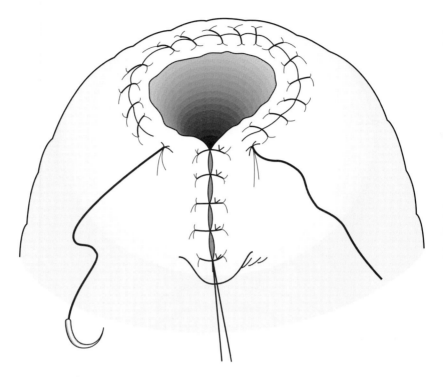

Fig. 13.12 After racket-handle closure of the bladder neck, the mucosal eversion suture makes the bladder neck easily identifiable.

Vesicourethral anastomosis

Chromic catgut is a much better suture material to use for the anastomosis as it slips easily and does not result in tearing, which may occur with braided suture material. All previous anastomotic techniques that have been described have used four or six sutures which have been placed in each end of the anastomosis first and then tied all at once. The sutures tend to get in the way of each other and may lead to a defect in the anastomosis, especially posteriorly. If this happens, then the situation cannot be retrieved without removing sutures. In my view, part of the reason why bladder-neck contracture occurs is persistent leakage of urine around the anastomosis which induces fibrosis. Therefore, a watertight anastomosis needs to be obtained and proper apposition of mucosa to mucosa is vital. The potential for leakage in non-apposition is more likely to be a problem posteriorly.

I now carry out the anastomosis by placing and tying the first suture at the 6 o'clock (i.e. posterior) position (Fig. 13.13). It is most important to ensure

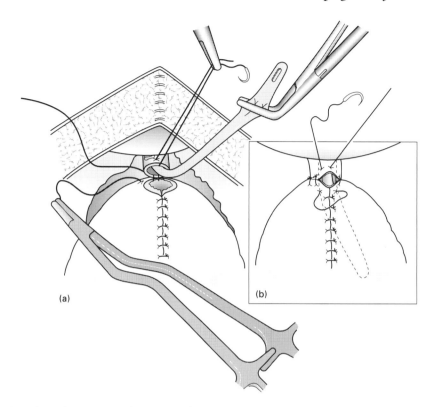

Fig. 13.13 Anastomotic closure. (a) Three interrupted sutures placed posteriorly. (b) The previously placed 12 o'clock suture used for the anterior

that the suture not only passes through the urethra itself but also involves the striated urethral sphincter layer. For this manoeuvre, the assistant plays an important role. With a pack and the assistant's left hand directly over the rectum and pushing posteriorly, the urethra and periurethral tissue can be well-seen. Pass a 20 French Foley catheter and bring it out through the wound and this will then allow the edge of the urethra to be seen. Using a Thompson–Walker needle holder and a 2–0 chromic suture, the first anastomotic stitch is placed from outside in, in the urethra at the 6 o'clock position. The assistant then removes his or her hand and the suture can be placed through the bladder neck inside out. That suture is tied down and the ends are cut. The next suture is placed at the 5 o'clock position and similarly tied and cut. A further suture is placed at the 7 o'clock position, and tied and cut as well. This then leaves three sutures in the posterior aspect of the anastomosis. One can then inspect this and see that there is proper apposition posteriorly and thus no chance of leakage here (Fig. 13.13). Several 2–0 chromic sutures can then be placed on the lateral sides of the anastomosis and tied. All these sutures are tied under direct vision so that you are sure that your anastomosis is in proper apposition.

This leaves only the anterior part of the anastomosis to complete. The 2–0 chromic suture that was previously placed in the anterior aspect of the urethra is used at this stage as a horizontal mattress suture through the bladder neck and urethra. Before tying this, a 20 French Silastic catheter is railroaded into the bladder and then the suture is tied. It may be necessary to place a 2–0 chromic stitch in the bladder neck just above this to make sure that it is watertight. The balloon is inflated with 30 ml and a whistle-tip syringe is used to fill the bladder with approximately 125 ml of water. If there is any leakage, it generally occurs anteriorly and can be closed. I believe that by performing the anastomosis under direct division with interrupted 2–0 chromic sutures placed and tied sequentially, the possibility of leakage is substantially eliminated and it ensures that the anastomosis is in proper approximation. Drain tubes are then placed down to the pelvis and brought out through stab incisions in each iliac fossa. The wound is now closed with 1 Dexon for the rectus sheath and staples for the skin.

Postoperative management

Patients can generally commence fluid intake in about 3 days. There is minimal leakage from the anastomosis and thus the drain tubes can usually be removed on the third or fourth day. Some patients may have persisting lymphatic drainage and it may be necessary to leave the drains in for a longer period.

The urethral catheters are removed on day 10 and the patient can then be discharged the following day. I find that most patients have urgency and urge incontinence over the first couple of days, but this settles rapidly. Urinary control is rapidly improved and stress incontinence is minimized. Most of my patients do not wear a pad (93.4%) and are not bothered by incontinence. The rest may wear one or two pads at most per day and are bothered by minimal stress incontinence with moderate exercise. As yet I have had no patients who have required artificial urinary sphincter implantation.

Lymphocoele formation can be a problem postoperatively and it has been noted that the incidence of lymphocoele has been markedly reduced by avoiding heparin. More recently, it has been proposed that using heparin in the upper arm or upper torso has resulted in the marked diminution of lymphocoele formation. It seems that subcutaneous heparin injected below the umbilicus may be taken up by the pelvic lymphatics and thus result in increased leakage of lymph. Since placing heparin in the upper arm, I have noticed a considerable diminution of lymphocoele formation, but my numbers are small.

Bladder-neck contractures historically were of the order of 30%. Walsh's modification with mucosal eversion has resulted in a marked diminution of bladder-neck contracture rates. In my own series, direct-vision sequential placing and tying of the anastomotic sutures have been associated with a current bladder-neck contracture rate of 3%. If bladder-neck contractures are going to occur, they generally do so in the first 3 months following surgery. These can be managed by urethral dilations but the scarring can be quite significant and may require an incision under general anaesthesia. I have not found in previous contractures that bladder-neck incision increases incontinence. It may, however, be necessary in the long term to dilate these bladder necks to keep them open.

Conclusions

Radical prostatectomy has become a much easier operation and certainly less threatening to the surgeon over recent years. A proper understanding of anatomy is most important, as is adequate surgical training in the technique. I feel it is of paramount importance that urologists who wish to carry out this operation train or visit centres where the procedure is performed frequently so that they use correct techniques right from the start. I do not think the operation should be performed by occasional prostatectomists, as the results will be less than optimal. Done well, the operation will leave both patient and surgeon happy with the long-term results.

References

* 1 Walsh PC & Donker PJ. Impotence following radial prostatectomy: insight into aetiology and prevention. *Urol* 1982; **128**: 492.
* 2 Walsh PC, Quinlan DM, Morton RA & Steiner MS. Radical retropubic prostatectomy, improved anastomosis and urinary continence. *Urol Clin North Am* 1990; **17**: 679–684.
* 3 Walsh PC. Radical retropubic prostatectomy. In: *Campbell's Urology*, 6th edn, Walsh PC, Retik AB, Stamey TA *et al.*, eds. Philadelphia: W.B. Saunders, 1992, pp. 2865–2886.
* 4 Catalona WJ. Nerve sparing radical retropubic prostatectomy. In: *Urologic Surgery*, 4th edn, Glen JF, Ed. Philadelphia: J.B. Lippincott, 1991, pp. 616–629.
* 5 Myers RP Improving the exposure of the prostate in radical retropubic prostatectomy: longitudinal bunching of the deep venous complex. *J Urol* 1989; **142**: 1282–1284.

* Reference of special interest.

14/Locally Invasive Prostate Cancer – Is There a Best Treatment?

R.J. Shearer

The recent increase in the incidence of prostatic cancer is predicted to continue well into the 21st century [1]. The difference between the USA and UK in the ratio of registration to deaths (6:1 in USA, 1.3:1 in UK) has led to speculation that the earlier stage at diagnosis (80% organ-confined at diagnosis, compared with 40% in the UK) leading as it does to early therapeutic intervention, provides an opportunity for curative treatment. However, the earlier stage at diagnosis in the USA has not been associated with a reduction in the death rate and the positive margin rate after radical prostatectomy suggests that many more patients have locally advanced (T3) disease than had been anticipated. There is as yet no firm evidence that early intervention is associated with an enhanced cure rate, and the difference in mortality in the USA may be no more than a manifestation of lead time and susceptibility bias in which an apparent benefit of treatment seems to result from preferentially selecting patients with early or slowly progressive disease and comparing them with patients with more aggressive disease.

The National Health Service Standing Group on Health Technology has identified assessment of prostate-specific antigen (PSA) and transrectal ultrasound (TRUS) as one of the priorities of health care research in the UK, and the rise in detection of early prostatic cancer will have a significant impact on work load and health economics. Limited evidence from screening studies indicates that even efforts to enhance early diagnosis result in a significant proportion of patients identified in screening programmes as having locally advanced disease. The introduction of the nerve-sparing or anatomical prostatectomy in 1983 [2] has been followed by a marked increase in the numbers of prostatectomies being undertaken. Every prostatectomy has a significant impact on resource utilization – the operation requires 2–3 h of operating theatre time, and a minimal stay in hospital of 3–4 days. However, staging investigations are insufficiently sensitive to detect extra prostatic invasion in all cases, and evidence is now accumulating that the margin-positive rate after total prostectomy is between 10 and 69%, and the need for further anticancer therapy within 4 years of prostatectomy is about 24%. In Detroit referral of prostate cancer for radiotherapy increased by 255%, while the number with metastatic disease remained constant, and decreased as a proportion of the whole from 55% in 1985 to 21% in 1992 [3]. An increase in the use of radiotherapy in the Netherlands has been reported, from 13% in 1875 to 31% in 1989 [4]. At the Royal Marsden Hospital, UK, there was a three- to fourfold increase in the number of patients referred for radical radiotherapy in the periods 1970–1979 and 1980–1989. This trend is continuing. There is therefore a considerable need to determine the optimum selection of patients for radical local treatment, and to decide on which therapeutic modality to employ, as well as the most effective and appropriate means of delivering treatment.

Accurate clinical staging of prostatic cancer remains a major problem. Even though TRUS-guided biopsy of the seminal vesicles is highly accurate [5], the overall staging accuracy of TRUS is 58% [6]. Magnetic resonance imaging (MRI), while providing an improvement in staging accuracy, still has a significant false-negative rate for detecting capsular invasion [5, 7]. Considerable attention is now being paid to methods of predicting which patients are likely to have capsular invasion or lymph node disease [8]. As these techniques become more sophisticated, there will be increasing selection of patients for radical surgery, with a consequent increase in the number of men deemed to have invasive disease, and for whom alternative therapy needs to be identified. A further difficulty arises in that management has traditionally been a difficult and controversial area with results that are often disappointing.

When considering therapeutic strategies for patients with locally advanced disease, the natural history of invasive prostate cancer needs to be considered as well as the natural history of the patient population involved. The Thames Cancer Registry evidence indicates that 88% of men presenting with prostate cancer in south-east England are aged 65 or over [1]. Evidence from screening/early detection studies suggested that early stage at diagnosis is associated with younger age, and it therefore follows that the overwhelming majority of men presenting with T3 disease will be over 65 years. Of the 750% increase in expenditure by Medicare on prostate cancer, 97.5% is accounted for by radiotherapy (unpublished data), indicating that the older patients are deemed unsuitable for surgery, presumably because of advanced disease.

Cure or palliation?

Data on the proportion of patients with locally invasive disease and involved lymph nodes are limited, but it is reasonable to assume that at least 40% of men with extraprostatic cancer will have nodal involvement. Patients with lymph node involvement have a chance of developing metastatic disease within 5 years of 80% or more [9] and are therefore beyond the scope of cure. Given the age range, however, therapeutic measures which result in a significant improvement in both local control and the development of metastases may be, in effect, curative, since they may delay progress until the patient has died of intercurrent disease.

Treatment options

Watchful waiting

While a strong case can be mounted for deferred treatment in early stage (T1/T2) prostate cancer, most patients with bulky T3 disease are symptomatic, and local progression is almost inevitable. It is rare for T3 prostatic cancer to be suitable for deferment of treatment, although in the older man with minimal symptoms this can be an option.

Radical surgery

Whatever the merits of radical anatomical prostatectomy in organ-confined prostate cancer, it is clear that it has no proven role in the management of T3 tumours. Cancer remains the dominant cause of death in patients with margin-positive disease, being 40% at 13.5 years [10], and the likelihood of PSA relapse at 10 years is between 46% for Gleason scores 2–6 and 58% for Gleason scores of 7 or more where there is established capsular penetration [11]. Identifiable local recurrence is less common than either distant progression or PSA relapse, although the low incidence (10%) of normalization of PSA after delayed radiotherapy to the prostate bed [11] suggests that most of these patients may have developed metastatic or lymphatic disease rather than local recurrence. In patients with clinically staged T3 disease, a retrospective review found a local recurrence-free rate of 90% at 5 years [12]. However, these were selected patients, and over half were treated with adjuvant hormone therapy, making interpretation of results difficult.

Neoadjuvant hormone therapy and radical surgery

The use of androgen deprivation or antiandrogens to downstage locally invasive prostate cancer prior to radical surgery is controversial. Labrie and coworkers in a randomized prospective trial have reported preliminary results indicating that the incidence of positive margins fell from 39 to 13% in a group of men treated by maximum androgen blockade for 3 months [13]. Others, however, have found minimal downstaging of stage T3 tumours [14, 15], and a number of studies are now underway to investigate further the role of neoadjuvant androgen deprivation, either alone or in combination with cytotoxic chemotherapy.

Radiotherapy

Radical radiotherapy is reserved for those patients presenting without evidence of metastases and with disease confined to the prostate or the prostate and immediately surrounding tissues. The decision to offer treatment is based on a judgement of the balance between the life expectancy of an individual patient and the chance of his disease progressing significantly during this period. The morbidity of treatment should also be considered. The likelihood of curative treatment is highest for small-volume tumours of Gleason grade < 7. As tumour bulk increases, so does the chance of seminal vesical or lymph node involvement [16]. When lymphadenopathy is demonstrated on computed tomography (CT) or magnetic resonance imaging (MRI) it is unrealistic to regard radical radiotherapy as a curative treatment, although radiotherapy can maintain local control in the majority of patients. Assessment of lymphadenopathy with CT or lymphography understages a significant number of patients, and is a major reason for the difficulties when comparing results of radical radiotherapy with radical surgery where pelvic lymph node staging is carried out. The initial enthusiasm for laparoscopic lymph node dissection has not been maintained with greater experience of the technique.

External-beam radiotherapy

Radical prostate irradiation should be carried out with a linear accelerator using at least 5–6 MeV for optimal dose distributions. At present, CT gives the most accurate localization of the prostate and seminal vesicles for radiotherapy planning using 5 mm slices for accurate localization of the upper aspect, and the apex of the gland. It is uncertain whether inclusion of pelvic lymph nodes in the treatment fields gives a survival or recurrence-free advantage. Some retrospective reviews have suggested a benefit for adjuvant lymph node irradiation [17–19], but reviews by the Patterns of Care study group and at the Royal Marsden Hospital have failed to demonstrate any convincing benefit for additional pelvic irradiation [20, 21] and it is not the current practice at the Royal Marsden to include pelvic nodes in the radiation fields.

The outcome for most patients is determined by the development of metastases. In a series from Stanford University, USA, disease recurrence occurred in 66% of patients at 10 years and 72% at 22 years. Local control can be obtained in most patients, however, with local recurrence rates varying from 19 to 31% at 10 years and 25–56% at 15 years [22–25]. Although radiotherapy may achieve long-term clinical local control of disease, the recent Medical Research Council (MRC) study comparing radiotherapy alone or in combination with orchidectomy with orchidectomy alone showed that radiotherapy gave no survival benefit over orchidectomy but that the orchidectomized patients had a longer disease-free interval, there being a delay in the development of metastases [26]. This suggests that many patients with locally advanced disease had subclinical metastases at the time of presentation.

Following radiotherapy, local failure can be demonstrated by clinical failure, posttreatment biopsy or posttreatment PSA elevation. There is now general agreement that a positive biopsy more than 12 months after radiotherapy suggests persistent disease which is associated with an increased risk of local failure [27, 28]. The incidence of biopsy-positive patients with T3 disease is between 20 and 64%, the most reliable indicator being digital rectal examination [28]. Studies of local failure have shown a correlation between local treatment efficacy and outcome, with 68–77% of patients with local failure developing metastases compared with 19–40% where treatment had achieved local control [29–31]. In one series of patients treated by interstitial radiotherapy, the time to development of distant metastases was on average longer for patients with local failure [29], thus suggesting that some metastases may develop from local tumour recurrences. It is therefore reasonable to attempt to control the local tumour provided that the morbidity of treatment is acceptably low. A number of strategies have been developed to try and improve local control, including conformal radiotherapy, interstitial radiotherapy, particle beam therapy and the neoadjuvant use of androgen deprivation therapy prior to radical external-beam radiotherapy.

Conformal radiotherapy

Conventional external-beam radiotherapy uses three or more beams shaped by straight-edged collimators in the head of the linear accelerator which therefore produces rectangular beams, resulting in the production of cuboid or cylindrical high-dose radiation volumes. The intended target organ (prostate and seminal vesicles with or without pelvic lymph nodes) does not conform to such a geometrical shape, and consequently a significant volume of normal tissue is included in the radiation field. Recent advances, using accurate three-dimensional reconstruction from CT images, improvements in three-dimensional computational dose calculations and the use of multileaf collimators, have resulted in the ability to make significant reductions in irradiated volume.

In a series of 138 men treated at the Royal Marsden Hospital, the total volume irradiated to the 90% isodose was reduced by 42%, the rectal volume by 46% and bladder volume by 41%. There has, however, been only a relatively slight and not significant reduction in acute side-effects, though there was an overall shortening of the time of acute reactions [32]. Late radiation reactions are dose-limiting and data on the effect of conformal techniques on late reactions are awaited, as are data on local control and survival.

A further potential advantage of conformal radiotherapy is that it may allow dose escalation. Conventional radiotherapy for prostate cancer treats to a tumour dose of 55–64 Gy. A number of dose escalation studies have been undertaken [33, 34], with meticulous planning and immobilization techniques. Doses of 75 Gy have been well-tolerated, and currently doses over 80 Gy are being delivered. Further National Cancer Institute-sponsored studies are planned.

Interstitial radiotherapy

Several studies have reported the results of interstitial brachytherapy using I^{125}, Ir^{192} or Au^{198}. Five-year recurrence-free rates between 43 and 94% have been reported, but the complication rate is high, and dose calculations are difficult to ensure with consistency [35–39].

Particle beam therapy

The ultimate method of improving radiation dose distributions is to use particle therapy (protons or pions). Irradiation delivered in this way has a highly advantageous dose distribution as energy is deposited in a peak over a small area, allowing a high dose to be delivered to the target area with a sharp fall in dose to the surrounding tissues. Results of a randomized study comparing photon and proton beam boost treatment are awaited. This study has produced data on the dose relationships for complications with an increase in rectal bleeding from 16 to 34% as the dose increased from 67.2 to 75.6 Gy [40].

Neutron beams have no inherent advantages for dose distribution but they have a higher linear energy transfer which may lead to an increased efficacy against hypoxic radioresistant tumours. A comparative study comparing mixed-beam irradiation (40% neutron with 60% proton) with photon therapy has reported improved local control and survival with mixed-beam therapy [41]. A comparison of pure neutron with photon radiation therapy has shown advantages for neutrons in terms of local control and PSA normalization, with clinical or biochemical failure occurring in 32 and 45% of the photon arm compared to 11 and 17% in the neutron arm [42]. Studies at other tumour sites have shown that neutron beam therapy may be associated with marked increases in normal tissue toxicity. Prostate cancer is no exception, with late treatment toxicity occurring in 11% of the neutron group, compared with 3% of the photon group. These complications are technique-dependent, and the technology to produce accurate particle-beam therapy is extremely expensive. Unless very clear survival advantages can be demonstrated with minimalization of toxicity, it is unlikely that particle beam therapy will gain wide acceptance.

Neoadjuvant androgen deprivation and radiotherapy

Local control of tumour by radiotherapy, judged clinically or on biopsy, becomes less certain with increasing tumour stage and, as discussed, local control may become a discriminant for the development of metastases and cancer-related death. Neoadjuvant androgen deprivation offers a potential advantage in two ways. Combined treatment may lead to increased cell kill (androgen deprivation probably causes apoptosis, while radiotherapy induces mitotic cell death). Initial shrinkage of prostatic volume can lead to favourable modification of the radiation treatment volume. This may favourably affect the therapeutic ratio either by reducing the radiation sequelae for a standard radiation dose or by permitting dose escalation, which should increase tumour control probability while maintaining acceptable levels of complications. Additionally, adjuvant hormone therapy may have an advantage in spatial cooperation – an improvement in therapeutic results which is achieved by one modality treating disease spatially missed by the other [43]. Such benefit has been demonstrated for the use of adjuvant hormone therapy in breast cancer [44, 45], but has not been adequately addressed in prostate cancer.

Studies at the Royal Marsden Hospital have used luteinizing hormone releasing hormone (LHRH) agonists for 3–6 months before radical radiation therapy. In an initial pilot study, 20 or 23 patients showed a reduction in volume of approximately 50%, from a median pretreatment volume of 66 ml (range 40–130 ml) to a median of 30 ml (range 13–47 ml) after androgen deprivation [46]. Further reduction in rectal and bladder sparing from the radiation fields was achieved by conformal radiotherapy techniques. The measurement in this study clearly showed that the two techniques were complementary, and a total of 79 patients have now been treated in this way. In this group pretreatment PSA levels were 1–280 ng/ml (median 30 ng/ml), with 71% having PSA > 10 ng/ml. After treatment with LHRH agonists, median PSA was 1 ng/ml and 83% had PSA < 10 ng/ml. Three months after radiotherapy (androgen deprivation ceasing at the completion of radiation, PSA levels had continued to fall until only 2% were > 10 ng/ml, and 80% were less than 2 ng/ml. At 18 months, biochemical control was maintained in the majority, with PSA < 2 ng/ml in 70%, but failures were becoming apparent with PSA > 10 ng/ml in 17% of patients. Further follow-up is being undertaken in these patients with particular reference to patterns of failure.

Further studies to address the issues of dose escalation in conjunction with conformal radiotherapy using three-dimensional radiotherapy techniques are starting. Large prospective trials are evaluating combined modality treatment in North America and Europe.

After a median follow-up of 41 months of 457 men in RTOG protocol 8610 there has been a significant reduction in the number of local recurrences from 29% in the control group to 16% in the study group. Results of RTOG protocol 8531 and EORTC protocol 22863 are awaited. These studies evaluate adjuvant androgen deprivation commenced concurrently with the start of radiation therapy. The current RTOG trial (9202) evaluates treatment with initial neoadjuvant LHRH agonist and radical radiotherapy with a subsequent randomization to continuing LHRH therapy for 2 years of discontinuing androgen deprivation.

Radical surgery and adjuvant radiotherapy

Many surgeons advocate low-dose radiotherapy for margin-positive disease after radical prostatectomy, on the grounds that it may improve local control with the lowest additional morbidity. There is, however, no objective evidence to support this hypothesis, and adjuvant radiation therapy does not produce a survival advantage [47].

Hormonal therapy

The Medical Research Council study [26] showed an advantage in disease-free survival, and in the onset of metastases, though not in overall survival from androgen deprivation in T3 patients. It is therefore reasonable to consider androgen deprivation as an effective palliative treatment in T3 prostate cancer. However, the cost is inevitable impotence, and in the younger, sexually active patient this constitutes a serious contraindication. The possible increased benefit from maximum androgen blockade (combined LHRH analogue and antiandrogen) in M1 patients with good performance status and low tumour burden suggests that this modality may have a place in the management of locally advanced disease. There are, however, no studies which can lend any statistical support to this concept.

Intermittent hormone therapy has often been postulated as a possible means of management of prostate cancer, but has not been evaluated.

Treatment of symptoms

The mainstay of management of obstructive urinary symptoms or retention in patients with bulky T3 disease has been, and remains, transurethral prostatectomy. Androgen deprivation by producing significant volume shrinkage does reduce obstructive symptoms, and has been shown to result in satisfactory voiding in 80% of patients in retention treated by LHRH analogue [48].

Palliative radiation therapy in patients in whom hormone therapy has failed to bring about local control is often effective.

Conclusions

There is no 'right' treatment for locally advanced prostate cancer, and the choice of therapy for an individual patient will depend upon his particular circumstances, including the extent of his disease, Gleason grade and life expectancy. At the present time, the theoretical advantages offered by neoadjuvant androgen deprivation and radiotherapy make this the treatment of choice in many patients, though the outcome of the several large trials will help to place combination therapy in context.

References

1 *Cancer in South East England 1990*. Thames Cancer Registry 1993.
* 2 Walsh PC, Lepor H & Eggleston JC. Radical prostatectomy with preservation of sexual function: anatomical and pathological considerations. *Prostate* 1983; **4**: 473.
3 Dearnaley D. Personal communication.
4 de Jong B, Crommelian M, van der Heijden LH & Coebergh J-WW. Patterns of radiotherapy for cancer patients in south-eastern Netherlands, 1975–1989. *Radiother Oncol* 1994; **31**: 213–221.
5 Terris MK, McNeal JE, Freiha FS & Stamey TA. Efficacy of transrectal ultrasound guided seminal vesicle biopsy in the detection of seminal vesicle invasion by prostate cancer. *J Urol* 1993; **149**: 1035–1039.
6 Rifkin MD, Zerhouni EA, Gatsonis CA *et al*. Comparison of magnetic resonance imaging and ultrasonography in staging early prostatic cancer. *N Engl J Med* 1990; **323**: 621–626.

* Reference of special interest.
** Reference of outstanding merit.

7 Chelsky MJ, Schnall MD, Seidmon EJ & Pollack HM. Use of endorectal surface coil magnetic resonance imaging for local staging of prostate cancer. *J Urol* 1993; **150**: 391–395.

8 Partin AW, Yoo J, Carter HB, Pearson JD, Chan DW, Epstein JI & Walsh PC. The use of prostate specific antigen, clinical stage, and Gleason score to predict pathological stage in men with localized prostate cancer. *J Urol* 1993; **150**: 110–114.

** 9 Hanks GE, Diamond JJ, Krall JM & Kramer S. A 10 year follow up of 682 patients treated for prostate cancer with radiation therapy in the United States. *Int J Radiat Oncol Biol Phys* 1987; **13**: 499–505.

10 Paulson DF. Impact of radical prostatectomy in the management of clinically localised disease. *J Urol* 1994; **152: 1826–1830.

11 Walsh PC, Partin AW & Epstein JI. Cancer control and quality of life following anatomical radical prostectomy: results at 10 years. *J Urol* 1994; **152**: 1831–1836.

12 Morgan WR, Bergstralh EI & Zincke H. Long-term evaluation of radical prostatectomy as treatment for clinical stage C (T3) prostate cancer. *Urology* 1993; **41**: 113–120.

13 Labrie F, Dupont A, Cusan L *et al.* Downstaging of early prostate cancer by combination therapy with Flutamide and Lupron. *Clin Invest Med* 1993; **16**: 499–509.

14 Oesterling JE, Andrews PE, Suman VJ, Zincke H & Myers RP. Preoperative androgen deprivation therapy: artificial lowering of serum prostate specific antigen without downstaging the tumor. *J Urol* 1993; **149**: 779–782.

15 MacFarlane MT, Abi-Aad A, Stein A, Danella J, Belldegrun A & de Kernion JB. Neoadjuvant hormonal deprivation in patients with locally advanced prostate cancer. *J Urol* 1993; **150**: 132–134.

*16 Hanks GE, Martz KL & Diamond JJ. The effect of dose on local control of prostate cancer. *Int J Radiat Oncol Biol Phys* 1988; **15**: 1299–1305.

17 Bagshaw MA. External radiation therapy of carcinoma of the prostate. *Cancer* 1980; **45: 1912–1921.

18 McGowan DG. The value of extended field radiation therapy in carcinoma of the prostate. *Int J Radiat Oncol Biol Phys* 1981; **7**: 1333.

19 Polysongsang S, Aron BS, Shehata WM *et al.* Comparison of whole pelvis versus small field radiation therapy for carcinoma of the prostate. *J Urol* 1986; **127: 10–16.

20 Leibel SA, Hanks GE & Kramer S. Patterns of care outcome studies: results of the national practice in adenocarcinoma of the prostate. *Int J Radiat Oncol Biol Phys* 1984; **10**: 401–409.

21 Dearnaley DP, Eeles R, Syndikus I *et al.* External beam radiotherapy for localised prostate cancer. Long term follow-up in 443 patients. *Radiat Oncol* 1992; **24**: S80.

*22 Goffinet DR & Bagshaw MA. Radiation therapy of prostate carcinoma: 30 year experience at Stanford University. In: *Treatment of Prostatic Cancer – Facts and Controversies.* Wiley-Liss, 1990, pp. 209–222.

23 Perez CA, Pilepich MV, Garcia D, Simpson JR, Zivunska F & Hederman MA. Definitive radiation therapy in carcinoma of the prostate localised to the pelvis; experience at the Mallinkrodt Institute of Radiology. *NCI Monogr* 1988; **7: 85–94.

24 Zagars GK, von Eschenback AC, Johnson DE & Oswald MJ. Stage C adenocarcinoma of the prostate: an analysis of 551 patients treated with external beam radiation. *Cancer* 1987; **60: 1489–1499.

25 Hanks GE, Diamond JJ, Krall JM, Martz KL & Kramer S. A 10 year follow up of 682 patients treated for prostate cancer with radiation therapy in the United States. *Int J Radiat Oncol Biol Phys* 1987; **13**: 499–505.

26 Fellows GJ, Clark PB, Beynon LL *et al.* Treatment of advanced localized carcinoma of the prostate by orchiectomy, radiotherapy or combined treatment. A Medical Research Council study. *Br J Urol* 1992; **70**: 304–309.

27 Freiha FS & Bagshaw MA. Carcinoma of the prostate: results of post-irradiation biopsy. *Prostate* 1984; **5**: 19–25.

28 Scardino PT & Wheeler TM. Local control of prostate cancer with radiotherapy: frequency and prognostic significance of positive results of postirradiation biopsy. *NCI Monogr* 1988; 7: 95–103.

29 Fuks Z, Leibel SA, Wallner KE *et al.* The effect of local control on metastatic dissemination in carcinoma of the prostate: long tem results in patients treated with I-125 implantation. *Int J Radiat Oncol Biol Phys* 1991, 21: 537–547.

*30 Zagars GK, von Eschenbach AC, Ayala AG, Schulthesis TE & Erman NE. The influence of local control on metastatic dissemination of prostate cancer treated by external beam megavoltage radiation therapy. *Cancer* 1991; **68**: 2370–2377.

31 Kuban DA, El-Mahdi AM & Schellhammer PF. Prognosis in patients with local recurrence after definitive irradiation for prostatic carcinoma. *Cancer* 1989; **63**: 2421–2425.

32 Tait D, Nahum A, Dearnaley DP *et al.* A randomised trial of conformal versus conventional radiotherapy: acute toxicity in patients treated with conventional fractionation. *Radiat Oncol* 1994; **32**(suppl 1): S114.

33 Leibel SA, Heimann R, Kutcher GJ *et al.* Three-dimensional conformal radiotherapy in locally advanced carcinoma of the prostate: preliminary results of a phase I dose-escalation study. *Int J Radiol Biol Phys* 1994; **28**: 55–65.

34 Sandler HM, Perez-Tomayo C, Ten Haken RK & Lichter AS. Dose escalation range for stage C (T3) prostate cancer: minimal rectal toxicity observed using conformal therapy. *Radiother Oncol* 1992; **23**: 53–54.

35 Weyrich TP, Kandzari SJ & Jain PR. Iodine 125 seed implants for prostatic carcinoma: five- and ten-year follow up. *J Urol* 1993; **41**: 122–6.

36 Donnelly BJ, Pedersen JE, Porter AT & McPhee MS. Iridium-192 brachytherapy in the treatment of cancer of the prostate. *Urol Clin North Am* 1991; **18**: 481–483.

37 Stromberg J, Martinez A, Benson R *et al.* Improved local control and survival for surgically staged patients with locally advanced prostate cancer treated with up-front low dose rate iridium-192 prostate implantation and external beam irradiation. *Int J Radiat Oncol Biol Phys* 1993; **28**: 67–75.

38 Holzman M, Carlton CE & Scardino PT. The frequency and morbidity of local tumour recurrence after definitive radiotherapy for stage C prostate cancer. *J Urol* 1991; **146**: 1578–1582.

39 Scardino PT, Frankel JM, Wheeler TM *et al.* The prognostic significance of post-irradiation biopsy results in patients with prostatic cancer. *J Urol* 1986; **135**: 510–515.

40 Benk VA, Adams JA, Shipley WU *et al.* Late rectal bleeding following combined X-ray and proton high dose irradiation for patients with stage T3–T4 prostate carcinoma. *Int J Radiol Oncol Biol Phys* 1993; **26**: 551–557.

41 Laramore GE, Krall JM, Thomas FJ *et al.* Fast neutron radiotherapy for locally advanced prostate cancer. *Am J Clin Oncol* 1993; **16**: 164–167.

42 Russell KJ, Caplan RJ, Laramore GE *et al.* Photon versus fast neutron external beam radiotherapy in the treatment of locally advanced prostate cancer: results of a randomized prospective trial. *Int J Radiat Oncol Biol Phys* 1994; **28**: 47–54.

43 Steel GG. Combined radiotherapy–chemotherapy: principles. In: *The Biological Basis of*

Radiotherapy, Steel GG, Adams GE, Horwich A, eds. Oxford: Elsevier Science, 1989, pp. 267–269.

44 Early Breast Cancer Trialists' Collaborative Group. Systemic treatment of breast cancer by hormonal, cytotoxic or immune therapy (part I). *Lancet* 1992; **339**: 1–15.

45 Early Breast Cancer Trialists' Collaborative Group. Systemic treatment of early breast cancer by hormonal, cytotoxic or immune therapy (part II). *Lancet* 1992; **339**: 71–85.

*46 Shearer RJ, Davies JH, Gelister JSK & Dearnaley DP. Hormonal cytoreduction and radiotherapy for carcinoma of the prostate. *Br J Urol* 1992; **69**: 521–524.

47 Paulson DF, Moul JW & Walther PJ. Radical prostatectomy for clinical stage T1–2 N0M0 prostatic adenocarcinoma: long-term results. *J Urol* 1990; **144**: 1180–1184.

48 Hampson SJ, Davies JH, Charig CR & Shearer RJ. LHRH analogues as primary treatment for retention in patients with prostatic carcinoma. *Br J Urol* 1993; **71**: 583–586.

15/Endocrine Treatment – Has it Reached its Limits?

P.H. Graversen and P. Iversen

Introduction

More than 50 years ago Huggins and Hodges [1] demonstrated the androgen dependence of prostatic adenocarcinoma and the beneficial effects of androgen deprivation by either orchidectomy or oestrogens. Many studies confirmed the remarkable symptomatic relief in most patients and, compared to historical controls, an increased survival was assumed until the publication of the first study by the Veterans Administration Cooperative Urological Research Group (VACURG) in 1967, which also questioned the need for early institution of therapy.

Within the last two decades a number of new pharmacological agents for androgen deprivation have been introduced. Although more therapeutic options have led to greater patient compliance, none of the new drugs, either alone or in combination, have resulted in major therapeutic breakthroughs in terms of cancer control. Treatment of advanced prostate cancer is still palliative, and the age-adjusted death rate of prostate cancer increases in many countries [2].

The optimal use of endocrine therapy in patients with prostate cancer is not a settled issue. Old problems like the optimal timing of therapy are still unsolved, and new (and some revived) concepts like chemoprophylaxis, nonsteroidal antiandrogen monotherapy, intermittent androgen deprivation, neoadjuvant and adjuvant therapy need to be further evaluated.

Endocrine regulation of the prostate

The prostate gland and the endocrine regulation of its growth have been extensively studied [3]. Androgens are clearly essential since the gland cannot develop, grow, differentiate or function without them. The major circulating androgen in men is testosterone (T), which is almost exclusively of testicular origin, but weak androgens are also secreted by the adrenal glands. Release of T from the testes is regulated by the hypothalamic–pituitary–gonadal axis (Fig. 15.1). The pituitary is stimulated by the pulsatile release of luteinizing hormone releasing hormone (LHRH) from the hypothalamus to release

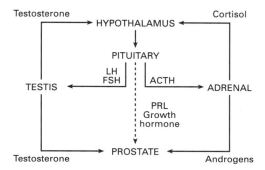

Fig. 15.1 Endocrine factors regulating prostatic growth and function. LH; luteinizing hormone; FSH, follicle-stimulating hormone; ACTH, adrenocorticotrophic hormone; PRL, prolactin.

luteinizing hormone (LH) and follicle-stimulating hormone (FSH). The Leydig cells of the testes are stimulated by LH to secrete T, which in turn regulates LH release by a negative feedback action.

Approximately 97% of the circulating T is bound to either sex hormone-binding globulin (SHBG) or to albumin but because of dissociation the biologically 'active' fraction is much greater. The unbound fraction enters prostate cells by diffusion and is converted into dihydrotestosterone (DHT) by the activity of 5α-reductase (Fig. 15.2). DHT is the mediator of the physiological events caused by androgens after its binding to the androgen receptor proteins which appear to be primarily nuclear-bound [4]. The activated receptor complex interacts with DNA sequences enabling transcription of specific genes and production of specific messenger RNAs, which in turn code for specific biological responses, such as the regulating processes of secretory protein production (e.g. prostate-specific antigen (PSA), prostatic acid phosphatase (PAP), growth factors, and also for the suppression of programmed cell death. Several other substances, such as prolactin, growth hormone and oestrogens, influence the growth of prostatic tissue but their actions and importance are at present not fully understood [3, 4].

Adrenocorticotrophic hormone regulates the production of steroid hormones in the adrenal cortex. Adrenal hormones with androgenic effects (primarily androstenedione and dehydroepiandrosterone) are metabolized into potent androgens in peripheral tissues, including the prostate. The importance of adrenal androgens in the prostate is controversial. Labrie *et al.* [5] and others claim that the adrenal androgens are responsible for as much as 15–50% of the total DHT present in the prostate cell. Conversely, others have found adrenal androgens not to cause significant prostatic growth [4, 6], and

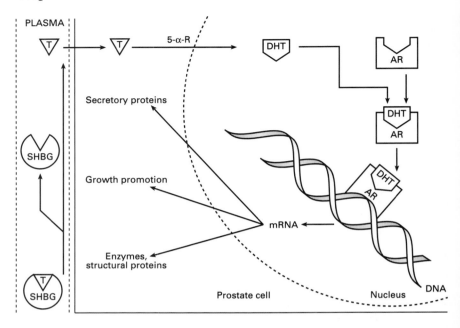

Fig. 15.2 Androgen action in prostatic cell. T, testosterone; SHBG, sex hormone-binding globulin; 5α-R, 5α-reductase; DHT, dihydrotestosterone; AR, androgen receptor.

clinical data differ as to the importance of adrenal androgens in endocrine manipulation of prostatic cancer.

Androgen deprivation

Stimulated by androgens, DNA synthesis and cell proliferation are initiated in immature prostatic cells (positive gene regulation). When the prostate reaches mature size, a negative regulation shuts down DNA synthesis and cell proliferation [7]. The number of cells is then maintained, and evidence suggests that androgens repress a specific genetic program, thereby preventing programmed death of prostatic cells [4, 7]. Following androgen deprivation this genetic program is activated and the programmed cell death, apoptosis, occurs as an active process caused by the appearance of specific proteins within the cell, and the size of the prostate is reduced to a basic level. The androgen withdrawal therefore has a double effect, i.e. triggering of apoptosis and inhibition of DNA synthesis and cell proliferation (for further information on apoptosis, see Chapter 4).

In the clinical situation, androgen deprivation is still the cornerstone in the management of advanced prostate cancer. The majority of patients respond favourably to androgen deprivation:

1   In all, 70–80% will experience symptomatic relief, such as reduced bone pain, increased performance status and a general improvement with increased sense of well-being.

2   Approximately 50% will show an objective response, such as reduced size of primary and metastatic tumours, fall in serum markers (PSA, PAP) and decreased urethral and/or ureteral obstruction. Complete remissions with normalization of all objective signs of malignancy are encountered in few patients.

The extent and duration of response following initiation of endocrine therapy in patients with advanced prostate cancer depend on several pretreatment prognostic factors, including T-category, histological grade, pain and performance status, serum alkaline phosphatase and serum T [8]. PSA has particular value as a 'dynamic' prognostic parameter, and the fall in PSA following the start of therapy seems to be the single most powerful predictor of outcome [9]. Patients with good prognostic factors will do well for a longer period than patients with bad prognostic factors. However, endocrine treatment is palliative in nature and relapse occurs if the patient survives competing causes of death. The median survival in metastatic patients treated with androgen deprivation is in the order of $2–2\frac{1}{2}$ years.

Some 20–30% of men with advanced prostate cancer will not respond clinically to androgen deprivation. The lack of initial response and the eventual relapse of initial responders are not completely understood. Clinical observations and experimental research suggest that prostate cancer is a biologically heterogeneous tumour composed of androgen-dependent, androgen-sensitive and androgen-independent populations of cells [10, 11]. Androgen deprivation therapy results in death of the androgen-dependent cells and in androgen-sensitive cells, growth and cellular functions are suppressed. However, eventually overgrowth of the androgen-independent cell clones will lead to progression of the tumour. Thus, in this 'clonal selection model', response to androgen withdrawal depends upon the ratios of these three cell types in the individual tumour. In a rat model [12] the androgen-independent clonal population seemed to be pre-existing but there was also evidence of genetic instability, resulting in generation of androgen-independent lines. In another rat model [11], it was suggested that androgen withdrawal affects the stem cell composition of the tumour, i.e. the androgen-independent line of cells surviving androgen deprivation is a consequence of the ability of a smaller number of initially androgen-dependent stem cells to adapt to a changed hormonal environment. This hypothesis supports the use of *intermittent endocrine therapy* (see later).

Supported by experimental data, Labrie *et al.* [5] claimed that the reason why some patients did not respond to conventional androgen deprivation was that these patients had androgen-hypersensitive tumours. Following elimination of testicular androgens, these tumour cells could continue growth and cellular functions in the presence of androgens of adrenal origin.

This debate on tumour biology and the clinical implications continues. However, in the clinical routine no specific hormonal or receptor measurements are currently available that allow discrimination between androgen-dependent, androgen-sensitive and androgen-independent prostatic cancer cells, which will help to identify the subset of patients who will not respond to endocrine therapy. The exact mechanisms of androgen deprivation 'escape' of human prostate cancer are still poorly understood. Intense research is ongoing in the hope that arresting or influencing the process can be made a target for a new therapeutic strategy.

Endocrine treatment options

In management of patients with prostate cancer, androgen deprivation is achieved by surgical ablation of the androgen source, antigonadotrophic action, blockade of androgen receptors and combinations (Table 15.1). Hypophysectomy and adrenalectomy have both been used as surgical ablative procedures – both are now obsolete. Another principle – pharmacological inhibition of steroid hormone synthesis – may be attained with drugs like aminogluthetimide and ketoconazole. However, these drugs are toxic and with no advantages and are not used in routine handling of patients.

Bilateral orchidectomy

Surgical removal of the testes is still considered to be the 'gold standard' in endocrine manipulation of prostate cancer. Removal of the primary source of circulating T (orchidectomy) is the most rapid method for reducing serum T and castrate range is reached within 24 h. Tissue levels of DHT are correspondingly decreased as a result. Once the procedure is performed, compliance is not a factor of concern and in old, debilitated patients this is an advantage. In patients with severe symptoms and imminent danger of spinal cord compression because of bone metastases, orchidectomy is preferable. The primary drawback of orchidectomy is the psychological impact.

Table 15.1 Endocrine treatment options.

Option	Endocrine action	Side-effects
ANDROGEN WITHDRAWAL		
Surgical	Removal of source of testosterone	Surgical complications Psychological impact Hot flushes Loss of libido and potency
Medical		

Oestrogens
  Oral
    Diethylstilboestrol
    Ethinyloestradiol
	Negative feedback on the hypothalamus
	Possible direct cytotoxic effect
		Gynaecomastia
		Nausea, vomiting
		Fluid retention, oedema
		Loss of libido and potency
		Venous thrombosis
		Pulmonary embolus
		Myocardial infarction

Parenteral
    Polyoestradiolphosphate
    Diethylstilboestrol phosphate
		As the oral agents but most likely without cardiovascular side-effects

LHRH agonists
  Leuprorelin
  Goserelin
  Buserelin
	Downregulation of pituitary LHRH receptors	Hot flushes
		Loss of libido and potency
		Gynaecomastia
		Flare phenomenon

ANDROGEN BLOCKADE		
Antiandrogens		
Steroidal Cyproterone acetate	Competes for the androgen receptor Progesterone-like antigonadotrophic activity	Loss of libido and potency Gynaecomastia Cardiovascular morbidity

Non-steroidal
  Flutamide (f)
  Nilutamide (n)
  Casodex® (C)
	Competes for the androgen receptor	Diarrhoea (f)
		Hepatic function abnormalities, reversible (f)
		Dark adaptation difficulty (n)
		Alcohol intolerance (n)
		Interstitial pneumonitis (n)
		Breast tenderness (n, f, C)
		Gynaecomastia (n, f, C)

COMBINATION TREATMENT See Chapter 16		

LHRH, luteinizing hormone releasing hormone.

LHRH agonists

Many studies have found treatment with LHRH agonists to be comparable to surgical castration with regard to efficacy (Table 15.2). Like endogenous LHRH, synthetic agonists stimulate the pituitary to release LH. However, continuous stimulation by potent synthetic agonists with a longer half-life than endogenous LHRH results in downregulation of pituitary LHRH receptors and a paradoxical suppression of circulating levels of LH and sex steroids. Castrate range of T is reached by the 15th day and maintained for the duration of therapy [13]. The initial stimulatory effect of LHRH agonists occurring during the first week of treatment may be associated with objective and subjective signs, called the flare phenomenon. This may result in temporary deterioration of symptoms: about 10% of patients will experience increase in bone pain and obstructive symptoms. More rarely, flare may precipitate serious manifestations of advanced disease like spinal compression and obstruction of ureters – death has even occurred.

Antiandrogens or oestrogens given during the initial period of LHRH agonist therapy counteract the flare. Recently, synthetic and potent LHRH antagonists have been introduced [13, 14]; these antagonists act on the same receptor sites as LHRH and cause an immediate inhibition of the release of LH, FSH and sex steroids. Whether LHRH antagonists have clinical potential either alone or in combination with LHRH agonists to prevent flare awaits further experimental and clinical research.

LHRH agonists are polypeptides and cannot be administered orally. Although nasal spray and daily subcutaneous injections have been employed, depot preparations for monthly injections are most commonly used. Depots which will enable administration only every 2 or 3 months are being introduced [15], and will add further to the acceptance of LHRH agonists.

Oestrogens

The antigonadotrophic effect of oestrogen has been used in the treatment of prostate cancer since Huggins's discoveries. Among the oestrogens available for both oral and parenteral administration (Table 15.1), diethylstilboestrol (DES) has been the most widely used. A daily oral dose of 5 mg or 3 mg reliably reduces serum T levels to castrate ranges, while the effect of 1 mg is less certain. Both experimental and clinical evidence suggests that oestrogen therapy may be superior to castration in terms of efficacy (Table 15.2), maybe because of a direct effect on the tumour [16]. However, apart from adverse feminizing effects, an unacceptable cardiovascular toxicity, first recognized in the VACURG studies

Table 15.2 Prospective, randomized studies comparing endocrine treatment options.

Investigator	Treatment design	No. of patients	Follow-up (median)	Results Progression-free survival (Median time)	Survival
Peeling [32]	Orchidectomy versus goserelin	144 148	24 months	40 weeks 27 weeks NS	104 weeks 115 weeks NS
Johansson et al. [18]	Orchidectomy versus oestrogens	76 74	96 months	49% 64% P = 0.04 } rate at 5 years	47% 51% NS
Haapiainen et al. [33]	Orchidectomy versus oestrogens	131 146	>60 months	54% 68% P < 0.05 } rate at 5 years	34% 31% NS
Waymont et al. [34]	Goserelin versus DES (3 mg/day)	124 126	43 months	14.5 months 11.4 months P = 0.06	27.4 months 27.7 months NS
Béland et al. [35]	Orchidectomy versus orchidectomy + nilutamide	96 98	18–48 months	12 months 12 months NS	18.9 months 24.3 months NS
Janknegt et al. [36]	Orchidectomy versus orchidectomy + nilutamide	216 207	35 months	14.9 months 20.8 months P = 0.005	24.2 months 27.3 months NS
Iversen et al. [37]	Orchidectomy versus goserelin + flutamide	133 129	30 months	16.3 months 16.6 months NS	27.6 months 22.8 months NS
Keuppens et al [38]	Orchidectomy versus goserelin + flutamide	163 164	18 months	11 months 17 months P = 0.004	29.5 months 31 months NS
Denis et al. [39]	Orchidectomy versus goserelin + flutamide	148 149	60 months	46 weeks 71 weeks P = 0.003	27.1 months 34.4 months P = 0.02
Crawford et al. [40]	Leuprorelin versus leuprorelin + flutamide	300 303		13.9 months 16.5 months P = 0.039	28.3 months 35.6 months P = 0.035

DES, diethylstilboestrol; NS, not significant.

[17] and since confirmed by others [18], has brought the use of oral oestrogens into disrepute. The dose-dependent cardiovascular side-effects of oral oestrogens seem to be caused by an altered production of coagulation factors, in particular increased factor VII and X and decreased antithrombin III [19] as a result of a first-pass effect of portal blood with high oestrogen concentration. However, recent studies have shown that the liver function remains unchanged in patients treated with *parenteral* oestrogens and that this treatment entails no increased risk of thrombosis or cardiovascular disease [20].

Thus, there is a renewed interest in the use of oestrogens. A multicentre study (SPCG 5) conducted by the Scandinavian Prostatic Cancer Group comparing polyoestradiol phosphate (Estradurin®) 240 mg intramuscularly every 4 weeks (every 2 weeks for the first 2 months) with total androgen blockade has currently recruited more than 450 patients out of 900 planned.

Antiandrogens

Antiandrogens are defined as substances which compete for the androgen receptor, thereby inhibiting the action of androgens at their target site. Antiandrogens are administered orally and can be divided into two groups [7]: steroidal and non-steroidal.

Steroidal antiandrogens, e.g. cyproterone acetate (CPA), have a dual mechanism of action. They compete with T and DHT for the androgen receptor but also possess progesterone-like antigonadotrophic activity, leading to decreased secretion of LH and FSH with a consequent decline in T production. Similar to orchidectomy, LHRH agonists and oestrogens, treatment with steroidal antiandrogens results in loss of sexual function and these antiandrogens are not considered alternatives to previously discussed monotherapies. CPA is effective in preventing flare in conjunction with LHRH agonist treatment and can be used to suppress hot flushes following orchidectomy or LHRH agonist treatment.

Non-steroidal or pure antiandrogens interact with the androgen receptor and block the intracellular effects of T and DHT. Flutamide, nilutamide and Casodex® (bicalutamide) belong to this group of antiandrogens. The negative feedback of androgens at the hypothalamic level is also blocked, resulting in reflex increments of LH, T and DHT levels.

Monotherapy with non-steroidal antiandrogens is the only current endocrine treatment modality which does not lead to loss of sexual function. This has obvious implications for quality of life, especially in younger patients with a strong desire to preserve potency. However, the marked rise in serum T is disturbing because it may 'overcome' the blockade of androgen receptors by the antiandrogen [7]. Currently, no paraclinical method exists to monitor the blockade.

Clinically, non-steroidal antiandrogens have been used in long-term combination with either surgical or medical castration, as well as antiflare therapy when initiating treatment with LHRH agonists. Flutamide is being used as monotherapy in selected patients, but in fact, the efficacy of flutamide or nilutamide as monotherapy has not been compared to standard endocrine treatment in large randomized studies with sufficient statistical power [21]. Casodex®, in a daily dose of 50 mg, has been compared with orchidectomy or LHRH agonist treatment in three large international trials. A pooled analysis of almost 1200 patients demonstrated shorter progression-free and overall survival for patients treated with Casodex®, thus substantiating the fear that the androgen blockade with antiandrogen monotherapy may be insufficient at the dose of 50 mg [22]. None the less, because Casodex® was extremely well-tolerated, studies with higher doses were undertaken and data on fall in PSA after 3 months' therapy suggested improved efficacy, similar to castration. Currently, large studies with Casodex® 150 mg daily compared to castration are maturing. There is no doubt that a well-tolerated therapeutic modality, equally effective as castration but preserving sexual function, would constitute a major step forward.

In prostate cancer patients progressing following therapy with flutamide, either alone or in combination with orchidectomy or LHRH agonist, a *flutamide withdrawal response* has been reported by several authors following discontinuation of flutamide [23]. This phenomenon is explained by a change in the androgen receptor resulting in a stimulation by the antiandrogen. Logically, withdrawal response must be anticipated with other antiandrogens as well. However, the clinical implications of this for the future use of anti-androgens are far from clear.

Combinations

A possible role of adrenal androgens in prostatic cancer was already speculated in the 1940s, but results following bilateral adrenalectomy were disappointing with severe morbidity. However, following the appearance of antiandrogens the concept has received renewed attention. During the last decade, the concept of *total, combined, complete or maximal androgen blockade* has been extensively studied and discussed. The principle – elimination of testicular androgens by orchidectomy or LHRH agonists combined with an anti-androgen – is discussed in Chapter 16.

Another combination of endocrine therapies has lately attracted interest.

While *5 α-reductase inhibitors* do not have a role as monotherapy in prostate cancer, they may be of significant value in combination with non-steroidal antiandrogens. In principle, the combination is rational. While the first inhibits the formation of the most active androgen DHT, the latter blocks the androgen receptors. Further, the combination holds the possibility of maintained sexual function and low toxicity. Preliminary studies are encouraging and larger comparative studies are underway [24].

Timing of treatment

The indication for initiation of androgen deprivation in the management of prostate cancer is clear and near absolute in patients with spinal compression, ureteral obstruction and/or painful osseous metastases. Otherwise, no clear consensus exists on when to start hormonal therapy. While it is clear that endocrine therapy is palliative in nature and therefore should be administered with quality of life in the individual patient as first priority, it is also apparent that we do not have enough knowledge about the optimal timing and indications. Should such therapy be *immediate*, and commenced as soon as prostate cancer is diagnosed, although it is clear that the patient may be beyond curative reach, or should it be *deferred* until symptoms appear.

In the 1960s a large number of patients with advanced prostate cancer were randomized in the VACURG study [17] to immediate endocrine therapy versus placebo followed by deferred endocrine treatment when they became symptomatic. No difference in survival was demonstrated. With today's standard, the study had several methodological and analytic flaws, and a later reanalysis actually found that younger patients with poorly differentiated tumours gained some benefit from immediate endocrine therapy [25]. None the less, for many years this study formed the scientific basis for withholding endocrine therapy until symptoms appear, thus avoiding adverse effects and loss of sexual function for as long as possible.

However, a number of developments have renewed interest in immediate or at least *early* endocrine therapy. For instance more patients are diagnosed with early disease; new and well-tolerated treatment modalities like GnRH agonists and non-steroidal antiandrogens have increased patient compliance; interest in multimodal therapy has grown; and the introduction of PSA has enabled better monitoring of the disease process.

Apart from the fact that immediate endocrine therapy in some patients may satisfy a psychological need for therapeutic action instead of expectancy only, a number of questions should be answered before immediate endocrine therapy is advocated in general.

1 Will immediate endocrine therapy prolong the time to progression, and if so, does this translate into longer survival?

2 Will immediate endocrine therapy, by reducing the tumour burden, increase the effect of other therapies, i.e. surgery, irradiation, chemotherapy or other systemic treatment?

3 Will immediate endocrine therapy identify patients not responding to or failing androgen deprivation earlier than with deferred therapy? If so, will the patient's better general condition result in improved effectiveness of an often toxic second-line therapy?

Time to progression and survival

Concerning the first question, several uncontrolled and non-randomized studies have indicated a longer progression-free and overall survival associated with immediate endocrine therapy [26]. Large randomized trials are underway in both Europe and the USA. Preliminary data [27] strongly indicate a longer progression-free survival, while a longer overall survival has not yet been proven to result from immediate endocrine therapy.

If immediate therapy carries a clear advantage over deferred therapy, a logical consequence would be to investigate the effect of early endocrine therapy in early, organ-confined prostate cancer, especially in elderly patients not suited for surgery, while realizing that such treatment would have to be given for many years. Several cooperative groups are currently preparing protocols for such studies.

Neoadjuvant endocrine treatment

With regard to the second question, the concept of neoadjuvant endocrine therapy was introduced as early as 1944 [28] but has recently gained new momentum with the employment of reversible forms of androgen deprivation. While the ultimate goal for this concept must be improved prospects for cure with longer progression-free and overall survival, the more immediate aims of neoadjuvant endocrine therapy, usually given for 3 months before surgery [29] or radiation in patients with localized or locally advanced prostate cancer, are to reduce the tumour burden – *downsize* and possibly *downstage* (stage reduction) and *downgrade* the cancer. Subsequent surgery may be facilitated, and in the case of radiotherapy, tumour cell kill may be enhanced with fewer adverse effects due to reduced target volume.

Several uncontrolled and non-randomized studies have suggested that neoadjuvant therapy may induce stage reduction and in some cases down-

grading or even disappearance of the malignancy has been described. Prospective randomized studies are needed and several are underway in the USA
[30] and in Europe. At present, a cautious conclusion based on available
evidence is that neoadjuvant endocrine therapy does indeed downsize and to
some extent facilitates radical prostatectomy and reduces blood loss. Further,
prostate-specific antigen (PSA) measurements after 3 months of endocrine
therapy seem to hold important prognostic information about whether or not
the cancer is organ-confined. On the other hand, downstaging and down-
grading have not been convincingly demonstrated, and, most important, we
will have to wait for many years before any conclusions regarding progression-
free and overall survival can be drawn.

Secondary chemotherapy

Cytotoxic chemotherapy has traditionally been administered in later stages of
disease, when patients are generally weakened and therefore the true effectiveness of such treatment is difficult to ascertain. If the hormonal-refractory
patients are identified at an earlier point in the course of disease they may well
be able to tolerate more intensive chemotherapy with the possibility of
improved response rates. The introduction of PSA has meant that progression
following initial endocrine therapy can be demonstrated much earlier than
before, since a rise in PSA precedes both symptomatic and other objective
signs of progression, typically by 6 months. Several trials with a wide range of
second-line therapeutic modalities are ongoing or being planned in patients
with such early 'PSA progression'.

Intermittent endocrine therapy

Intermittent therapy adds further to the controversy surrounding the timing of
endocrine treatment. The cell death process induced by androgen withdrawal
is incomplete and surviving tumour cells progress to an androgen-independent
state. Bruchovsky and associates [11] found evidence that this progression is a
consequence of a lack of androgen-induced differentiation of stem cells in the
primary tumour with resultant loss of apoptotic potential; new growth factors
substituting for androgens and stimulating tumour growth may also be generated. Therefore, if androgen stimulation of the surviving stem cells were
resumed in a cyclic form, this could allow the tumour to repopulate with
androgen-sensitive cells with recovery of apoptotic potential and hence the
possibility of retreatment by androgen withdrawal [7, 31]. Potential benefits of
this intermittent therapy might include prolongation of the androgen-

dependent state of the tumour and, maybe, a better quality of life with recovery of libido and potency. While the principle has been tried before in the treatment of advanced prostate cancer, the use of PSA to monitor the cancer has formed the basis for a revived enthusiasm. Studies employing this principle are underway (see Chapter 4).

Chemoprevention

When debating the issue of timing, chemoprevention may be considered as the extreme use of early endocrine manipulation. As discussed, androgens play an important role in the development and progression of prostate cancer. The most powerful androgen in men is DHT, synthesized from T through the action of the enzyme 5α-reductase in the prostatic cell. 5α-reductase inhibitors competitively inhibit this enzyme and are capable of reducing prostate volume and serum PSA. The observations of the absence of prostate cancer in pre-pubertally castrated men, in men with 5α-reductase deficiency and in men with androgen-insensitive syndrome have given rise to the hypothesis that sup-pression of DHT with a 5α-reductase inhibitor before the development of clinically evident cancer may decrease the incidence of prostate cancer. A large chemopreventive study, prompted by the USA National Cancer Institute, with planned inclusion of 18 000 healthy males 55–70 years of age, randomizing between a 5α-reductase inhibitor (5 mg finasteride) or placebo, is presently recruiting in the USA.

Do patients have a choice?

In advanced-stage prostate cancer there is no other treatment with a 40–60% objective and a 70–80% subjective response rate and therefore in most symptomatic patients the decision to initiate endocrine therapy is not difficult. On the other hand, because of the current lack of precise knowledge about timing of therapy, the asymptomatic patient has an option. The patient should carefully be informed about the advantages of a possible longer progression-free survival, which should be weighed against the side-effects that endocrine treatment most often confers.

Once the decision to initiate endocrine therapy has been taken, the choice of therapeutic modality depends upon a number of variables.

1 *Previous cardiovascular disease.* Such patients should not be treated with oestrogens.

2 *Pharmacological aspects.* Patients considered to be endangered by immi-nent spinal compression or ureteral obstruction should not receive LHRH

agonists as monotherapy.

3 *Adverse effects.* Patients should be informed about the adverse effects that may be expected from various treatments.

4 *Patient compliance.* In mentally weakened patients, orchidectomy is preferable, and regimens including regular administration should be avoided.

5 *Patient preference.* Many patients are well-informed, especially about the possibility of potency preserving treatment with non-steroidal antiandrogens or the potential benefits of maximal androgen blockade.

6 *Cost.* In many countries, the patient will have to pay for at least part of the treatment. Considering that some of the pharmacological regimens are very costly, this aspect cannot be disregarded.

While the variety of treatment options has significantly complicated the information which must be given to the patient with prostate cancer, it has most certainly added to our ability as physicians to tailor an optimal treatment for the individual patient, keeping in mind that the best possible quality of life remains as the most important aim in a palliative treatment.

As discussed, the optimal use of endocrine manipulation in prostate cancer is not a settled issue, and intensive ongoing research will most probably bring further improvements in the near future.

References

* 1 Huggins C, Hodges CV. Studies on prostate cancer I: the effect of castration, of oestrogen and of androgen injection on serum phosphatases in metastatic carcinoma of the prostate. *Cancer Res* 1941; **1**: 293–297. [The first report showing the efficacy of endocrine therapy; or historical interest.]
* 2 Carter HB & Coffey DS. The prostate: an increasing medical problem. *Prostate* 1990; **16**: 39–48. [The authors demonstrate that prostate cancer constitutes a growing major health care problem.]
** 3 Griffiths K, Davies P, Eaton CL, Harper ME, Turkes A & Peeling WB. Endocrine factors in the initiation, diagnosis, and treatment of prostatic cancer. In: *Endocrine Dependent Tumors*, Voigt K-D & Knabbe C, eds. New York: Raven Press, 1991, pp. 83–130. [A comprehensive review of the endocrine regulation of the prostate with reference to current and future treatments.]
** 4 Coffey DS. The molecular biology, endocrinology, and physiology of the prostate and seminal vesicles. In: *Campbell's Urology*, Walsh PC, Retik AB, Stamey TA & Vaughan ED Jr, eds. Philadelphia: W.B. Saunders, 1992, pp. 221–266. [A comprehensive review of molecular biology, endocrinology and physiology of the prostate with a thorough reference list.]
* 5 Labrie F, Belanger A, Dupont A, Luu-The V, Simard J & Labrie C. Science behind total

* Reference of special interest.
** Reference of outstanding merit.

androgen blockade: from gene to combination therapy. *Clin Invest Med* 1993; **16**: 475–492. [Review of the rationale of total androgen blockade and arguments for its use.]

6 Oesterling JE, Epstein JI & Walsh PC. The inability of adrenal androgens to stimulate the adult human prostate: an autopsy evaluation of men with hypogonadotrophic hypogonadism and panhypopituitarism. *J Urol* 1986; **136**: 1030–1034. [Convincingly argues for the view that the adrenal glands are unable to stimulate prostatic growth.]

* 7 Bruchovsky N. Androgens and antiandrogens. In: *Cancer Medicine*, 3rd edn, Holland JF, Frei III E, Bast RC, Kufe DW, Morton DL & Weichselbaum RR. Philadelphia: Lea & Febiger, 1993, pp. 884–896. [A review of the biological effects of androgens and antiandrogens and the clinical application of the antiandrogens.]

* 8 Chisholm GD, Hedlund PO, Adolfsson J *et al*. The TNM system of 1992. Comments from the TNM working group. *Scand J Urol Nephrol* 1994; **162**: 107–114. [Classification and discussion of prognostic parameters in metastatic prostate cancer.]

9 Matzkin H, Eber P, Todd B, van der Zwaag R & Soloway MS. Prognostic significance of changes in prostatic-specific markers after endocrine treatment of stage D2 prostatic cancer. *Cancer* 1992; **70**: 2302–2309. [The authors show that pretreatment PSA level predicted disease progression and posttreatment normalization of PSA was prognostic of prolonged progression-free survival.]

10 Isaacs JT, Schulze H & Coffey DS. Development of androgen resistance in prostatic cancer. *Prog Clin Biol Res* 1987; **234A**: 21–29. [Experimental studies giving evidence for the existence of a mixture of hormone-dependent and hormone-independent cells before the initiation of hormonal treatment.]

11 Bruchovsky N, Rennie PS, Coldman AJ, Goldenberg SL, To M & Lawson D. Effects of androgen withdrawal on the stem cell composition of the Shionogi carcinoma. *Cancer Res* 1990; **50**: 2275–2282. [Experimental study that suggests that androgen deprivation 'escape' is a consequence of the ability of stem cells to adapt to the changed hormonal environment.]

*12 Isaacs JT & Coffey DS. Adaptation versus selection as the mechanism responsible for the relapse of prostatic cancer to androgen ablation therapy as studied in the Dunning R-3327-H adenocarcinoma. *Cancer Res* 1981; **41**: 5070–5075. [Experimental study suggesting that relapse of prostate cancer after androgen withdrawal is caused by growth of pre-existing clones of androgen-independent tumour cells.]

13 Conn PM & Crowley WF Jr. Gonadotrophin-releasing hormone and its analogues. *N Engl J Med* 1991; **324: 93–103. [An expert review of GnRH physiology and general considerations of therapy with GnRH agonists.]

14 Pinski J, Yano T, Miller G & Schally AV. Blockade of the LH response induced by the agonist D-Trp-6-LHRH in rats by a highly potent LH-RH antagonist SB-75. *Prostate* 1992; **20**: 213–224. [Experimental study of GnRH antagonists and a discussion of the potential clinical employment.]

15 Dijkman GA, Debruyne FMJ, Fernandez del Moral P *et al*. A randomised trial comparing the safety and efficacy of the Zoladex 10.8–mg Depot, administered every 12 weeks, to that of the Zoladex 3.6-mg Depot, administered every 4 weeks, in patients with advanced prostate cancer. *Eur Urol* 1995; **27**: 43–46. [This study shows the efficacy and safety of the long-acting depot formulation of Zoladex.]

*16 Ferro MA. Use of intravenous stilbestrol diphosphate in patients with prostatic carcinoma refractory to conventional hormonal manipulation. *Urol Clin North Am* 1991; **18**: 139–143. [Review of literature showing experimental evidence of direct cellular cytotoxicity of oestrogens and clinical efficacy in patients with otherwise hormone-refractory disease.]

*17 Byar DP. The Veterans Administration Cooperative Urological Research Group's studies of cancer of the prostate. *Cancer* 1973; **32**: 1126–1130. [The epoch-making VACURG studies showing the excess incidence of cardiovascular deaths following DES treatment and suggesting that delayed hormonal therapy has no adverse effects on survival.]

*18 Johansson J-E, Andersson S-O, Holmberg L & Bergström R. Primary orchidectomy versus oestrogen therapy in advanced prostatic cancer – a randomized study: results after 7 to 10 years of followup. *J Urol* 1991; **145**: 519–523. [This study with long-term follow-up shows oestrogen therapy to be more efficient than orchidectomy in terms of time-to-progression but also with excess incidence of cardiovascular morbidity and mortality.]

19 Henriksson P, Blombäck M, Bratt G, Edhag O & Eriksson A. Activators and inhibitors of coagulation and fibrinolysis in patients with prostatic cancer treated with oestrogen or orchidectomy. *Thromb Res* 1986; **44**: 783–791. [Oral oestrogens cause an increased production of coagulation factors responsible for the increase in cardiovascular side-effects.]

20 Stege R & Sander S. Endocrine treatment of prostatic cancer. A renaissance for parenteral estrogen. *Tidsskr Nor Laegeforen* 1993; **113**: 833–835. [Study showing that parenteral oestrogens cause no change in liver function and therefore probably no increase in cardiovascular side-effects.]

21 Delaere KPJ & Van Thillo EL. Flutamide monotherapy as primary treatment in advanced prostatic carcinoma. *Semin Oncol* 1991; **18**: 13–18. [A study of flutamide monotherapy and a review of previous studies, concluding that clinical results are encouraging but efficacy unsettled.]

22 Iversen P. Update of monotherapy trials with the new anti-androgen, Casodex (ICI 176,334). *Eur Urol* 1994; **26**(suppl 1): 5–9. [Casodex (50 mg/day) was shown to be inferior to castration, yet was very well-tolerated and further studies at higher doses are in progress.]

*23 Kelly WK & Scher HI. Prostate specific antigen decline after antiandrogen withdrawal: the flutamide withdrawal syndrome. *J Urol* 1993; **149**: 607–609. [This article shows that discontinuation of antiandrogen therapy may trigger a sustained decline in PSA values and may be an appropriate first step before more toxic therapies.]

*24 Fleshner NE & Trachtenberg J. Treatment of advanced prostate cancer with the combination of finasteride plus flutamide: early results. *Eur Urol* 1993; **24**(suppl 2): 106–112. [Pilot study, in which the combination of finasteride and flutamide was well-tolerated. Eight of 10 patients remained potent.]

*25 Sarosdy MF. Do we have a rational treatment plan for stage D-1 carcinoma of the prostate? *World J Urol* 1990; **8**: 27–33. [A reanalysis of the VACURG study I and II showing that those patients who received early oestrogen treatment did better than those with deferred treatment; new randomized studies of the timing of treatment are very much needed.]

26 Kozlowski JM, Ellis WJ & Grayhack JT. Advanced prostatic carcinoma. Early versus late endocrine therapy. *Urol Clin North Am* 1991; **18: 15–24. [A comprehensive review of early versus late endocrine treatment, strongly supporting early androgen deprivation.]

*27 van den Ouden D, Tribukait B, Blom JHM *et al.* Deoxyribonucleic acid ploidy of core biopsies and metastatic lymph nodes of prostate cancer patients: impact on time to progression. *J Urol* 1993; **150**: 400–406. [Interim analysis of a prospective, randomized study of early versus delayed endocrine treatment, showing that early treatment was associated with significantly longer time-to-progression.]

28 Vallett BS. Radical perineal prostatectomy subsequent to bilateral orchiectomy. *Del Med J* 1944; **16**: 1–7.

*29 Witjes WPJ, Horenblas S, Oosterhof GON, Schaafsma HE & Debruyne FMJ. Neoadjuvant therapy in prostate cancer – is it of any use? *Eur Urol* 1993; **24**: 433–437.

*30 Labrie F, Cusan L, Gomez-L *et al*. Down-staging of early stage prostate cancer before radical prostatectomy: the first randomized trial of neoadjuvant combination therapy with flutamide amid a luteinizing hormone-releasing hormone agonist. *Urology* 1994; **44**: 29–37.

*31 Akakura K, Bruchovsky N, Goldenberg SL, Rennie PS, Buckley AR & Sullivan LD. Effects of intermittent androgen suppression on androgen-dependent tumors: apotosis and serum prostate-specific antigen. *Cancer* 1993; **71**: 2782–2790.

32 Peeling WB. Phase III studies to compare gloserelin (Zoladex) with orchidectomy and with diethylstilboestrol in treatment of prostatic carcinoma. *Urology* 1989; **33**(suppl 5): 45–52.

33 Haapiainen R, Ranniko S, Ruutu M *et al*. Orchidectomy versus oestrogen in the treatment of advanced prostate cancer. *Br J Urol* 1991; **67**: 184–187.

34 Waymont B, Lynch TH, Dunn JA *et al*. Phase III randomised study of Zoladex versus stilboestrol in the treatment of advanced prostate cancer. *Br J Urol* 1992; **69**: 614–620.

35 Béland G, Elhilali M, Fradet Y *et al*. A controlled trial of castration with and without nilutamide in metastatic prostatic carcinoma. *Cancer* 1990; **66**: 1074–1079.

36 Janknegt RA, Abbou CC, Bartoletti R *et al*. Orchiectomy and nulutamide or placebo as treatment of metastatic prostatic cancer in a multinational double-blind randomised trial. *J Urol* 1993; **149**: 77–83.

37 Iversen P, Christensen MG, Friis E *et al*. A phase III trial of Zoladex and flutamide versus orchiectomy in the treatment of patients with advanced carcinoma of the prostate. *Cancer* 1990; **66**: 1058–1066.

38 Keuppens F, Denis L, Smith P *et al*. Zoladex and flutamide versus bilateral orchiectomy. A randomized Phase III E O R T C 30853 study. *Cancer* 1990; **66**: 1045–1057.

39 Denis LJ, Whelan P, Carneiro de Moura J *et al*. Goserelin acetate and flutamide versus bilateral orchiectomy: A phase III E O R T C trial (30853). *J Urol* 1993; **42**: 119–129.

40 Crawford ED, Eisenberg MA, McLeod DG *et al*. A controlled trial of leuprolide with and without flutamide in prostatic carcinoma. *N Eng J Med* 1989; **321**: 419–424.

16/Endocrine Treatment – Should it be Total (Maximal) Blockade?

L. Denis

Introduction

Modern treatment for prostate cancer was conceived by Huggins *et al.* [1] more than 50 years ago and is based upon research and investigations that showed the key role played by androgens in the control of normal and neo-plastic growth of the prostate. In a series of studies on treatment of prostate cancer, Huggins *et al.* established the effect of castration on the tumour and the benefit to the patient which could follow, but they were very careful to label this effect as palliative treatment. Based on these landmark studies, endocrine treatment and surgical castration in particular became the 'gold standard' for first-line treatment of symptomatic prostate cancer. The under-lying principle was to stop prostate cancer cells from stimulation by the available androgens so that arrest of growth and regression of tumour would occur over a period of time to induce a clinical remission, or stabilization or no change of disease. The results were impressive but not perfect, because stan-dard endocrine treatment showed objective remission in 40–60% of cases with 60–85% of subjective remissions [2].

Consequently, the search for more effective endocrine treatment was on, and a myriad of medical treatments led by the orally active diethylstilboestrol (DES) have been tested in clinical practice to find better or 'a best' form of endocrine treatment. Traditionally, these have relied upon withdrawal of androgens from the environment of prostate cancers by surgical or medical castration but more recently antiandrogens that block androgen action directly within prostate cells have been available. However, it has always been a source of concern that after castration androgens of adrenocortical origin remain present and could have a small, but significant, stimulatory effect on prostate cancer cells. This has led to the concept of total androgen blockade whereby treatment by castration is combined with an antiandrogen acting within prostate cancer cells to block adrenal androgens. Steroidal antiandrogens exert dual endocrine action for they inhibit the release of luteinizing hormone but also block intracellular binding of 5α-dihydrotestosterone (DHT) to its receptor in prostatic cells. The most important steroidal antiandrogen in use is cyproterone acetate (CPA), as medroxyprogesterone acetate and chlormadinone acetate are no longer popular. The pure antiandrogens that have recently been developed are non-steroidal, such as flutamide, nilutamide and bicalutamide, and they exert their influence by directly blocking the androgen receptor. Many different treatments have been tested; Table 16.1 lists those still used in daily clinical practice for first-line treatment.

Table 16.1 Current first-line endocrine treatment.

Androgen withdrawal
Bilateral orchidectomy (subcapsular)
Luteinizing hormone releasing hormone agonists (LHRH A)
Oestrogens
    Diethylstilboestrol 1 mg
    Estramustine phosphate

Androgen blockade
Antiandrogens
    Steroid: cyproterone acetate
    Pure: flutamide, bicalutamide, nilutamide

Combination treatment: maximal androgen blockade
Castration (surgical/medical) and pure antiandrogens

Endocrine basis of total androgen blockade

A major innovation in endocrine therapy for prostate cancer has been the introduction of luteinizing hormone releasing hormone agonists (LHRH A) which, on chronic administration, have been proved to be as effective as surgical castration in the management of symptomatic prostate cancer [3]. However, it is frequently ignored that the effects of endocrine agents are dose-dependent so that not all efforts to achieve castration result in castrate levels of serum testosterone (T) and not all efforts to block androgenic stimulation have similar responses. For example, in the randomized trials of the Veterans Administration Cooperative Urological Research Group (VACURG), 0.2 mg daily of DES did not reduce serum T to castrate levels [4], nor did 200 mg daily of medroxyprogesterone in the randomized trials of the European Organization of Research and Treatment of Cancer (EORTC) [5].

Equally ignored is the fact, previously known to Huggins, that the adrenals secrete large amounts of steroids, some of which can be transformed into active androgens. It has been demonstrated that steroids of adrenal origin can be converted by prostatic tissues *in vitro* and *in vivo* into T and DHT [6]. These observations explain the fact that high concentrations of DHT have been measured in prostate cancer tissue after castration [7]. At the present time, there is agreement that serum T levels are reduced by 90–95% after proper castration but that the tissue concentration of DHT, which is the most potent androgen affecting the prostate, is decreased by only 50–60%. This biological situation suggests that neutralization of the action of these androgens by inhibitors of androgen biosynthesis or by blockade of receptors by an antiandrogen might increase the response rate to endocrine treatment and benefit men suffering from prostate cancer. The critical level above which growth is not arrested in a human cancer cell line (PC82) is equivalent to the tissue concentration of T and DHT found in castrated men [8]. However, Geller and Candari demonstrated that 7 of 38 castrated patients showed DHT levels over this critical threshold [9].

These were the concepts upon which Huggins and Scott introduced surgical adrenalectomy as early as 1945, and hypophysectomy at a later stage, to obtain secondary remissions in patients with prostate cancer suffering relapse after initial endocrine treatment [10]. The high surgical mortality and morbidity rates coupled with a short duration of response decreased the enthusiasm for these procedures despite objective and subjective responses that were reported in some small phase II studies.

However, introduction of antiandrogens as second-line hormonal treatment followed the same concept and additional clinical responses ranging from 6 to 15% patients were confirmed [11]. This concept had already been promoted by Bracci using CPA [12] and was later expanded by Labrie *et al.* using nilutamide initially and flutamide later [13]. Thus, the concept of total androgen blockade was born.

Clinical results of total androgen blockade

The positive and enthusiastic reports about total androgen blockade from Bracci and Labrie created much interest from several clinical groups. The term total androgen blockade was first adopted but afterwards was baptized more realistically as complete androgen blockade or deprivation by the US intergroup study (CAB–CAD) and maximal androgen blockade (MAB) by the urological group of the EORTC. In this review, MAB will be preferred.

A landmark trial to evaluate the clinical credibility of MAB was introduced in North America (INT0036) in 1985. This was a phase II randomized, double-blind, placebo-controlled trial designed to compare time to progression and survival in patients with metastatic prostate cancer treated either with leuprorelin (1 mg subcutaneously per day) and placebo or by MAB with leuprorelin (1 mg/day) and flutamide (250 mg t.i.d.). A total of 603 patients were studied. Despite a higher incidence of diarrhoea and gastrointestinal disturbances in the group receiving MAB, the results with regard to progression-free survival (16.5 months for MAB versus 13.9 months for medical castration with placebo) and increased median length of survival (35.6 versus 28.3 months) were statistically in favour of the combination treatment [14]. These differences were particularly evident for patients with minimal metastatic disease and good performance status but statistical power was lacking to validate these results. Indeed, the statistical power aimed to detect a 40% improvement in median survival time from 3 to 4.2 years and a 30% improvement in the median progression-free survival time from 65 to 85 weeks.

In the meantime, the EORTC had launched three randomized trials on MAB treatment in patients with M1 disease prostate cancer (Table 16.2).

The first trial (EORTC 30805 – study coordinator M.R.G. Robinson) evaluated three arms of treatment. These were: (i) bilateral orchidectomy; (ii) DES 1 mg t.i.d.; and (iii) bilateral orchidectomy with CPA 50 mg t.i.d. There were 351 patients in this study. Unlike the North American study (INT0036), in this trial there were no significant differences observed between any treatment arm with regard to time to progression or overall survival resulting from two analyses, of which the second dates from 1988 [15].

The second trial (EORTC 30843 – study coordinator H.J. de Voogt) was an open three-arm study in which 368 patients were randomized to treatment by: (i) bilateral orchidectomy; (ii) the LHRH analogue buserelin (400 µg t.i.d. intranasally) with CPA 50 mg t.i.d. for 14 days; and (iii) buserelin 400 µg t.i.d.

Table 16.2 Scheme of three consecutive European Organization of Research and Treatment of Cancer (EORTC) phase III studies on maximal androgen withdrawal.

30805: Study coordinator M. Robinson
Bilateral orchidectomy
Bilateral orchidectomy + CPA 50 mg t.i.d.
DES 1 mg daily

30843: Study coordinator H. de Voogt
Bilateral orchidectomy
Buserelin 400 µg + CPA 50 mg t.i.d. 14 days
Buserelin 400 µg + CPA 50 mg t.i.d.

30853: Study coordinator L. Denis
Bilateral orchidectomy
Zoladex® (gloserelin) + flutamide 250 mg t.i.d.

CPA, cyproterone acetate; DES, diethylstilboestrol.

with CPA 50 mg t.i.d. continuously. The mean follow-up time was 2 years and no significant differences between these treatment arms regarding time to progression, survival and cancer deaths were observed [16].

These disappointing results made most clinicians sceptical about the clinical idea of MAB and led the EORTC group to embark on a third phase III two-arm trial (EORTC 30853). As bilateral orchidectomy was judged to be the 'gold standard' for endocrine treatment of advanced prostate cancer, in this study its effectiveness was compared with MAB given as goserelin depot 3.6 mg injected subcutaneously once monthly with flutamide 250 mg t.i.d. in patients with metastatic disease and good performance status. This trial accrued 327 patients from March 1986 to May 1988 and its statistical power aimed to detect a 50% difference in median time to progression and survival and 20% difference in the response rate. Extensive quality control was established to monitor changes in both objective and subjective parameters of progression and six *ad hoc* independent committees were set up to monitor pathology, endocrine results, bone scan evaluation, response criteria, quality of life and prostate-specific antigen (PSA) evaluation.

This study set out to disprove the clinical importance of MAB in view of previous EORTC and other trials, but the results decided otherwise. As early as 1989, statistically significant different responses between the two treatment regimens had been noted as well as increased time to progression for patients receiving the combination treatment. With regard to response, elevated acid phosphatase levels normalized in 57% of patients treated by orchidectomy in comparison with normalization in 70% of men treated by MAB ($P = 0.005$). Furthermore, in patients treated by MAB in this trial, subjective progression was delayed by 35 weeks ($P = 0.009$), objective progression was delayed by 48 weeks ($P = 0.008$) and median duration of survival was prolonged by 7.3 months [17]. These observations are similar to the data from INT0036. The advantages of MAB in the EORTC 30853 trial in terms of P values, hazard ratios and confidence intervals after a median follow-up of 5 years are shown in Table 16.3.

However, by the time these mature data had been determined, a number of small trials had been published showing no advantage to MAB treatment. There was, therefore, considerable disillusion and confusion among clinicians because no study had reported the excellent results of the earlier Phase II studies of Labrie *et al.* [13].

Consequently, it was decided to undertake a meta-analysis and an international group was created in 1989, followed by two workshops in 1990 and 1992 (Table 16.4). The findings of a third workshop were published in 1993 [18].

Table 16.3 EORTC 30853 – advantages for MAB treatment.

Parameter	*P* value	Hazard ratio	95% CI
Time to:			
Subjective progression	0.009	0.67	0.50–0.90
Objective progression	0.008	0.64	0.46–0.89
First progression	0.002	0.64	0.49–0.84
Death	0.02	0.73	0.56–0.95
Death from cancer	0.007	0.67	0.49–0.90

CI, confidence interval.

Table 16.4 Workshops leading to the organization of an overview (meta-analysis) on maximum androgen blockade treatment in prostate cancer.

1989	Atlanta: American Cancer Society (ACS) Comparability of four trials
1990	Paris: European Organization of Research and Treatment of Cancer (EORTC) Feasibility of an overview
1992	Paris: International Prostate Health Council (IPHC) Organizing an overview

In 1994, the results of the overview analysis were presented by Dalesio to a satellite meeting of the European Association of Urology in Berlin. She concluded that the evidence from the overview did not support the hypothesis that MAB is associated with a reduction of mortality from locally advanced or metastatic prostate cancer when compared with treatment by castration alone. However, the confidence intervals were so large that it was not possible to differentiate between no effect and a small effect. This created a further wave of confusion which was unnecessary because the problems arising from the overview analysis had been carefully analysed in the conclusions of the third workshop [19]. It had been emphasized that prognostic factors had been largely ignored in the overview, with the result that widely different cohorts of patients had been analysed as a single group. A further problem arose from the number of events not shown in the analysis that compromised the final conclusion. Last but not least, an elegant computer model system devised by Blumenstein demonstrated that most trials had been underpowered and that most trials lacked maturity at the time of the overview analysis [20].

Two fundamental observations emerged from the overview analysis and from increasing clinical experience with MAB. The first was that no study which had used CPA as a combination therapy had shown benefit in favour of

MAB. The second observation concerns the flutamide withdrawal syndrome in which serum PSA decreases after withdrawal of an antiandrogen in patients in whom PSA increases after an extended period of remission [21].

In conclusion, at the present time all the clinical trials which have used a pure antiandrogen in sufficiently large numbers of patients show some benefit in response, time to objective progression and sometimes survival [22]. The question of the size of the clinical advantage is also clinically relevant.

Indications for MAB treatment

There is consensus that endocrine treatment using an LHRH A in patients with widespread metastatic prostate cancer is enhanced by addition of an antiandrogen in the first 14 days of treatment to avoid a clinical flare-up of the disease [23].

The subgroups that benefit most from MAB treatment are those with good prognostic factors and minimal metastatic disease. In particular, the difference in time to progression can exceed 18 months. Unfortunately, conclusive statistical evidence is lacking due to small numbers of patients in the trials. Therefore, the statistical analysis of a 1300-patient trial (INT0105) is eagerly awaited to solve these issues. Meanwhile, experience to the present time suggests that MAB in general offers limited benefits and is of minimal advantage to those patients with poor prognostic factors. More benefit is likely for patients with a good prognosis.

We favour quality of life as the guiding principle for treatment of individual patients. While MAB should be the standard control arm in new clinical trials of treatment, for individual patients a tailored treatment regimen based on the patient's choice is acceptable provided that this is closely supervised. This would appear to be the view of the majority of urologists, judging from the international meeting held in Paris in 1994. When questioned in a panel discussion, 89% voted for MAB as primary treatment for patients with M1 prostate cancer. However, 21% restricted their preference for use of MAB to patients suffering from symptomatic disease and 25% to patients with good prognostic factors [23]. Still, it appears that most urologists practise palliative tailored treatment inasmuch as 61% would suggest antiandrogen monotherapy in preference to MAB in clinical situations where patients emphasize potency as a treatment outcome.

Cost-effectiveness of MAB treatment

The cost of MAB treatment has to be balanced between the health advantage gained and the toxicity, together with the cash expense of antiandrogens added to castration. The overall toxicity of antiandrogens can reach up to 10% of treated cases with mostly gastrointestinal problems and, rarely, increases of liver enzymes. Both of these adverse effects are reversible after withdrawal of the drugs.

The financial cost of MAB treatment has been calculated at US$ 2250 per year per patient. Recent studies have suggested that MAB is as expensive as other life-prolonging treatments such as renal dialysis [24]. However, common sense should guide a clinician's recommendations for treatment and it was of great interest that 68% of the urologists present at the Paris meeting in 1994 let the initiation of MAB treatment be influenced by the age of individual patients.

Conclusion

MAB aims to be the 'gold standard' of treatment for patients with M1 prostate cancer but more supporting data are needed to define its precise place in different cohorts of patients, especially in those with earlier stages of the disease. Experience to date suggests that there is a case to recommend MAB to patients with good performance status and minimal metastatic disease.

References

1 Huggins C, Stevens RE & Hodges CV. Studies of prostatic cancer 2. The effects of castration on advanced carcinoma of the prostate gland. *Arch Surg* 1941; **43**: 209–228.

2 Denis L & Mahler C. Prostatic cancer: an overview. *Rev Oncol* 1990; **3**: 665–677.

* 3 Turkes AO, Peeling WB & Griffiths K. Treatment of patients with advanced cancer of the prostate. Phase III trial, Zoladex against castration; a study of the British Prostate Group. *J Steroid Biochem* 1987; **27**: 543–549.

* 4 Bailor JC & Byar DP. Estrogen treatment for cancer of the prostate: early results with 3 doses of diethylstilbestrol and placebo. *Cancer* 1970; **26**: 257–261.

5 Pavone-Macaluso M, de Voogt HJ, Viggiano G *et al.* Comparison of diethylstilbestrol, cyproterone acetate and medroxyprogesterone acetate in the treatment of advanced prostatic cancer: final analysis of a randomized phase III trial of the EORTC Urological Group. *J Urol* 1986; **136**: 624–631.

6 Harper ME, Pike A, Peeling WB & Griffiths K. Steroids of adrenal origin metabolized by human prostatic tissue *in vivo* and *in vitro. J Endocrinol* 1974; **60**: 117–125.

7 Farnsworth WE & Brown JR. Androgens of the human prostate. *Endocrinol Res Common* 1976; **3**: 105–117.

8 van Weerden WM, van Kreuningen A, Moerings EPCM, de Jong FH, van Steenbrugge GI & Schröder F. Assessment of the critical level of androgen for growth response of transplantable human prostatic carcinoma (PC82) in nude mice. *Urol Res* 1991; **19**: 1–5.

* Reference of special interest.

9 Geller J & Candari CD. Comparison of DHT levels in prostate cancer metastasis and primary prostatic cancer. *Prostate* 1989; **15**: 171–179.

10 Huggins C & Scott WW. Bilateral adrenalectomy in prostatic cancer: clinical features and urinary excretion of 17-ketosteroids and oestrogens. *Ann Surg* 1945; **122**: 10–31.

11 Labrie F, Dupont A, Giguere M *et al*. Benefits of combination therapy with flutamide in patients relapsing after castration. *Br J Urol* 1988; **61**: 341–346.

12 Bracci U. Anti-androgens in the treatment of prostatic cancer. *Eur Urol* 1979; **5**: 303–306.

13 Labrie F, Dupont A & Bélanger A. A complete androgen blockade for the treatment of prostate cancer. In: *Important Advances in Oncology*, de Vita VT, Hellman S, Rosenberg SA, eds. Philadelphia: JB Lippincott 1985, 193–200.

*14 Crawford ED, Eisenberger MA, McLeod DG *et al*. A controlled trial of leuprolide with and without flutamide in prostatic carcinoma. *N Engl J Med*, 1989; **321**: 419–424.

15 Robinson MRG. EORTC protocol 30805: A phase III trial. In: *Management of Advanced Carcinoma of the Prostate and Bladder*, Pavone-Macaluso M & Smith PH, eds. New York: Alan Liss, 1988; pp 101–110.

16 de Voogt HJ, Klijn JGM, Studer U *et al*. and members of the EORTC GU group. Orchidectomy versus buserelin in combination with cyproterone acetate, for 2 weeks continuously, in the treatment of metastatic prostatic cancer. Preliminary results of EORTC trial 30843. *J Steroid Biochem Mol Biol* 1990; **37**: 965–969.

*17 Denis LJ, Whelan P, Carneiro de Moura JL *et al*. and members of the EORTC GU Group and EORTC data center. Goserelin acetate and flutamide versus bilateral orchidectomy: a phase III EORTC trial (30853). *Urology* 1993; **42**: 119–129.

18 Denis L & Murphy GP. Third international workshop on randomized trials on maximal androgen blockade in M1 prostate cancer patients. *Cancer* 1993; **72**: 3781–3895.

*19 Denis L & Murphy GP. Overview of phase III trials on combined androgen treatment in patients with metastatic prostate cancer. *Cancer* 1993; **72**: 3888–3895.

20 Blumenstein BA. Some statistical considerations for the interpretation of trials of combined androgen therapy. *Cancer* 1993; **72**: 834–840.

21 Scher H & Kelly WK. Prostate specific antigen decline: its impact on clinical trials in hormone-refractory disease. *J Clin Oncol* 1993; **11**: 1566–1572.

22 Crawford ED & DeAntoni EP. Combined androgen blockade: an idea whose time has come. In: *Proceedings of the 4th International Symposium on Recent Advances in Urological Cancer*. Murphy G, Khoury S, Chatelain C & Denis L, eds. Paris: SCI 1995; pp 260–268.

23 Denis L. Adding anti-androgen to castration: is the controversy resolved? In: *Proceedings of the 4th International Symposium on Recent Advances in Urological Cancer*. Murphy G, Khoury S, Chatelain C, Denis L, eds. Paris: SCI, pp. 273–278.

24 Bennett CL, McLeod DG & Hillner BE. Estimating the cost-effectiveness of total androgen blockade for stage D2 prostate cancer. *Proc Am Meeting ASCO* 1994; **13**: A724.

Part 4
Monitoring Progress and Secondary Treatment

17/Detection of Relapsed Disease – Is Prostate-Specific Antigen Enough?

D.M. Bolton

Introduction

Since methods of hormonal manipulation to treat prostate cancer became available approximately 50 years ago, identification of relapsed or progressive prostate carcinoma has always played a crucial role during the posttreatment observation of this condition. Although techniques to detect persistence of disease and disease progression are now far more sophisticated than in earlier times, the principle underlying posttreatment surveillance remains the same – identification of increasing tumour volume in an attempt to determine the prognosis of the individual patient.

Traditionally urologists have relied upon digital rectal examination (DRE) to identify local progression of prostate carcinoma after radiation therapy or local recurrence after radical prostatectomy, and upon relatively non-specific modalities such as serum alkaline phosphatase, serum prostatic acid phosphatase and skeletal X-rays in order to detect occult or symptomatic distant metastases. With the evolution of biochemical and imaging technologies has come the availability of additional more advanced techniques for identifying prostate carcinoma in particular circumstances, such as serum prostate-specific antigen (PSA) determination, nuclear scintigraphy, computed tomography (CT), transrectal ultrasonography (TRUS) and magnetic resonance imaging (MRI). Each of these diagnostic methods has a valuable and distinct role to play in the detection of relapsed disease, but appropriate use and recognition of their limitations to provide the best possible treatment outcome for patients with prostate carcinoma remain one of the major challenges in the contemporary management of this condition.

Serum prostate-specific antigen determination

Since its initial applications to prostatic adenocarcinoma were identified [1], this antigenic protein component of human seminal plasma has come to play a prominent and crucial role in almost all aspects of the detection and management of prostate cancer. However, in no area of prostate cancer treatment has it achieved such a pre-eminent role as in the detection and monitoring of relapsed disease.

PSA is produced almost exclusively by the epithelial cells of the prostate gland, and thus lends itself almost ideally to posttreatment surveillance of those therapies that seek to remove all prostatic tissue, such as radical prostatectomy by retropubic or transperineal approaches. If a surgical cure has been achieved following such therapy, the serum PSA level should fall to undetectable levels, and except for rare reports of clinical recurrence without detectable serum levels [2], almost all men with recurrent or persistent disease should record a detectable serum concentration of this protein. Clinicians have now become familiar with the concept of serial PSA determinations after radical prosta-tectomy to document undetectable levels so as to determine the success of surgery in achieving a curative resection, and this remains the only diagnostic situation where an *absolute* serum PSA level will identify with certainty the long-term prognosis of an individual's prostatic carcinoma.

The serum PSA determination also plays a major but less precise role in the surveillance of prostate cancer after treatment by external-beam or implantable radiation therapy, and after institution of androgen deprivation therapy (previously often referred to as hormonal manipulation therapy). As PSA is produced and liberated into the serum by prostatic epithelium from normal glandular tissue, and from tissue of benign prostatic hyperplasia within the transition zone of the prostate gland in particular, a residual posttreatment serum level of PSA can be expected after treatment by these methods. Usually a serum PSA level taken soon after the completion of radiation therapy or after the institution of androgen deprivation therapy will demonstrate reduction of serum PSA concentration to a lower plateau level. This minimum posttreat-ment level has been termed the PSA nadir [3].

The level of the PSA nadir may function as both an important indicator of the response to treatment of prostatic carcinoma and as a baseline for deter-mining the likelihood of tumour progression after initial therapy. Although a low serum PSA level may not accurately reflect tumour burden, particularly in treatment with androgen deprivation, a nadir PSA which falls to within the normal range is usually associated with a prolonged remission of disease (Fig. 17.1). Similarly, an increasing serum PSA concentration heralds the onset of tumour progression after radiation, and of hormone insensitivity after androgen deprivation therapy.

Tumour recurrence after radical prostatectomy and tumour progression after radiation therapy as predicted by serial elevations of serum PSA above the nadir level are well-documented to precede detection of recurrent prostatic carcinoma by other traditional methods. This has led to the concept of *bio-chemical failure* of therapy, prior to the advent of any clinical evidence of

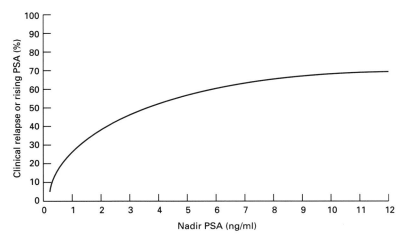

Fig. 17.1 Probability of clinical relapse or rising prostate-specific antigen (PSA) as a function of nadir PSA value after external-beam radiation therapy. After Zagars [22].

tumour after attempted curative methods of treatment have been employed. The variation in lead detection time has been estimated at between 5 months [4] and 3–7 years [5], depending upon the stage and grade of carcinoma concerned and upon the method of initial therapy. None the less, the identification of posttreatment PSA progression does not itself provide an absolute prediction of survival outcome, and does not allow differentiation between the local persistence of tumour and the existence of development of distant microscopic metastases. Similarly, a rise in PSA from nadir levels does not in itself provide a picture of the biological aggression of the individual carcinoma concerned. Much doubt also exists about the optimum method for managing such persistent or progressive carcinoma that may be identified only on the basis of PSA testing.

A feature of serum PSA increments above the nadir level which may provide insight into the likely behaviour of an individual carcinoma is the posttreatment *PSA doubling time*. When expressed more simply as a rate of increase of serum PSA per time elapsed, this tumour progression is often referred to as the *PSA velocity*. Serum PSA doubling times after radical retropubic prostatectomy where persistent tumour has been identified have been shown to increase at a far greater rate (median doubling time 4.3 months) for those patients who ultimately progressed to distant metastases than for those in whom a clinical local recurrence failed to progress to distant metastases or in whom a serum PSA elevation remained the only evidence of persistent disease (median doubling time 11.7 months) [6]. A short postradical prostatectomy PSA doubling time has been suggested as a criterion by which to select those patients with margin positive tumours at surgery for postoperative treatment with external-beam radiation therapy to the prostatic bed.

PSA doubling times have also been shown to be predictive for the time to clinical disease relapse following radiation therapy, with a high tumour grade correlating strongly with a reduced doubling time and a shorter time to clinical relapse (Fig. 17.2). Interestingly, the rate of decline of serum PSA during treatment by external-beam radiotherapy has also been identified as a strong positive predictor of relapse-free survival in those patients with an elevated baseline PSA value ($P < 0.0001$) [7]. As stated above, in all such studies the recognition of biochemical failure of therapy on the basis of a rising serum PSA level appears to precede clinical evidence of recurrent disease by months to years.

The usefulness of serum PSA determinations as a method for identifying relapsed disease after primary treatment has been further enhanced by the more recent development of ultrasensitive PSA assays. Such assays include the Yang Pros-Check, Abbott IMx, Tosoh AIA-PACK PA and the Nichols Institute PSA assays. The residential cancer detection limit for these four ultrasensitive assays has been stated as 0.06, 0.01, 0.07 and 0.05 ng/ml respectively [9] and these lower detection limits have permitted much earlier detection of

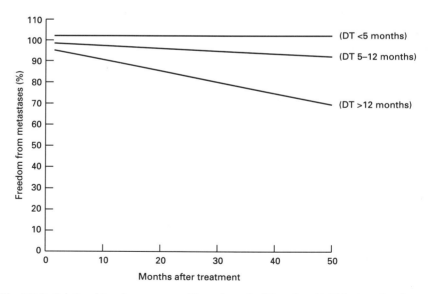

Fig. 17.2 Relationship of prostate-specific antigen doubling time (DT) in months after radiotherapy to freedom from metastases in management of prostate cancer. After Pollack *et al.* [8].

persistent disease following attempted curative therapy than has been available from routine radioimmunoassays for PSA. Because of the lower serum concentrations at which persistent carcinoma may now be identified, it has been estimated that approximately one-third more persistent carcinomas may be identified within the first 8 months after surgery than with traditional assays [10]. Assays for the serum concentration of the complex of PSA with α_1-antichymotrypsin have also been suggested as having potential in this regard for greater sensitivity in the earlier detection of biochemical failure after surgery [11]. Clearly, more widespread usage of these assays has the potential to affect both our knowledge of the incidence of relapsed prostatic carcinoma, and indeed the established figures for cure after radical prostatectomy and radiation therapy.

The predictive value of serum PSA determinations in identifying those patients at higher risk of harbouring residual prostatic carcinoma despite initial attainment of undetectable serum PSA levels after radical prostatectomy may be further enhanced by techniques to identify the serum half-life of PSA in such circumstances. It has been suggested that residual prostatic adenocarcinoma prolongs the half-life of PSA by contributing to minute serum concentrations of this protein [12]. The half-life of serum PSA in patients who appear to have undergone curative resection of prostatic carcinomas has been calculated as 1.6 days. This period is considerably shorter than that calculated in reports on general patient populations regardless of the stage of any carcinoma present and the outcome of any treatment undertaken, where the accepted serum half-life of PSA is over 4.6 days. This latter figure also implies that determination of serum PSA values at less than 1 month after attempted curative surgery for prostatic carcinoma is of little value in the detection or exclusion of residual malignant tissue [13]. The standard serum PSA level at 3 months after definitive treatment has been demonstrated to be a reliable prognostic factor for future tumour recurrence, particularly following external-beam radiation therapy [14].

Typically, an extremely small, but often biochemically detectable amount of PSA in serum may arise by secretion from the urethral mucosa and the periurethral glands. Determination of the extent of the contribution of this form of PSA to serum levels or to samples taken by urethral swabs after surgery or radiotherapy has not been shown to correlate with likelihood of tumour persistence or with long-term prognosis [15]. More likely, however, is that PSA of this origin serves to explain those cases where low levels of PSA are evident after apparently curative therapy, and yet no clinical evidence of recurrence can be identified even after long-term surveillance.

Transrectal ultrasonography

One investigation which does appear, in conjunction with serum PSA level determination, to increase the yield of identification of tumour recurrence after attempted curative treatment of prostate adenocarcinoma is TRUS and ultrasound-directed biopsy. This technique appears from clinical studies to be more efficacious in this regard than DRE of the prostate bed in association with serum PSA [16]. Ultrasound findings which are considered to be suspicious for local tumour persistence include any unusual hypoechoic tissue adjacent to the bladder neck, retrotrigone or anastomotic site, and TRUS-guided biopsy of such lesions has now effectively replaced traditional trans-urethral methods of biopsy. Although the value of radiation therapy to such local tumour persistence after radical prostatectomy remains debatable, this combination of techniques appears to offer the greatest likelihood of positive detection of residual carcinoma which may be targeted for local treatment after attempted curative therapy and where posttreatment PSA levels have sequentially risen. In conjunction with its established preoperative role to detect and stage prostate cancer, where cancer detected by DRE has repeatedly been demonstrated to be more pathologically advanced and more likely to be non-organ-confined at radical prostatectomy than that identified on the basis of serum PSA elevation and subsequent TRUS-directed sextant prostate biopsy [17], this application clearly identifies TRUS as a technique of key importance in the contemporary management of prostatic adenocarcinoma.

The likelihood that this combination of procedures will be eventually found to yield a positive and treatable result may also be estimated to a significant degree of accuracy early in the postoperative period simply by careful and detailed examination of the excised specimen following radical prosta-tectomy. This fundamental aspect of surgical assessment is often now neglected in view of the sophisticated biochemical and imaging procedures available to the clinician, yet in the immediate postoperative period this procedure remains the most accurate guide to long-term prognosis. Using actuarial analysis, the 10-year likelihood of freedom from PSA relapse was identified in one study as 85% for men with organ-confined disease, 82% where focal capsular penetration was evident, 54% with established capsular penetration and low Gleason score (2–6) and 42% with high Gleason score (7 or higher) under the same circumstances, and 43% where seminal vesicle involvement is apparent [18]. Neural sheath involvement has also been identified as a potentially poor prognostic factor for biochemical and clinical failure following margin-negative radical prostatectomy, as has a non-diploid assessment of the primary tumour on nuclear protein flow-cytometry. Such information, which appears consistent with our treatment experience with clinically localized prostatic carcinoma, should not be overlooked in an attempt to provide optimal posttreatment surveillance for all patients after radical surgery. It may be that less expensive, time-consuming and costly follow-up protocols can be utilized for certain patients after attempted curative surgery for prostate cancer who appear at a relatively lower risk for tumour recurrence.

It would appear then on the basis of contemporary published experience that in this era of precise evaluation and surveillance of biochemical failures with serum PSA determinations, together with the potential for precise imaging of local recurrences using TRUS in conjunction with traditional digital examination of the prostatic bed, that other diagnostic tools would have little role to play in the detection of relapsed disease. Certainly this is so in the early phase of follow-up after apparently successful radical prostatectomy or radiation therapy for localized disease. However in most other situations where surveillance of prostate cancer is undertaken, these additional forms of assessment continue to have a substantial role to play.

Nuclear isotopic bone scanning

Isotopic bone scanning, traditionally undertaken using technetium-99m methylene diphosphonate because of its high bone–soft-tissue distribution ratio and the rapidity of imaging permitted, retains a significant role in the detection of metastatic disease. Although isotopes will be concentrated in all areas of increased bone turnover and not metastatic lesions alone, this investigation will usually permit exclusion of bone secondary tumour deposits if the scan is negative for focal areas of increased activity. Such areas, when identified, can be further investigated to confirm or exclude the presence of metastases using conventional bone radiography. In the detection of relapsed disease isotopic bone scanning currently has a valuable role to play in excluding the need for pelvic lymph node sampling where this is under consideration before instituting additional or initial radiotherapy for localized or locally recurrent prostate carcinoma, and in determining a time for the institution of androgen deprivation therapy where an observant approach to such treatment has been undertaken, again either after initial attemptive curative therapies have failed or as a *per primam intentionem* treatment strategy. Isotopic bone scanning has effectively replaced bone marrow aspiration as a method for identifying occult bone metastases. However, bone marrow biopsy may occasionally still be used in conjunction with skeletal radiography to exclude the presence of secondary deposits at equivocal sites of increased isotope uptake on nuclear scans.

Pelvic lymph node sampling

In the detection of relapsed disease pelvic lymph node sampling may also serve
to exclude regional metastases, and so prevent the institution of local radiotherapy to the prostate gland or the postresection prostate bed following
radical prostatectomy, where no benefit in terms of disease control is likely to
be obtained. The clinical application of this diagnostic procedure has become
more widespread in recent years since the development of laparoscopic surgical
techniques (see Chapter 12). Although this operation finds its greatest use for
initial staging of prostate carcinoma in the period after initial presentation
when an individual patient's treatment plan is being developed, the low
morbidity and minimal hospitalization involved have resulted in an expansion
of the clinical indications for which it is now considered. Amongst such more
recently popularized indications include the staging of locally persistent disease
after radical prostatectomy where a perioperative lymph node sampling has not
been undertaken due to the choice of a transperineal approach to the gland or
in view of a low PSA at the time of surgery, which is an increasing trend in
those patients with low PSA prostate carcinoma presenting with clinical stage
T1c disease.

Lymphangiography has effectively been discarded as a method of identification of regional metastases, as traditionally this investigation has identified
such lesions in only approximately 50% of affected patients due to its inability
to identify micrometastases and to image the hypogastric and presacral lymph
node chains.

Computed tomography scanning

CT scanning retains a significant role in the detection of relapsed prostatic
adenocarcinoma. Although also unable to identify accurately instances of
micrometastatic disease in pelvic lymph nodes, it does allow for guided sampling using fine-needle aspiration technology of any enlarged lymph nodes
identified. It also provides for detection of extraprostatic spread of carcinoma
of prostatic bed tumour recurrence after radical surgery with a degree of
sensitivity accepted approximately to equal that of TRUS. Distortion of the
capsular plane and thickening in the periprostatic connective tissues are the
hallmarks of extraglandular progression of tumour, and when used with the
aim of identifying relapsed disease there is less likelihood of confusion of these
features with postbiopsy haemorrhage artifact which may be present after the
initial staging of disease in an individual patient. Local recurrences after radical
prostatectomy will usually present as a soft-tissue density mass in the region of

the vesicourethral anastomosis. As with all imaging techniques with a role to play in the detection of treatment failures, CT scanning should be performed only on the basis of suspicion of failure aroused by clinical examination or on the basis of an elevated surveillance PSA, and not as an investigation in the routine follow-up of patients after attempted curative treatment. CT of localized skeletal sites may also be used to help exclusion of metastatic disease at the site of increased tracer activity on isotopic bone scan.

Magnetic resonance imaging

MRI of the prostate gland is a technique which has been available to clinicians managing prostate adenocarcinoma since the early 1980s. However, it has yet to find an established place in the detection of relapsed cases of this disease. This is largely due to the degree to which CT and TRUS have become integral methods of investigating instances of elevated PSA after initial treatment or following primary observation therapy. These techniques have an advantage over MRI by their greater availability, lower cost and the absence of the need for use of a rectal coil in order to provide optimum imaging. Local or lymph node recurrences also cannot be biopsied under MRI direction using conventional techniques. None the less, excellent visualization of local disease relapse is obtainable using magnetic resonance methods, and this imaging modality may occasionally function as an accessory to others in the assessment of possible tumour recurrence.

Newer imaging techniques

Additional imaging techniques with obvious clinical potential for usage in the identification of relapsed adenocarcinoma of the prostate are also appearing on the horizon. These include radioimmunoscintigraphy using indium-111 labelled CYT-356 (7E11-C5.3-glycyl-tyrosyl-(N,e-diethylenetriaminepenta-acetic acid)-lysine [19]. This agent has been demonstrated as being able to identify with an encouraging degree of sensitivity occult sites of recurrent prostate cancer in patients who had previously undergone radical prostatectomy and in whom a persistently elevated serum PSA level was apparent. Although the specificity of this investigation is not yet equivalent to that seen with conventional isotopic bone scanning, and the injection to imaging period is far more prolonged at between 2 and 4 days, this technique possesses great potential for future application in the detection and treatment of recurrent, small-volume prostate cancer.

Serum prostatic acid phosphatase

The role of serum acid phosphatase (PAP) level determination in the identification of recurrent prostatic carcinoma remains controversial. This enzyme, first associated with prostate cancer metastases in 1938 [20], was one of the first tumour markers in any branch of clinical oncology and for many decades formed the cornerstone of assessment of the extent and curability of an individual patient's prostate carcinoma. The later discovery of a more specific prostatic component of this enzyme titre, inhibitable by tartrate and preferentially hydrolysing certain substrates such as β-glycerophosphate and thymolphthalein monophosphate, added further to its role as the dominant factor in assessing the prognosis of clinically organ-confined prostate cancer [21]. Although serum levels of PAP may occasionally be raised as a result of prostatitis, prostatic infarction, and even rarely obstructive benign prostatic hyperplasia, the enzyme is able to enter far more easily into the circulation from cells of prostate adenocarcinoma, in much the same manner as PSA. Elevation of serum concentration of a PAP above the normal range was for many years accepted as virtual proof of metastatic disease, even where no clinical evidence of such spread could be identified.

With the widespread availability of PSA, the role for serum PAP level determination has become marginalized even for staging prostate cancer, and it is now rarely used in the surveillance of this condition after the institution of primary therapy by any means. Many authors consider that it is obsolete in all aspects of prostate cancer management, yet some weight is added to the argument for its continued usage by the repeated identification of a core group of patients (estimated at around 8% of the total number of men with metastatic prostate cancer) who can be identified as having disseminated disease in the absence of an elevated PSA, yet where serum PAP levels are above the normal range. Most of these tumours are poorly differentiated and do not secrete PSA into the serum at levels detectable by conventional assays. Furthermore, it is also accepted that an elevated serum level of PAP is a marker for a poorer treatment outcome in patients with metastatic prostate carcinoma, so that regular assay of PAP is only useful for prognostic assessment. Serum alkaline phosphatase level determinations, whilst only likely to be elevated beyond the normal range in many patients with prostatic carcinoma, are even less sensitive than PAP concentrations and certainly are substantially less useful in this regard than the more recently developed investigations such as PSA and isotopic bone scanning, and thus this test has largely been eliminated as a diagnostic modality in the detection of relapsed and metastatic disease in patients known to suffer from prostatic adenocarcinoma.

Conclusion

Although clinicians have many investigational options available to detect relapsed adenocarcinoma of the prostate gland, serum PSA determinations remain the most sensitive method to identify residual or relapsing disease. When an elevated PSA has been established, more invasive studies may be considered depending upon the results of clinical examination and the pathological features of the initial tumour. However, the frequency with which posttreatment PSA assays are undertaken for surveillance purposes may be variable and usually depends upon the treatment philosophy of individual clinicians.

Many authors advocate routine measurement of serum PSA levels 3-monthly following commencement of treatment, whether this is attempted cure or palliation. If serum levels of this enzyme remain suppressed and stable 12 months after therapy, the frequency of PSA assessments may eventually be reduced to 6- and then to 12-monthly. Should detectable levels of PSA be detected after radical prostatectomy, the aggressiveness of investigations to detect locally persistent disease may depend upon the confidence of the attending clinician in the ability of radiation therapy directed to the prostatic bed to prolong survival. Detailed clinical information of benefit from this form of treatment has yet to be accepted by many clinicians.

Should serum PSA levels increase progressively after local radiation or androgen deprivation treatment, the option exists for further investigation of the pelvis by TRUS, CT or MRI to identify recurrent disease that might be treatable. However, when serum PSA is increasing sequentially without evidence of local recurrence, most authors would advocate androgen deprivation treatment before symptomatic relapse of the disease in order to minimize complications from tumour metastasis, especially pathological fracture, but also disasters such as ureteric obstruction and paraplegia from spinal cord compression. When endocrine therapy has failed biochemically in a patient managed by a policy of deferred hormone manipulation, routine use of isotope bone scans and other radiographic imaging could help reduce the frequency of these major and disabling complications.

We live in an era of cost-consciousness, so that clinicians also have responsibility for following an acceptably cost-effective plan to undertake surveillance for relapsed disease. This would include the potential benefit that might be gained from detailed imaging of a local tumour recurrence, especially if no active treatment may follow, or when there may be no proof that treatment would delay the time to symptomatic progression or to prolong survival.

Therefore, at the present time serial measurement of serum PSA provides the fundamental structure for follow-up and detection of relapsed disease in men suffering from organ-confined or metastatic prostate cancer. This is clinically effective, of minimal discomfort to patients and is cost-conscious.

References

1 Nadji M, Tabei SZ & Castro A. Prostatic-specific antigen: an immunohistologic marker for prostatic neoplasms. *Cancer* 1981; **48**: 1229–1232.
2 Takayama TK, Kreiger JN, True LD & Lange PH. Recurrent prostate cancer despite undetectable prostatic specific antigen. *J Urol* 1992; **148**: 1541–1542.
* 3 Ploch NR & Brawer MK. How to use prostatic specific antigen. *Urology* 1994; **43**(suppl): 27–35.
* 4 Kaplan LD, Cox RS & Bagshaw MA. Prostate specific antigen after external beam radiotherapy for prostatic cancer: followup. *J Urol* 1993; **149**: 519–522.
* 5 Montie JE. Follow-up after radical prostatectomy or radiation therapy for prostate cancer. *Urol Clin North Am* 1994; **21**: 673–676.
6 Trapasso JG, deKernion JB, Smith RB & Dorey F. The incidence and significance of detectable levels of serum prostate specific antigen after radical prostatectomy. *J Urol* 1994; **152**: 1821–1825.
** 7 Chauvet B, Felix-Faure C, Lupsacka N *et al*. Prostate-specific antigen decline: a major prognostic factor for prostate cancer treated with radiation therapy. *J Clin Oncol* **12**: 1402–1407.
** 8 Pollack A, Zagars GK & Kavadi VS. Prostate specific antigen doubling time and disease relapse after radiotherapy for prostate cancer. *Cancer* 1994; **74**: 670–678.
9 Prestigiacoma AF & Stamey TA. A comparison of 4 ultrasensitive prostate specific antigen assays for early detection of residual cancer after radical prostatectomy. *J Urol* 1994; **152**: 1515–1519.
10 Takayama TK, Vessella RL, Brawer MK, Notebook J & Lange PH. The enhanced detection of persistent disease after prostatectomy with a new prostate specific antigen assay. *J Urol* 1993; **150: 374–378.
11 Stenman UH, Hakama M, Knekt P, Aromaa A, Teppo L & Leinonen J. Serum concentrations of prostate specific antigen and its complex with alpha-one antichymotrypsin before diagnosis of prostate cancer. *Lancet* 1994; **344**: 1594–1598.
12 Semjonow A, Hamm M & Rathert P. Elimination kinetics of prostate-specific antigen in serum and urine. *Int J Biol Markers* 1994; **9**: 15–20.
13 van Straalen JP, Bossens MM, de Reijke TM & Sanders GT. Biological half-life of prostate-specific antigen after radical prostatectomy. *Eur J Clin Chem Clin Biochem* 1994; **32**: 53–55.
*14 Zagars GK & Pollack A. The serum prostate-specific antigen level 3 months after radiotherapy for prostate cancer: an early indicator of response to treatment. *Radiother Oncol* 1994; **30**: 121–127.
15 Takayama TK, Vessella RL, Brawer MK *et al*. Urinary prostate specific antigen levels after radical prostatectomy. *J Urol* 1994; **151**: 82–87.
16 Foster LS, Jojodia P, Fournier G Jr, Shinohara K, Carroll P & Narayan P. The value of prostate specific antigen and transrectal ultrasound guided biopsy in detecting prostatic

* Reference of special interest.
** Reference of outstanding merit.

fossa recurrences following radical prostatectomy. *J Urol* 1993; **149**: 1024–1028.

17 Mettlin C, Murphy GP, Lee F *et al*. Characteristics of prostate cancer detected in the American Cancer Society national prostate cancer detection project. *J Urol* 1994; **152**: 1737–1740.

*18 Walsh PC, Partin AW & Epstein JI. Cancer control and quality of life following anatomical radical retropubic prostatectomy: results at 10 years. *J Urol* 1994; **152**: 1831–1836.

19 Kahn D, Williams RD, Seldin DW *et al*. Radioimmunoscintigraphy with 111 indium labelled CYT-356 for the detection of occult prostate cancer recurrence. *J Urol* 1994; **152**: 1490–1495.

20 Gutman AB & Gutman EB. 'Acid' phosphatase occurring in the serum of patients with metastasising carcinoma of the prostate gland. *J Clin Invest* 1938; **17**: 473–479.

21 Henneberry MO, Engel G & Grayhack JT. Acid phosphatase. *Urol Clin North Am* 1979; **6**: 629–642.

*22 Zagars GK. Prostate specific antigen as an outcome variable for T1 and T2 prostate cancer treated by radiation therapy. *J Urol* 1994; **152**: 1786–1791.

18/Treatment of Relapsed Disease – What is the Choice?

S.D. Fosså and P.H. Smith

Introduction

Treatment of advanced prostate cancer with hormones reduces the androgenic stimulation of prostate cancer cells. Androgen ablation will result in subjective improvement for 70–80% of patients and an objective response can be expected in 30%, lasting for median intervals of 24 months in men with M1 disease and about 36 months in N + M0 patients. When prostate cancer becomes refractory to control by hormonal means, disease progression occurs, so that palliative treatment is often necessary. However, such treatment cannot cure patients of prostate cancer and the primary objective is therefore improvement of symptoms such as pain, fatigue, paresis and micturition problems. Prevention or delay of morbidity and prolongation of life are secondary objectives

Progression of disease

Accurate monitoring of advanced prostate cancer by clinical methods is not easy because it is usually not possible to obtain measurements of metastatic tumours in this malignancy.

In practical terms, progression of disease has to be regarded as either an objective or a subjective event.

Objective progression

Objective progression may be recorded if there is demonstrable evidence of local reactivation of disease, new metastases and/or an increase in serum levels of biochemical markers.

Pelvic relapse becomes evident when there is an increase in volume or upstaging of tumour within the pelvic area. This may be detected by digital palpation or imaging with transrectal ultrasound or magnetic resonance imaging (MRI), and/or evidence of additional involvement of pelvic regional lymph nodes demonstrated by computed tomography (CT) or MRI. These changes may lead to problems with micturition, pain or lower limb oedema that require local palliation.

Metastatic progression should only be considered to have occurred with development of new soft-tissue metastases or of new persisting hot spots that appear on bone scans, sometimes with subsequent radiological changes.

With *biochemical progression* there is an increase of serum levels of prostate-specific antigen (PSA) and other biochemical parameters such as alkaline phosphatase and lactate dehydrogenase (LDH). However, serum PSA is not raised in about 20% of patients with hormone-refractory disease which may be due to an unexplained direct effect of androgen ablation on PSA expression of prostate cancer cells that is independent of the antitumour effect of the treatment [1]. Increases of alkaline phosphatase and LDH levels in serum may also mirror disease activity but are too non-specific to justify changes in the treatment of the individual patient.

Subjective progression

Subjective progression in men with hormone-refractory prostate cancer may occur before relapse can be demonstrated objectively. For instance, difficulty or adverse changes in the pattern of micturition may develop without mea-surable growth of the primary tumour. Deterioration of general health, anaemia, increasing bone pain and fatigue may become a clinical problem several weeks or even months before there is objective evidence of progression of metastatic disease.

Timing of treatment after progression

In hormone-refractory prostate cancer, commencement of palliative treatment depends upon the symptoms and wishes of the patient and his family, the severity of the toxicity associated with the planned treatment and the effec-tiveness of the therapy. It is not known whether early treatment of a relapsing patient is more effective than therapy that is delayed. Until the results of current randomized clinical trials are available, most clinicians will tend to postpone therapy until patients with relapsing prostate cancer develop symp-toms. The doctor and the patient should be aware that any benefit from treatment of hormone-refractory prostate cancer will be transient (weeks to months) and that prolongation of life has, so far, not been achieved by any therapeutic modality that is currently available [2].

Locoregional treatment for pelvic relapse

When prostate cancer in the pelvis escapes from hormonal control, its natural

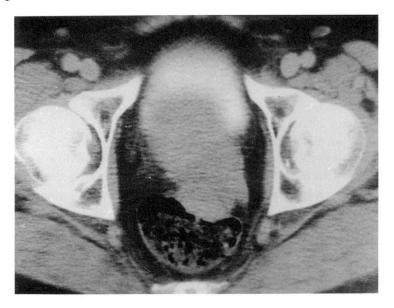

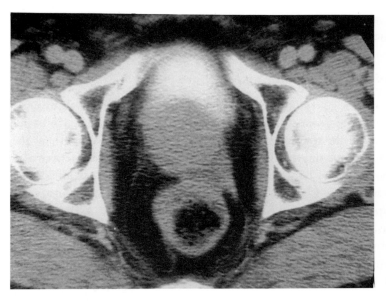

Fig. 18.1 (*Above and opposite*) Significant reduction in tumour size and rectal wall infiltration after palliative radiotherapy (60 Gy/6 weeks) to the primary tumour. The patient had used a luteinizing hormone-releasing hormone analogue for 3 years prior to irradiation. (*Top*) Before radiotherapy; (*bottom*) after radiotherapy.

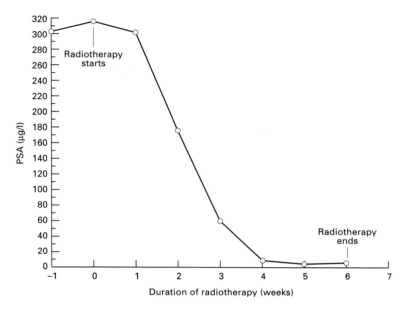

Fig. 18.1 (*continued*) Serum prostate-specific antigen (PSA) during the course of radiotherapy.

course may extend over several years, especially when distant metastases are either absent or minimal. It is therefore important to achieve worthwhile long-standing local palliation in these patients. Palliative surgery such as transure-thral prostatectomy (TURP), laser beam treatment and cryotherapy may give effective relief of symptoms from obstructed micturition. Pelvic radiotherapy (50–60 Gy) may produce a significant diminution in tumour volume, may prevent rapid regrowth of the cancer and often reduces pelvic pain due to local infiltration by the tumour (Figs 18.1 and 18.2). However, many patients may have obstructive symptoms and if these are not improved or resolved following primary therapy, or if they recur despite previous resolution, then a clearance TURP is always appropriate. However, the results of TURP in these patients are less satisfactory than in men with benign prostatic hyperplasia (BPH) because the urethra in men with prostate cancer is more rigid and this makes it more difficult to resect a satisfactory amount of tumour. Furthermore, when prostate cancer extends distal to the verumontanum, it may infiltrate the external sphincter mechanism. Consequently, incontinence following TURP is more frequent when undertaken for locally advanced prostate cancer than for BPH.

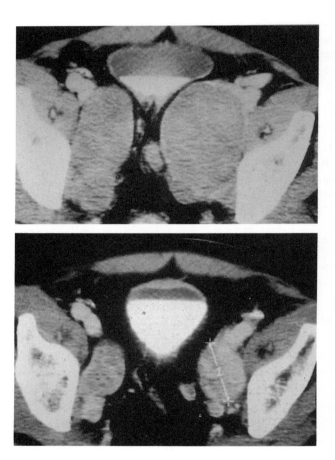

Fig. 18.2 Biopsy-proven pelvic lymph node metastases from prostate cancer before (above) and 3 months after (below) palliative radiotherapy (50 Gy/5 weeks).

Systemic therapy

Should the level of serum testosterone be greater than in the castrate range in patients receiving primary antiandrogen therapy for hormone-escaped disease, treatment should be changed to medical or surgical castration. Discontinuation of antiandrogen when used alone may be followed by a decrease in serum PSA (the antiandrogen withdrawal effect) and this phenomenon has been described for both flutamide [3] and Casodex® [4]. Similarly, when antiandrogen is withdrawn in men escaping hormonal control by total androgen blockade, serum PSA is reduced in 30–50% of patients.

It has been debated whether it is safe to discontinue androgen-suppressive therapy in patients undergoing clinical progression from hormone refractory prostate cancer. Most clinicians are reluctant to recommend such a policy, particularly in younger patients, as the serum levels of testosterone and PSA will increase after discontinuation of luteinizing hormone releasing hormone (LHRH) therapy (Fig. 18.3). This indicates that, even in patients with disease progression from hormone-refractory prostate cancer, hormone-dependent prostate cancer cells have remained and, in particular, have retained their ability to proliferate when stimulated by androgens. However, the clinical impact of such stimulation is unknown. In a retrospective study, the survival of relapsing patients in whom prior androgen suppression had been discontinued was similar to those in whom androgen deprivation had been continued [5].

Secondary orchidectomy is occasionally effective when serum testosterone levels have remained above the castrate range during primary androgen-suppressive treatment. Oral corticosteroids reduce adrenal corticosteroid

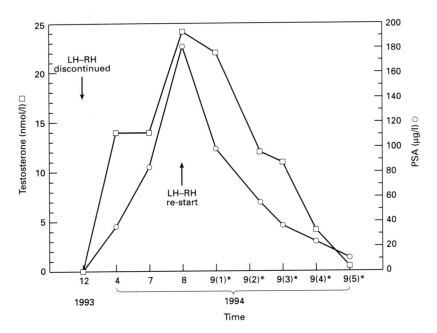

Fig. 18.3 Serum testosterone and prostate-specific antigen (PSA) in a 58-year-old patient with progressing hormone-resistant prostate cancer with bone metastases who discontinued treatment with a luteinizing hormone releasing hormone analogue after 2 years' use, but restarted the treatment 6 months after because of increasing bone pain. *Multiple blood samples taken during September 1994. LH, luteinizing hormone; RH, releasing hormone.

production and yield a subjective response in 10–30% of patients associated with decrease in serum PSA [6–8]. Aminoglutethimide and ketoconazole reduce synthesis of corticosteroids by the adrenals and aminoglutethimide also inhibits peripheral conversion of corticosteroids to androgen. Both drugs have shown some benefit when administered to men with hormone-resistant prostate cancer [9–11]. However, treatment with aminoglutethimide and with ketoconazole requires simultaneous administration of corticosteroids to prevent Addisonian-like crisis, and it is often difficult to distinguish the clinical effect of these drugs from that of corticosteroids. Non-steroidal antiandrogens may give a 30% subjective and biochemical response if total androgen blockade has not been used previously [12–14]. More recently, the imidazole derivative R75 251 (Liarazole, Janssen Pharmaceutical) has been shown to suppress adrenal corticoid synthesis, with benefit for some patients with hormone-refractory prostate cancer [15]. Corticosteroids are not needed with this drug, which is a particular advantage over aminoglutethimide and ketoconazole. In recent years, high-dose oestrogen has become a popular form of treatment for relief of skeletal pain [16].

There is a limited role for chemotherapy in relapsing prostate cancer, whether given as monotherapy or in combination: the objective response rates (using World Health Organization criteria) are most often less then 20% (Table 18.1), even though a decrease in serum PSA levels may be achieved in 30% of patients. Problems with toxicity and feasibility prevent widespread application of cytostatics for most patients with hormone-resistant prostate cancer, but the most effective drugs are probably Adriamycin, epirubicin and mitomycin [17, 18]. Combination chemotherapy has not been proved to be more effective than single-drug treatment.

Estramustine phosphate (EM) is a combination of nitrogen mustard and oestradiol and it has a special place among cytostatic agents. This drug, in theory, acts both as a high-dose oestrogen and as a cytostatic drug by interfering with the formation of the mitotic spindle. However, only limited effectiveness has been reported for EM therapy in patients with hormone-refractory prostate cancer [14, 19] but combinations of EM with vinblastine or EM with VP-16 have been claimed to be of benefit in about 50% of patients with hormone-refractory prostate cancer [20, 21].

Attempts to influence the clinical course of hormone-refractory prostate cancer have been made by inhibition of growth factors. In this respect, the drug most often used has been the antiparasitic compound Suramin [22, 23]. Objective response rates of 30% have been reported accompanied by greater than 50% reduction of serum PSA in 50–70% of patients. Another drug that affects cellular growth factors is somatostatin and this has occasionally been

Table 18.1 Experience of the EORTC GU-group with single-drug chemotherapy in measurable hormone-resistant prostate cancer.

Drug (dose schedule)	Response		
	No. of patients evaluated	No. of responding patients (WHO criteria)	Response rate (95% CI)
Methyl-glycoxal Bis-guanylhydrazone Methyl-GAG (500 mg/weekly)	30	3	10% (1–21)
Vindesine (3 mg/m² weekly)	27	5	19% (4–34)
Mitomycin C (15 mg/m² per 6 weeks)	31	5	29% (13–45)
Epirubicin (12 mg/m² weekly)	33	9	12% (1–23)
Methotrexate (40 mg/m² biweekly)	24	4	7% (–4–12)
Epirubicin (100 mg/m² per 3 weeks)	39	9	23% (10–36)

WHO, World Health Organization; CI, confidence interval.

reported to be effective in the treatment of hormone-refractory prostate cancer [24].

Radiotherapy of bone metastases

External-beam radiotherapy can be given to limited parts of the skeleton or to large fields as, for example, by hemibody irradiation. Fractionated hemibody irradiation is more effective than single-dose application [25]. Single-fraction small field irradiation (8 Gy) to bone metastases is as effective as multiple-fraction radiotherapy (3 Gy × 10) [26]. However, for treatment of spinal compression or imminent pathological fracture, most radiation oncologists prefer to give multiple fractions. Symptomatic relief achieved by palliative radiotherapy to bone metastases is claimed to be of the order of 50–70%. Nevertheless, the overall pain-relieving benefit of radiotherapy is less obvious in patients with very advanced skeletal metastases in whom new areas of pain often develop outside the field of radiation, frequently during or immediately after treatment [27].

Chapter 18

In recent years, the administration of radioactive isotopes, such as strontium and samarium, has become popular both as a treatment for existing pain and also in attempts to avoid new bone pain [28, 29]. Relief from metastatic bone pain is experienced in about 60% of patients. When given in conjunction with local radiotherapy, new bone pain in non-irradiated areas is delayed by 15 weeks [29]. Except for transient moderate haematological toxicity, intravenous isotope treatment is tolerated well and can be repeated after 3 months if necessary.

Progression as an emergency situation

The most frequent emergency situation in patients with hormone-resistant prostate cancer is paraplegia caused by tumour compression of the spinal cord [30, 31]. Neurological symptoms associated with this dreaded development are often preceded by increasing back pain, which should alert clinicians towards early diagnostic and therapeutic action. Meningeal metastases can cause cerebral symptoms [32] and soft-tissue extension of skull metastases not uncommonly cause cranial nerve palsies that result in symptoms such as visual disturbance or difficulty with speech or swallowing.

Should neurological symptoms arise, immediate treatment with high-dose dexamethasone (4 mg × 4 daily orally) should be commenced to attempt reduction of oedema at the area of spinal cord or cranial nerve compression. Surgical intervention to decompress the spinal cord may be considered but has, in general, not proved to be more effective than radiotherapy to the area of the lesion. The final outcome of treatment for spinal cord compression depends upon the extent of neurological deficit that exists before treatment is commenced. For instance, in a completely paralysed person expectation for resolution of the neurological deficit would be minimal, whereas significant improvement of functional status may occur if some muscular activity has remained when treatment is commenced.

Rapidly developing uraemia may necessitate urinary diversion if life expectancy is reasonable, especially if the obstructing primary tumour has not been irradiated previously. Imminent or established pathological fracture in weight-bearing long bones should be considered for orthopaedic surgery. Metastases in pelvic or retroperitoneal lymph nodes which induce deep leg vein thrombosis and inferior vena caval obstruction should be treated by irradiation after initial anticoagulation. In these cases, chemotherapy may also assist in reduction of tumour mass and venous obstruction.

Chronic problems

The most frequent challenge in the management of patients escaping from hormonal control is maintenance of a good quality of life for as long as possible. Freedom from pain and preservation of social contact with family members and friends are the most important quality-of-life issues [33]. Treatment of pain requires sufficient provision of effective analgesics in addition to administration of appropriate systemic anticancer regimens and palliative radiotherapy. Doctors and their patients must realize that daily use of even several hundred milligrams of morphine may be needed to achieve adequate relief of pain but side-effects from high-dose morphine regimens, such as severe constipation, must be avoided. Bisphosphonates may decrease pain from skeletal metastases as they may decrease osteoclast activity [34]. Other patients may develop malaise sometimes associated with anaemia and treatment with high-dose corticosteroids or progesterone derivatives can help improve their general condition [35, 36]. Intermittent blood transfusion may also be helpful.

Prognosis

Duration of survival of patients undergoing relapse from hormonal control is strongly correlated with the criteria for diagnosis of relapse. This is a lead-time effect. For instance, if relapse is defined only as the time at which patients have developed symptoms irrespectively of the level of PSA, subsequent survival is usually 8–10 months less than in those in whom relapse has been defined on biochemical grounds only, such as increase of serum PSA.

The median survival after symptomatic relapse is 6–8 months; this is independent of treatment [37, 38]. Prognostic factors have identified performance status and time from initial hormone treatment to relapse as the most important parameters predicting survival. Serum levels of LDH, alkaline phosphatase and creatinine are also associated with prediction of survival, whereas serum PSA has only a limited role [39]. On the other hand, when serum PSA decreases during systemic treatment of relapse, subsequent survival is better than in those patients in whom there is no reduction of PSA [40].

Conclusions

So far there is no evidence that any currently available treatment regimens will prolong life once prostate cancer has escaped from hormone control. In these men the role of PSA as a tumour marker indicating hormone-refractory disease is less helpful than during primary endocrine treatment.

Systemic treatment is transiently effective in 20–30% of patients. Secondary hormone treatment should be tried before using cytostatic agents or growth inhibitors, which are often toxic. External-beam radiotherapy, intravenous isotope irradiation, orthopaedic surgery and palliative transurethral resections of the prostate should be used to deal with specific local problems. Imminent spinal cord compression should be considered as an emergency situation that requires immediate intervention.

Doctors and their patients should be aware of the reality of the situation. Such patients can only be offered palliative treatment in which the principal goals are relief of pain and maintenance of quality of life for a limited period.

References

** 1 Leo ME, Bilhartz DL, Bergstrahl EJ & Oesterling JE. Prostate specific antigen in hormonally treated stage D2 prostate cancer: is it always an accurate indicator of disease status? *J Urol* 1991; **145**: 802.

* 2 Eisenberger MA, Simon R, O'Dwyer PJ, Wittes RE & Friedman MA. A reevaluation of nonhormonal cytotoxic chemotherapy in the treatment of prostatic carcinoma. *J Clin Oncol* 1985; **3**: 827–841.

** 3 Scher HI & Kelly K. Flutamide withdrawal syndrome: its impact on clinical trials in hormone-refractory prostate cancer. *J Clin Oncol* 1993; **11**: 1566–1572.

4 Small EJ & Carroll PR. Prostate-specific antigen decline after casodex withdrawal: evidence for an antiandrogen withdrawal syndrome. *Urology* 1994; **43**: 408–410.

** 5 Hussain M, Wolf M, Marshall E, Crawford ED & Eisenberger M. Effects of continued androgen-deprivation therapy and other prognostic factors on response and survival in phase II chemotherapy trials for hormone-refractory prostate cancer: a Southwest Oncology Group report. *J Clin Oncol* 1994; **12**: 1868–1875.

6 Patel SR, Kvols LK & Hahn RG. A phase II randomised trial of megestrol acetate or dexamethasone in the treatment of hormonally refractory advanced carcinoma of the prostate. *Cancer* 1990; **66**: 655–658.

* 7 Fosså SD & Paus E. Reduction of serum prostate-specific antigen during endocrine or cytotoxic treatment of hormone-resistant cancer of the prostate. *Eur Urol* 1994; **26**: 29–34.

** 8 Tannock I, Gospodarowicz M, Meakin W, Panzarella T, Stewart L & Rider W. Treatment of metastatic prostatic cancer with low-dose prednisone: evaluation of pain and quality of life as pragmatic indices of response. *J Clin Oncol* 1989; **7**: 590–597.

9 Eichenberger T & Trachtenberg J. Effects of high-dose ketoconazole on patients who have androgen-independent prostatic cancer. *CJS* 1989; **32**: 349–352.

10 Gerber GS & Chodak GW. Prostate specific antigen for assessing response to ketoconazole and prednisone in patients with hormone refractory metastatic prostate cancer. *J Urol* 1990; **144**: 1117–1179.

*11 Labrie F, Dupont A, Belanger A *et al.* Anti-hormone treatment for prostate cancer relapsing after treatment with flutamide and castration. Addition of aminoglutethimide

* Reference of special interest.
** Reference of outstanding merit.

and low dose hydrocortisone to combination therapy. *Br J Urol* 1989; **63**: 634–638.

*12 Labrie F, Dupont A, Giguere M *et al.* Benefits of combination therapy with flutamide in patients relapsing after castration. *Br J Urol* 1988; **61**: 341–346.

13 Fosså SD, Hosbach G & Paus E. Flutamide in hormone-resistant prostatic cancer. *J Urol* 1990; **144**: 1411–1414.

*14 deKernion JN, Murphy GP & Priore R. Comparison of flutamide and Estracyt in hormone-refractory metastatic prostatic cancer. *Urology* 1988; **31**: 312–317.

15 Mahler C & Denis L. Management of relapsing disease in prostate cancer. *Cancer* 1992; **70**: 329–334.

16 Ferro MA. Use of intravenous stilbestrol diphosphate in patients with prostatic carcinoma refractory to conventional hormonal manipulation. *Urol Clin North Am* 1991; **18**: 139–143.

17 Delaere KPJ, Leliefeld H, Peulen F, Stapper EW, Smeets J & Wils J. Phase II study of epirubicin in advanced hormone-resistant prostatic cancer. *Br J Urol* 1992; **70**: 641–642.

18 Jones WG, Fosså SD, Bono AV *et al.* and members of the EORTC Genito-Urinary Tract Cancer Co-operative Group. Mitomycin-C in the treatment of metastatic prostate cancer: report on an EORTC phase II study. *World J Urol* 1986; **4**: 182–185.

19 Newling DWW, Fosså SD, Tunn UW, Kurth KH, de Pauw M & Sylvester R. Mitomycin C versus estramustine in the treatment of hormone resistant metastatic prostate cancer: the final analysis of the European Organization for Research and Treatment of Cancer, Genitourinary Group prospective randomised phase II study (30865). *J Urol* 1993; **150**: 1840–1844.

20 Seidman AD, Scher H, Petrylak D, Dershaw DD & Curley T. Estramustine and vinblastine: use of prostate specific antigen as a clinical trial end point for hormone refractory prostate cancer. *J Urol* 1992; **147**: 931–934.

21 Pienta KJ, Redman B, Hussain M *et al.* Phase II evaluation of oral estramustine and oral etoposide in hormone-refractory adenocarcinoma of the prostate. *J Clin Oncol* 1994; **12**: 2005–2012.

22 Myers C, Cooper M, Stein C *et al.* A novel growth factor antagonist with activity in hormone-refractory metastatic prostate cancer. *J Clin Oncol* 1992; **10**: 881–889.

23 Eisenberger MA, Reyno LM, Jodrell DI *et al.* Suramin, an active drug for prostate cancer: interim observations in a phase I trial. *J Natl Cancer Inst* 1993; **85**: 611–621.

24 Parmar H, Charlton CDA, Phillips RH *et al.* Therapeutic response to somatostatin analogue, BIM 23014, in metastatic prostatic cancer. *Clin Exp Metastasis* 1992; **10**: 3–11.

25 Zelefsky MJ, Scher HI, Forman JD, Linares LA, Curley T & Fuks Z. Palliative hemiskeletal irradiation for widespread metastatic prostate cancer: a comparison of single dose and fractionated regimens. *Int J Radiat Oncol Biol Phys* 1989; **17: 1281–1285.

*26 Price P, Hoskin PJ, Easton D, Austin D, Palmar SG & Yarnold JR. Prospective randomised trial of single and multifraction radiotherapy schedules in the treatment of painful bony metastases. *Radiother Oncol* 1986; **6**: 247–266.

*27 Fosså SD. Quality of life after palliative radiotherapy in patients with hormone-resistant prostate cancer: single institution experience. *Br J Urol* 1994; **74**: 345–351.

28 Bolger JJ, Dearnaley DP, Kirk D *et al.* and members of the UK Metastron Investigator's Group. Strontium-89 (Metastron) versus external beam radiotherapy in patients with painful bone metastases secondary to prostatic cancer: preliminary report of a multicenter trial. *Semin Oncol* 1993; **20: 32–33.

29 Porter AT, McEwan ABJ, Powe JE *et al.* Results of a randomised phase-III trial to evaluate the efficacy of strontium-89 adjuvant to local field external beam irradiation in the management of endocrine resistant metastatic prostate cancer. *Int J Radiat Oncol Biol Phys* 1993; **25: 805–813.

30 Zelefsky MJ, Scher HI, Krol G, Portenoy RK, Leibel SA & Fuks ZY. Spinal epidural tumor in patients with prostate cancer. *Cancer* 1992; **70**: 2319–2325.

*31 Rosenthal MA, Rosen D, Raghavan D *et al.* Spinal cord compression in prostate cancer. A 10-year experience. *Br J Urol* 1992; **69**: 530–533.

32 Blomlie V, Lehne G, Lien HH, Windern M & Fosså SD. Meningeal tumour infiltration in hormone resistant prostate cancer demonstrated with magnetic resonance. *Eur J Cancer* 1993; **9**: 1357.

*33 Fosså SD, Aaronson NK, Newling D *et al.* and the members of the EORTC GU group. Subjective response to treatment of hormone resistant metastatic cancer. *Eur J Cancer Clin Oncol* 1990; **26**: 1133–1136.

34 Vorreuther R. Biophosphonates as an adjuvant to palliative therapy of bone metastases from prostatic carcinoma. A pilot study on clodronate. *Br J Urol* 1993; **72**: 792–795.

35 Daniel F, MacLeod PM & Tyrrell CJ. Megestrol acetate in relapsed carcinoma of the prostate. *Br J Urol* 1990; **65**: 275–277.

36 Fosså SD, Jahnsen JU, Karlsen S, Øgreid P, Haveland H & Trovåg A. High-dose medroxyprogesterone acetate versus prednisolone in hormone-resistant prostatic cancer. *Eur Urol* 1985; **11**: 11–16.

*37 Petrylak DP, Scher HI, Li Z, Myers CE & Geller NL. Prognostic factors for survival of patients with bidimensionally measurable hormone-refractory prostatic cancer treated with single-agent chemotherapy. *Cancer* 1992. **70**: 2870–2878.

*38 Fosså SD, Dearnaley DP, Law M, Gad J & Newling DW. Prognostic factors in hormone-resistant progressing cancer of the prostate. *Ann Oncol* 1992; **3**: 361–366.

*39 Fosså SD, Wæhre H & Paus E. The prognostic significance of prostate specific antigen in metastatic hormone-resistant prostate cancer. *Br J Cancer* 1992; **66**: 181–184.

*40 Kelly WM, Scher HI, Mazamdar M, Vlamis V, Schwartz M & Fosså SD. Prostate specific antigen as a measure of disease outcome in metastatic hormone refractory prostate cancer. *J Clin Oncol* 1993; **4**: 607–615.

19/Screening for Early Prostate Cancer – Is it Possible or Justifiable?

F. Calais da Silva

Introduction

The incidence and mortality of prostate cancer are increasing faster than can be attributed simply to the increasing age of the population. One response to these statistics has been increasing demands of screening programmes. Is early detection possible and would early treatment help?

In this context, screening involves the examination of asymptomatic men in order to classify them as likely or unlikely to have prostate cancer. Men who appear likely to have the disease are investigated further to arrive at a final diagnosis and those who are found to have the disease are treated. The organized application of early diagnosis and treatment activities in large groups is often described as population screening. The goal of screening is to reduce mortality from the disease among the people screened by early treatment of the cases of prostate cancer discovered. Screening calls attention to the likelihood of disease before symptoms appear. Population screening offers the potential to reduce mortality but large-scale randomized studies are required to prove their efficacy. Before embarking on trials to evaluate their efficacy there are a number of criteria which should be fulfilled: these were outlined by Wilson and Jungner [1]. These criteria have been able to withstand the test of time and their application to the current situation with prostate cancer is a useful way to seeing how far the present circumstances go towards meeting criteria for establishing a screening programme, at least on an experimental basis.

Criteria for screening

Is prostate cancer an important public health problem?

Prostate cancer is undoubtedly a common and major public health problem and is one which seems to be set to increase. During 1978–1982 in the European Community (EC), with some geographical variations, its incidence amounted to 55 per 100 000, with a mortality of 22.6 per 100 000, a cumulative lifetime risk of 3.9% to the age of 74 years and a cumulative mortality of 1.2%. This amounts to 84 889 new cases and 35 084 deaths per year [2]. Worldwide, in 1980 it was estimated that 250 000 new incident cases were diagnosed and the 85 000 new cases in the member states of the EC represented 13% of all cancers diagnosed in men (excluding non-melanoma skin cancer) [3]. In Europe, prostate cancer is the second commonest incident form of cancer in men after lung cancer and accounts for one-tenth of male cancer deaths in many countries.

Therefore, the association of prostate cancer with age has enormous implications for the future. Assuming that age-specific incidence rates remain fixed at 1980 levels, the number of cases of prostate cancer in men aged over 65 in the EC will rise through 80 000 in 1990 to 92 000 in the year 2000. Even if age-specific incidence rates remain stable, the problem of prostate cancer seems sure to increase in absolute terms simply because of the ageing of the population. Life expectancy at birth in many western countries is still increasing and half of the boys born today can expect to reach the age of 80 years.

This has major implications for the future burden of prostate disease, including cancer. Half of the male population can soon expect to attain an age when 88% of them will have histological evidence of benign prostatic hyperplasia (BPH) [4] and at least half will have symptoms compatible with the presence of BPH [5]. Assuming no change in the age-specific risk of contracting prostate cancer, the number of cases of prostate cancer in the EC countries among men aged 65 and over will increase from 79 000 in 1990, to 92 000 in 2000, 102 000 in 2010, reaching 120 000 in 2020 – an increase of 50% in 30 years. At the present time in the EC there is more than three times the number of incident prostate cancers than of cervix cancers, which is the object of several national screening programmes [3].

Is there an effective treatment for localized disease?

Approximately one-half of patients diagnosed with prostate cancer present with locally advanced and/or metastatic disease at the time of first diagnosis. The prognosis of patients with advanced prostate cancer, even with the most aggressive treatment, is poor. Cure is elusive, with a median time to progression of 18 months and a median survival of metastatic patients of 24 months.

Results obtained with either radical prostatectomy or radiotherapy for localized disease are favourable. Median survival has been shown to be longer than 15 years in patients with stage B disease [6]: the observed crude survival rates parallel the normal survival curve [7]. Thus, the search for early-stage prostate cancer could, potentially, lead to a reduction in the mortality rate from this condition.

Are facilities for further diagnosis and treatment available?

At present, the health services of most countries would be stretched by the increased number of men, both true cases and false-positives, needing further work-up resulting from the implementation of a population-wide screening programme. An incidental consequence would be the increased number of men with BPH diagnosed as having a pathological disease: some of these would also consume additional health care resources requiring treatment for asymptomatic deterioration of renal function. This concerns only a small group of patients but half of those diagnosed with BPH would have symptoms that require medical treatment if they are bothersome.

However, in the context of a randomized screening trial based within one or two geographical regions of a country, the resources necessary to cope with the increased workload resultant from a screening programme could be found. Such an investment could result in longer-term savings.

Is there an identifiable latent or early symptomatic stage of prostate cancer?

Locally confined prostate cancer is a well-defined early stage of the disease; it is usually asymptomatic and is frequently diagnosed during the course of treatment for BPH: tumours found unexpectedly by the pathologist following prostatectomy for BPH are called incidental prostate cancer. Between 8 and 14% of all prostatectomy specimens can have evidence of malignancy and the incidence of all early lesions is strongly dependent on age [8].

Undoubtedly, there is a significant proportion of men who are asymptomatic, leading lives with a natural time course and who have latent prostate cancer. The great majority of such men will have a completely natural life since, of identified cases, only 12% progress and 3% die from T1a disease. The pathological grading is important and patients with incidental extensive disease (T1b) or higher histological grades are high-risk patients to develop clinical disease. Identification of these lesions which are neither palpable nor visible on transrectal ultrasound (TRUS) can only be made by a blind biopsy. The usual indication for such an approach is an elevated prostate-specific antigen (PSA). Restraint in blind multiple biopsies should be exercised to avoid overdiagnosis. While there is no doubt that some of these lesions are prognostically very favourable and do not require any treatment, identification of men with such lesions enrolled within a screening programme and informing them about the diagnosis may also cause some psychological trauma.

There is a hopeful development with recent reports of possible premalignant lesions of the prostate. These lesions, atypical adenomatous hyperplasia (AAH) and prostatic intraepithelial neoplasia (PIN), have been associated with cancers of the transitional [9] and peripheral zone [10] of the prostate, respectively. Identification of a premalignant lesion, particularly one which could be readily identified by a relatively simple test, would be of great consequence to prostate screening.

Are screening tests effective?

There is a range of possible tests which could be used in screening for prostate cancer, covering wide spectra of complexity, invasiveness, cost, acceptability and, indeed, efficiency in detecting prostate cancer [11]. These include digital rectal examination (DRE), PSA, TRUS and a random biopsy of the prostate.

The most recent published review of the literature on DRE [12] summarized the qualities of DRE as a screening test as sensitivity between 55 and 69%, specificity between 89 and 97%, positive predictive value between 11 and 26%, negative predictive value between 85 and 96%. Subsequently, a detection rate of 1.12% was found in a randomly selected population of men reacting to an invitation [13]. The positive predictive value of a suspect DRE was 30%. DRE has advantages in being inexpensive, non-invasive and with no measurable associated morbidity. However, the detection rate generally achieved by DRE alone (0.13–1.65%) appears to be low to recommend use of this test on its own [11].

Furthermore, the value of the test depends very much on the skills of the examiner and it remains to be demonstrated that routine annual screening by DRE can lead to reductions in prostate cancer mortality. Early assessments have given little encouragement [14] and the recent findings of Gerber and colleagues is particularly telling [15]. On the first screen, 73% of cancers were localized to the prostate with a 97% 5-year survival rate. However, on a second screen only 1 year later, 33% of cancers found were localized, producing a 5-year survival rate of 82%.

Imaging of the prostate gland can be achieved by ultrasound, computed tomography and magnetic resonance imaging [16]. TRUS has been the focus of most attention in a variety of settings: again, unfortunately, there has been no study capable of accounting for the important biases mentioned above. Waterhouse and Resnick [17] summarized the available literature by suggesting that TRUS has levels of sensitivity and specificity which are probably too low for a single-modality screening test. Sensitivity ranged from 71 to 92% for prostate cancer and from 60 to 85% for subclinical disease. Specificity values ranged from 41 to 79% and reported positive predictive values have frequently been around 30%.

It appears unlikely that any single modality has adequate sensitivity for use by itself in population screening. The sensitivity and positive predictive value appear to be better for TRUS than for DRE, although the relatively low specificity, the invasiveness and the cost of the test are particularly powerful arguments against the use of TRUS as a single-modality screening test and suggest that it may be more suitable as a second-stage test for men not cleared by a combination of PSA and DRE.

PSA has recently emerged as a test with promise in screening although, once again, the characteristics of the test as a screening tool have yet to be investigated satisfactorily. The estimated sensitivity appears to be around 70% and the positive predictive values vary between 26 and 52%. These, of course, can be optimized by changing the cut-off points in the definition of 'normal' values in the test.

PSA has several advantages and disadvantages as a screening test. On the positive side, the test is simple, lacks real invasiveness and is relatively low-cost (especially when compared to TRUS, or even DRE if you include the specialist's time in the cost).

Recently, several large-scale studies have been conducted to examine the role of PSA as a screening test for prostate cancer [18, 19]. At Washington University in St Louis, Catalona and associates evaluated 1653 healthy, asymptomatic men 50 years of age or older with a serum PSA determination; 37 men were diagnosed with cancer for an overall detection rate of 2.2% [18]. Brawer and colleagues at the University of Washington in Seattle, in their study of 1249 symptom-free men also 50 years of age or older and with no family history of prostate cancer, identified 32 patients with prostate cancer for a detection rate of 2.2% [20]. Labrie and associates evaluated the ability of PSA to detect prostate cancer in 1002 men between 45 and 80 years old who were randomly chosen from the electoral roles of Quebec City and its surrounding area using a cut-off point of 3 ng/ml (Tandem-R PSA assay), they observed a 4.6% prostate cancer detection rate [19]. All these values are somewhat better than the 1.3–1.5% reported for DRE [21]. In the Washington University study, 32% of the patients identified would have been missed if DRE alone were used. The Seattle group found that 38% of their cancers would not have been identified if DRE had been used to screen the population under consideration.

PSA can be improved, as noted above, by altering the definitions of the normal range. The single cut-off level for serum PSA measurement has recently come under scrutiny. Oesterling *et al.* [22] examined a randomly selected sample of 471 men aged 40–79 years from Olmsted County, Minnesota, USA, by serum PSA measurement, DRE, and TRUS. Regression models were used to assess the association between PSA concentration and age and the derived age-specific reference ranges. After analysing the data, the authors recommended an upper limit of normal for serum PSA using the Tandem-R PSA assay for men aged 40–49 years of 3.0 ng/ml; 50–59 years, 4.1 ng/ml; 60–69 years, 5.6 ng/ml; and 70–79 years, 7.6 ng/ml. These data must be corroborated by other investigators before age-specific reference ranges can be generally adopted. However, by decreasing the reference range in younger men, the sensitivity for the detection of prostate cancer will be increased, whereas by increasing the cut-off level in elderly men, the specificity will be increased, thereby reducing the number of unnecessary biopsies in elderly men. It is also possible when investigating men with large prostates to utilize PSA density. When the volume of the prostate is known by ultrasound, correction of elevated PSA levels is thought to be possible by dividing the PSA level by the estimated volume. However, the limited information available about this comes uniquely from clinical studies and cannot be applied to (asymptomatic) screening populations: the value of PSA for screening, whether adjusted for volume or otherwise, will require to be calculated in this same population (of asymptomatic men from the general population).

Are the tests acceptable to the population?

It is difficult to quote reliable, global estimations of acceptance/compliance in prostate screening studies: none has really been conducted so far. However, some information is available from the pilot programme undertaken in Antwerp (Denis and Standaert) which looked at DRE, PSA and TRUS.

During the first year, in 1991, attention was focused on the development of a smooth cooperation between the different partners involved in the screening process: the general practitioners, the city administration, the research centre, the organizing committee and the target group of men aged 60–74 years. Men were selected from the population registry and had to be informed and invited. They were asked to accept randomization procedure. To explain this procedure and to recruit eligible men, the target population as a first step received an informative letter. This was followed by a home visit by a social nurse who explained the whole study procedure and asked consent from each potential participant.

A total of 1949 men were screened, being 30% of the men asked to participate. When considering the combined results of 1992 and 1993 of the pilot studies in which three screening tests were applied, the best positive predictive value was obtained with the combination of all three tests, the positive predictive value being lowest with TRUS alone. It is interesting to note that the combination of PSA and DRE revealed a positive predictive value of the same magnitude as all three tests together.

Amongst the 32 biopsy-positive cases in which serum PSA was determined, 10 cases had a PSA value under 4 ng/ml; 7 cases ranged between 4 and 10 ng/ml. This resulted in an adjusted cancer detection rate of 7.2% amongst those with a PSA value between 4 and 10 ng/ml, compared to 46% for the higher and 1.2% for the lower PSA groups.

Despite the uncomfortable nature of the examination, a high proportion of men agreed to be screened again.

Is the natural history of prostate cancer known?

The high rate of prostate cancer noted in many autopsy series generates some concern about overdetection of clinically insignificant disease. However, cancer detection rates using PSA, DRE and TRUS are lower ($\sim$ 3–5%) than the incidence reported in autopsy series (e.g. 30–50%), suggesting that most diagnosed tumours are of higher volume. This may correspond to data showing relative PSA elevations only after tumours reach about $1 \, cm^3$ [23]. In order to be well-visualized by TRUS, tumours also need to have an approximately volume of $0.5–1.0 \, cm^3$ (i.e. 6–10 mm in average diameter). Given that approximately 60% of autopsy tumours are less than $0.5 \, cm^3$ [24], current early detection protocols using PSA, DRE and TRUS are unlikely to detect clinically insignificant lesions in most men. For palpable or visible lesions, better prognostic factors are still needed to discern the fraction of indolent tumours, especially in the older age groups.

The natural history of prostate cancer remains a controversial area due to the spectrum of disease stage and grade, along with varied interpretations of non-randomized studies estimating untreated progression rates. The recent review of the literature by Schroder and Boyle details the expected progression rates for localized disease [25]. Their conclusions are quite reasonable in suggesting observation for T1a cancer tumours and more aggressive therapy for T1b lesions due to their estimated progression rates of 13.5 and 4.75 years, respectively [26]. The median time to progression for T2 tumours is about 6 years but varies with subclassification [25]. Prognostic factors for individual patients with T2 tumours need improvement due to inconsistent tumour grading between biopsy and radical prostatectomy specimens. Biopsy specimens routinely underestimate tumour grade such that the greatest risk for overtreating T2 disease is when tumours are uniformly lower-grade (e.g. Gleason $\leqslant$ 6). Currently, patients with uniformly lower-grade tumours cannot be differentiated from those with undiagnosed higher-grade subpopulations. The potentially small fraction of patients with uniformly lower-grade tumours may also be prime candidates for observation since their progression rate may be closer to T1a disease than the median T2 rate. The probability of having uniformly low-grade tumours in PSA-based screening programme needs further evaluation in order to assess the true risk of progression for most clinically detectable cancers.

The possibility cannot, at present, be excluded that screening may upset this balance through diagnosing more cases of early prostate cancer, leading to more men being treated and to more deaths resulting from complications of the surgery either in the short or medium term. This is not an argument against the conduct of screening trials; indeed, it provides powerful reasons why they should be conducted before screening infiltrates into routine medical care.

Which patients should and should not be treated?

The only group of patients which can be safely excluded from treatment on the basis of a pretreatment evaluation are those who have well-differentiated focal prostate carcinoma.

Use of TRUS (as a diagnostic procedure) is now making it increasingly possible to preselect patients with localized, palpable disease and the possibility of overtreatment in this particular group, which could not be excluded in the immediate past, is now decreasing. This is an important advance in the development of screening tests for prostate cancer.

Is the cost of screening acceptable?

It is true to state that the costs involved in an evaluation of prostate screening in a large, randomized trial are much less than those which would be incurred and squandered if an unevaluated methodology, which was ineffective, became commonly accepted and implemented as a screening procedure by the medical profession. This is particularly true for TRUS and PSA.

The recent finding that two-thirds of members of the American Urological Association used PSA as a screening test in men up to the age of 80 is of considerable concern [27]. So also is the recent statement from the American Cancer Society recommending that the PSA be used annually in multiphasic health checks in men older than 55 years of age. It remains unknown if using PSA as a screening test will lead to a reduction in mortality from prostate cancer and the costs of the test, including the significant costs of working up those false-positives, would eat up a significant proportion of the entire health budget in many countries with an ageing population (see also Chapter 20).

Is effective treatment available and does management of cases in the early stages have a favourable impact on prognosis?

Radiotherapy and radical prostatectomy have been considered 'effective forms of treatment in physicians' attempts to cure tumors limited to the prostate for appropriately selected patients' [28]. The key phrase in that quote from the National Institutes of Health consensus development conference may be 'appropriately selected'. Cumulative patient risk factors for disease progression are difficult to quantify due to variable tumour grading, staging inaccuracies and age selection biases. Historical comparisons of different treatments are thus fraught with error and generate further debates about the relative merits of each therapy. However, the uncertainties about therapy could be confined to the need for therapy in patients with low-volume, low-grade disease, rather than suggesting a threatening risk–benefit ratio for patients with clinically significant disease.

Controversies about the benefits of early therapy could also be more focused towards the oldest age groups, or patients with comorbid medical conditions that preclude at least a 10-year life expectancy [29]. It has been estimated that the average decrease in life-years for patients with prostate cancer is only 9 years [30], since the average age at diagnosis is over age 70. For healthy patients younger than age 70, few would argue against the high probability of disease progression for higher-volume cancers (T1b or greater) with Gleason scores of 5 or above. Until we can identify the more indolent cancers which are well-suited for observation alone, refinements of potentially curative therapies should include lower morbidity and associated costs.

Practical problems related to screening

Quality of life

It is also clear that the criteria of Wilson and Jungner [2] neglect the question of whether screening adds positive value to the quality of life of participants. This point is at the same time very difficult to evaluate but may be of particular interest for prostate cancer since many men with prostate cancer will die from other causes. Furthermore, quality of life is taking on increasing importance in cancer therapy in general but particularly in prostate cancer. This is a disease which commonly affects elderly men and one of the benefits of the 20th century has been the apparent slowing down of ageing. On average, someone of 70 years today is fitter, healthier and has a better quality of life than someone of the same age 30 or 40 years ago. The remaining years of life of useful quality will be increasingly important and the prolongation of life of high quality will be an important consideration in decisions regarding disease therapy and, even in certain instances, diagnosis in the coming years.

It is also important to know whether the available screening procedures can detect potentially 'curable' cancers.

Life expectancy

About 50–60% of all cases of prostate cancer in the EC present with obvious metastases or are locally too advanced for potentially curative management. Of those cancers that seem to be limited to the prostate clinically, 25–35% will have lymph node metastases [31]. Of the remainder, another 25–35% will be too advanced for curative treatment and will turn out to be unresectable if surgery is attempted [32]. Those patients who present with metastatic disease and are treated with maximal endocrine treatment will have a median survival of 36 months [33]. On the other hand, patients with locally confined but palpable disease who are treated by either radiotherapy or radical prosta-tectomy will show 5-year survival rates of 75–85% and will enjoy a life expectancy comparable to that of an age-matched male population [34]. Against this background, therefore, it seems we should try to detect prostate cancer early and to reduce mortality by aggressive early management. This simplistic view is, however, untenable.

Aggressive potential of tumours

The challenge therefore is to identify aggressive tumours. Most (latent) car-cinomas of the prostate found at necropsy are focal, with a diameter of 1–2 mm and a volume of $0.005–0.05\,cm^3$. Tumours of this size are not identified clinically except incidentally in surgical specimens removed because of BPH. Half of such incidental tumours are focal. The generally accepted policy is not to treat these tumours unless they are detected in a very young patient [35]. Tumours detected by DRE, through raised values of PSA or by TRUS are usually $4–7\,cm^3$ in volume, and truly focal lesions are diagnosed in fewer than 4% of cases. The risk of identifying focal lesions on a large scale in any screening programme therefore seems negligible [36]. The overall detection rate of one-time screening is about 2.5%.

Treatment policy

Once a carcinoma has been detected, should it be treated? There are no valid randomized comparative studies of surveillance versus treatment. Historical comparisons between the results of the few surveillance studies of locally confined disease with results of treatment studies are not conclusive. Important prognostic factors such as T category, grade of differentiation, DNA, plasma values of PSA and age make comparisons difficult. Accordingly, there are no great differences in cancer-related and overall mortality between treatment and surveillance studies. This might be due to the ineffectiveness of treatment, to a slow rate of progression of tumours, to competing causes of death or, most likely, to a combination of all these factors. Radiotherapy and radical prostatectomy are effective in treating locally confined prostate cancer [28]. Clearly, therefore, some of the clinically detected locally confined tumours do not form an immediate threat to life. These tumours are, however, part of the lifetime incidence quoted above (3.9%), which suggests that overtreatment occurs in 2 out of 3 patients.

Which tests?

The sensitivity, specificity and positive predictive values of all three diagnostic tests (DRE, PSA and TRUS) are too low to justify their use [37]. The use of each alone would result in many unnecessarily worried men and unwarranted prostate biopsies. Unfortunately, we do not yet know the accuracy of the three tests in combination. The low specificity and positive predictive value is not, however, the only reason for not recommending the routine use of these tests. Early detection regimens should not be applied unless benefit is shown in terms of reduced mortality from cancer for randomized prospective trials. This has not yet been shown.

There is, however, considerable pressure in many parts of the world to apply these methods as screening tests. Pressure comes from patients but also from doctors. In the USA the American Urological Association recommend an annual DRE for men aged over 50. A recent survey has shown that most American urologists will also test for PSA in any patient in that age group who walks into their office [38]. In Germany, population screening for prostate cancer has been a policy since 1978, and in Belgium an insurance-supported annual check-up includes a DRE.

Yet screening should not be recommended as public health policy until clear benefit in terms of reduced mortality from cancer can be shown in prospective screening studies. Such studies need to be carried out urgently, but in the meantime it seems that both public and profession are ready to accept a considerable possibility of overtreatment.

Can screening be harmful?

Another problem is the possibility that screening may induce anxiety and psychological harm. There are two population groups to consider when assessing harm to persons who are screened: men who are free of disease and those with prostate cancer. Group 1 represents a large proportion of men who would undergo testing if we were to follow recent literature recommendations to perform PSA testing on all men older than 50 years [29]. For these men the harms of the actual venepuncture are obviously minimal but the consequences of false-positive results are potentially great. At a minimum, thousands (possibly millions) of men without disease would need to return for repeat testing and experience anxiety while they await the results. Thousands of men without disease would undergo needle biopsies, and some men with insignificant disease would undergo unnecessary prostatectomy and other procedures. The potential complications of these procedures are part of the resulting 'screening cascade'. One review estimated that radical prostatectomy alone has a 25% risk of impotence, 18% risk of urethral stricture, 6% risk of urinary incontinence, 3% risk of rectal injury and 1–2% risk of death [39].

The cascade of adverse effects would be a minor concern if false-positive results were uncommon but current evidence suggests that PSA screening of asymptomatic men would generate false-positive results on at least 2 men for every true case of cancer detected [18]. Moreover, these data come from studies of men who were not entirely representative of the patients for whom nationwide screening is recommended [40]. Low-risk men face a high probability of false-positive results. For example, an abnormal PSA test in a man with a 1% likelihood of having clinically significant prostate cancer is 50 times more likely to be false-positive than a true-positive. (Positive predictive value 1.9% assumes that sensitivity and specificity are 79 and 59% [39], respectively, and that pretest probability for clinically significant prostate cancer in this hypothetical case is 1%.)

In addition to its effects on men without disease, screening can also harm men with prostate cancer. Given current evidence from autopsy studies and natural history data, which suggest that half of older men have histological evidence of prostate cancer and that most of these are slow-growing tumours of little clinical significance [41], it can be predicted that widespread screening will produce a large cohort of men with clinically insignificant disease. (Indeed, increased screening has already generated an 'epidemic' of prostate cancer, with the incidence of new cases increasing by about 16% in 1989 to 1990 alone [42]). The ideal approach would be to inform these men at detection that they have a subtype of prostate cancer that is known to be clinically insignificant, thereby sparing them the complications of further intervention and the psychological burden of being labelled with cancer. However, our understanding of the biology of this disease is currently too primitive to make this distinction; we feel compelled to treat all diagnosed cases. As a result, we cannot know how many thousands of men will undergo unnecessary treatment and surgery as a result of nationwide screening.

Knowing the harms but now knowing the benefits of these interventions, how can we ensure that screening will result in more good than harm? At a minimum, are we not obligated to advise otherwise healthy patients of this situation before they undergo screening? These men have a right to know at the outset that there is incomplete information about the benefits and harms of treating prostate cancer and to make an informed choice about proceeding with screening [43].

Future status of screening

Should there be a randomized trial of screening? There are currently no great hopes of major advances in therapy and prospects for primary prevention are remote: risk factors for prostate cancer are poorly understood. Advance in tools introduced to diagnose prostate cancer without necessitating a biopsy have resulted in hopes that they could be successfully employed as screening procedures.

At present there is not enough evidence to advocate the implementation of widespread population screening programmes: the screening tests available, alone or in combination, have not been properly characterized (in terms of sensitivity and specificity) and none have been evaluated in randomized trials to determine whether they can lead to a reduction in the mortality rate of prostate cancer. However, the current situation goes a long way to meet the criteria established by Wilson and Jungner [2] to judge whether screening can be advocated on a trial basis.

There remains an urgent need for more information and a clearer understanding of the natural history of prostate cancer, including the possible association between AAH and PIN lesions and focal carcinoma. It is of fundamental importance to know which of the very small prostate cancers identified by transurethral resection of the prostate or random biopsy in a screened individual are important tumours (i.e. aggressive cancers caught at an early stage) and those which would have remained latent and not been at high risk of growing, metastasizing and causing death. The absence of this information is a barrier to propositions for even experimental studies of screening.

Having considered these and other factors we recommend that scientific evaluation of population screening for prostate cancer be undertaken. It is essential that some element of randomization of individuals forms the basis of this. Randomization of individuals is just as necessary in the present context as in clinical trials of cancer therapy.

There are other arguments which can be advanced for conducting large randomized screening trials. These offer important opportunities to investigate in a prospective manner the natural history of prostate cancer and other lesions by following those found incidentally at screening. It is difficult to think of another way in which this could be done at present in a cost-effective design. Furthermore, the delineation of undiseased controls could be of essential importance in the formulation of satisfactory comparison groups for epidemiological studies, not only of prostate cancer but also of BPH.

It is clear that at the present moment, the need is for randomized trials of prostate cancer screening: it must be shown that the screening tests can reduce mortality from the disease and not replace this reduction with premature deaths due to mortality following prostatectomy.

References

1 Wilson JMG & Jungner G. *Principles and Practice of Screening for Disease*. Public health paper No. 34. Geneva: WHO, 1969.
* 2 Móller Jensen O, Esteve J & Móller H. Cancer in the European Community and its member states. *Eur J Cancer* 1990; **26**: 1167–1256.
3 Jensen OM, Esteve J, Moller H & Renard H. Cancer in the European Community and its member states. *Eur J Cancer* 1990; **26**: 1167–1256.
4 Boyle P. Epidemiology of benign prostatic hyperplasia. *Prospectives* 1990; **1**: 1–4.
5 Guess H. Population studies in benign prostatic hyperplasia. *Prospectives* 1992; **2**: 1–4.
6 Gibbons RP. Total prostatectomy for clinically localized prostate cancer: long-term surgical results and current morbidity. *NCI Monogr* 1988; 7: 123–126.
* 7 National Cancer Institute. *Consensus Development Conference on the Management of Clinically Localised Prostate Cancer* NCI Monograph 7. Bethesda: NIH, 1988.
8 Schroder FH. The natural history of incidental prostatic carcinoma. *Proc Symp Incidental Prostatic Cancer* (in press).

* Reference of special interest.
** Reference of outstanding merit.

9 Bostwick DG & Srigley JR. Premalignant lesions. In: *Pathology of the Prostate*, Bostwick DG, ed. New York: Churchill Livingstone, pp. 37–59.

10 Mostofi FK, Davis CJ & Sesterhenn I. Pathology of carcinoma of the prostate. *Cancer* 1993; **70**: 235–253.

11 Bentvelsen FM & Schroder FH. Modalities available for screening for prostate cancer. *Eur J Cancer* 1993; **29A**: 804–811.

12 Resnick MI. Editorial comments: In: *Genitourinary Cancer*, Rattiff TL *et al.*, eds. Boston: Martinus Nijhoff, 1987; pp 94–99.

13 Pederson KV, Carlsson P, Varenhorst E, Loftman O & Berglund K. Screening for carcinoma of the prostate by digital rectal examinations in a randomly selected population. *Br Med J* 1990; **300**: 1041–1044.

14 Friedman GD, Hiatt RA, Quesenberry CP & Selby JV. Case-control study of screening for prostate cancer by digital rectal examination. *Lancet* 1991; **337**: 1526–1529.

15 Gerber JS, Thomson IM, Thisted R & Chodak GW. Disease specific survival following routine prostate cancer screening by digital rectal examination *JAMA* 1993. **269**: 61–64.

16 Rifkin MD, Dähnert W & Kurtz AB. State of the art: endorectal sonography of the prostate gland. *AJR* 1990; **154**: 691–700.

17 Waterhouse RL & Resnick MI. The use of transrectal prostatic ultrasonography in the evaluation of patients with prostatic carcinoma. *J Urol* 1989; **141**: 233–239.

18 Catalona WJ, Smith DS, Ratliff TL *et al.* Measurement of prostate-specific antigen in serum as a screening test for prostate cancer. *N Engl J Med* 1991; **324: 1156–1161.

19 Labrie F, Dupont A, Suburu R *et al.* Serum prostate specific antigen as pre-screening test for prostate cancer. *J Urol* 1992; **147**: 846–851.

20 Brawer MK, Chetner MP, Beatie J, Buchner DM, Vessella RL & Lange PH. Screening for prostatic carcinoma with prostate specific antigen. *J Urol* 1992; **147: 841–845.

21 Mettlin C, Lee F, Drago J & Murphy GP. The American Cancer Society national prostate cancer detection project: findings on the detection of early prostate cancer in 2425 men. *Cancer* 1991; **67: 2949–2958.

22 Oesterling JE, Jacobsen SJ, Chute CG *et al.* Serum prostate-specific antigen in a community based population of health men. *JAMA* 1993; **270: 860–864.

23 Brawn PN, Speights VO, Kuhl *et al.* Prostate-specific antigen levels from completely sectioned, clinically benign, whole prostates. *Cancer* 1991; **68**: 1592–1599.

24 McNeal JE, Kindrachuk RA, Freiha FS *et al.* Patterns of progression in prostate cancer. *Lancet* 1986; **1**: 60–63.

25 Schroder FH & Boyle P. Screening for prostate cancer – necessity or nonsense. *Eur J Cancer* 1993; **29A: 656–661.

26 Lowe BA & Listrom MB. Incidental carcinoma of the prostate: an analysis of the predictors of progression. *J Urol* 1988; **140**: 1340–1344.

27 Thompson IM & Zeidman EJ. Current urological practice: routine urological examination and early detection of carcinoma of the prostate. *J Urol* 1992; **148**: 326–329.

28 National Cancer Institute. Consensus development conference on the management of clinically localized prostate cancer. *NCI Monogr 7*. Bethesda: NIH, 1988.

*29 Mettlin C, Jones G, Averette H, Gusberg SB & Murphy G. Defining and updating the American Cancer Society guidelines for the cancer-related checkup: prostate and endometrial cancers. *CA Cancer J Clin* 1993; **43**: 42–46.

*30 Horm JW & Sondick EJ. Person-years of life lost due to cancer in the United States, 1970 and 1984. *Am J Public Health* 1989; **79**: 1490–1493.

31 Donohue RF, Mani JH, Whitesel JA *et al.* Stage D1 adenocarcinoma of prostate. *Urology* 1984; **23**: 118–121.

32 Van den Ouden D, Tribukait B, Blom JHM *et al.* Deoxuribonucleic acid ploidy of core biopsies and metastatic lymph nodes of prostate cancer patients – impact on time to progression? *J Urol* 1993; **150**: 400–406.

*33 Crawford ED, Eisenberger MA, Mcleod DG *et al.* A controlled trial of leuprolide with and without flutamide in prostatic carcinoma. *N Engl J Med* 1989; **321**: 419–424.

*34 Gibbons RP, Correa RJ Jr, Brannen GE & Weissman RM. Total prostatectomy for clinically localized prostatic cancer: long-term results. *J Urol* 1989; **141**: 564–566.

35 Walsh D & Patrick C. Radical prostatectomy in locally confined prostatic carcinoma. *Proc Chem Biol Res* 1990; **359**: 199–207.

*36 Scardino PT, Weaver R & Hudson MA. Early detection of prostate cancer. *Hum Pathol* 1992; **23**: 211–222.

37 Bentvelsen FM & Schröder FH. Modalities available for screening of prostate cancer. *Eur J Cancer* 1993; **29A**: 804–811.

*38 Thompson IM & Zeidman EJ. Current urological practice: routine urological examination and early detection of carcinoma of the prostate. *J Urol* 1992; **148**: 326–329.

39 Optenberg SA & Thompson IM. Economics of screening for carcinoma of the prostate. *Urol Clin North Am* 1990; **17**: 719.

40 Demark-Wahnefried W, Catoe KE, Paskett E, Robertson CN & Rimer BK. Characteristics of men reporting for prostate cancer screening. *Urology* 1993; **42**: 269.

41 Garnick MB. Prostate cancer: screening, diagnosis and management. *Ann Intern Med* 1993; **118**: 804.

*42 Reynolds T. Prostate cancer experts debate screening, treatment at workshop. *J Natl Cancer Inst* 1993; **85**: 1104.

43 Hahn DL & Roberts RG. PSA screening for asymptomatic prostate cancer. *J Fam Pract* 1993; **37**: 432.

20/Screening for Prostate Cancer – Is it Affordable?

W.B. Peeling, D.E. Neal and R.L. Byrne

Introduction

In the USA several leading personalities who have received treatment for prostate cancer have called for increased use of screening to detect the disease at an early stage. Different pressures exist in the UK where recent media publicity about prostatic disease is creating increasing concern that the National Health Service is not providing a screening service for early prostate cancer which many men (and their wives) regard as a basic right equal to screening of women for breast and cervical cancer. For politicians and health care administrators in all industrial countries a considerable challenge and dilemma is building up about central funding to provide national screening services for prostate cancer, but the central issue is the cost of mass screening. Every step in a screening process costs money which, when considered on a national scale, could exceed the political will of a government administration to give it support. Therefore, it is possible that the cost of mass screening could create a situation whereby epidemiological and clinical arguments about practical and ethical issues of screening would take second place to purely financial decisions about budget priorities. For example, in the UK screening currently costs £300–400 million ($450m–$500m) a year [1] and this allocation of money does not include screening for early prostate cancer. Is it realistic to expect government agencies to shoulder an additional burden of screening for prostate cancer, despite its high profile as a major male malignancy that is predicted to become the commonest male cancer within a few years?

Resource implications of screening for prostate cancer

What are the practical implications of screening for prostate cancer? First, there is identification of the population at risk and its volume. A specific test or group of tests applied to these men would yield either a positive or negative result. It is not yet known whether screen-negative men should be subjected to further testing at intervals, but all screen-positive men would require prostatic biopsy as a mandatory process. If a biopsy is negative, most men would remain under review but those with proven cancer would enter a treatment programme that would depend upon staging and other factors. Any therapy-related complications would need attention and finally the patient would require regular review and follow-up for many years.

Each step in this chain of screening carries a financial implication. To contact men at risk is a complex exercise that requires the cooperation of family practitioners and their staff if a community-based screening programme is being undertaken. Alternatively, contact may come from publicity through media channels. Either system can be time-consuming for staff, with considerable expense required for materials and postage or fees. The choice of screening tests has an important influence on costs. Should screening be by measurement of serum levels of prostate-specific antigen (PSA) alone, by serum PSA with digital rectal examination (DRE), and where does transrectal ultrasound (TRUS) examination of the prostate fit in, if used as a front-line screening test? According to the American Cancer Society National Prostate Cancer Detection Project (ACS-NPCDP):

1   DRE becomes one of the most expensive diagnostic options, especially if carried out by generalists who are not urologically trained.
2   Serum PSA assays are more expensive, with a decision level of 2 ng/ml rather than PSA concentrations of 4 ng/ml.
3   The marginal costs (cost per cancer detection over time) of TRUS either alone or in association with DRE and PSA are unduly high, especially when used for serial testing over 2–3 years [2].

Prostatic biopsy carries costs which include the expense of histological examination of the biopsy specimens.

For screen-positive men there are costs of treatment, whether this is by radical prostatectomy or irradiation, both of which can have complications that may require secondary treatment. There is even a cost implication for management by a surveillance policy, for these men will need regular reviews and will belong to younger age groups who would have an appreciable chance of eventual clinical progression of disease for which irradiation or endocrine treatment would be prescribed, neither of which is inexpensive. Furthermore, some screened men will, after biopsy, carry a diagnosis of prostatic intra-epithelial neoplasia (PIN) and will be entered into a surveillance scheme for detection of delayed cancers (see Chapter 2).

Estimated costs of mass screening

In the USA

Costing the process of screening can, therefore, be complex. In earlier studies of a stand-alone screening programme reported in 1984, it cost $6000 to detect each prostate tumour [3]. However, more recent calculations by Optenberg and Thompson based upon a clinical decision analysis model showed a very different pattern of costs if the whole package of screening and treatment was combined [4]. They calculated that charges for screening American men aged 50–70 years for prostate cancer by TRUS and any treatment that followed would be $23.6 billion in the first year, with charges from DRE totalling $3.8 billion, and charges from serum PSA assay as $27.9 billion when a decision point for biopsy was 4 ng/ml and $11.3 billion when it was 10 ng/ml. The resource implication of a national mass screening programme in the USA based on these estimates would be a shift of annual spending on prostate cancer from 0.06% ($255 million) to over 5% of the total US health care budget.

In the UK

It is obvious that costs of screening and treatment will differ from country to country and it would therefore be necessary for each country to calculate its own cost levels rather than extrapolate data from North America or elsewhere. In fact, apart from the USA, where hospital accountancy has been a major managerial tool for many years, there is little if any guidance from British, European or other experience from which to arrive at a reasonable estimate of mass screening costs for prostate cancer.

However, it is possible to examine on a theoretical basis some of the economic consequences that might follow establishment of a mass screening programme for prostate cancer in a health region of 8 000 000 people in the UK. There would be about 800 000 men aged between 50 and 68 years in that region who would be considered for screening. The costs for identification, contact and appointments for DRE and blood testing and examination of such a volume of men would be considerable. Of these, it is likely that 120 000 men could have prostate cancer (15% of men aged 50–68 years) and, if all men agreed to undergo screening, about 40 000 could be found to have a tumour (assuming detection rate for screening of 5%).

From previous data it is likely that only 70% would agree to screening (560 000 men). The costs of PSA testing alone would be £8 400 000. If 12% of men tested required TRUS and biopsy (67 200 men), the costs of this investigation, excluding staff time and costs of provision of computer facilities, would be £6 720 000. About 28 000 men would be found to have a tumour. As the average in-hospital costs of a radical prostatectomy would be of the order of £4000, treatment of 20 000 men who might request radical prostatectomy would cost £80 000 000. This sum of money is equivalent to the annual running costs of a medium/large hospital in the UK. Furthermore, these operations would be in addition to the routine workload of urological departments of that region and could not be achieved without considerable expansion of staff and in-patient facilities. For instance, assuming that the surgery would be undertaken by urologists who specialize in radical prostatectomy, and that each urologist carries out 10 radical prostatectomies per week for 40 weeks in the year, 50 urologists would be needed to cope with 20 000 radical prostatectomies arising from a mass screening programme in that region. Back-up staff such as consultant anaesthetists, nurses and secretarial/clerical workers would also be needed.

Using this imaginary scenario, the costs for PSA testing, TRUS biopsy and radical prostatectomy would be £95 120 000. These estimates exclude costs of staffing, administration, materials, treatment by other means such as irradiation, treatment of complications from surgery or radiotherapy and follow-up of patients. When these figures are expanded on a national scale to 14 regions, the cost for radical prostatectomy alone would escalate to £832 million and the cost of testing and biopsy with radical prostatectomy would become £1 317 680 000.

Diagnostic patterns of screening

It is likely that most cancers in the population at risk will be exposed during the first diagnostic trawl of a mass screening programme. The investigators of the ACS-NPCDP have data on 1449 men who were examined annually and reported that detection rates declined from 5.4% in the first year to 2.4% in the second year and 1.0% in the third year [5]. Another recent study showed that the incidence of prostate cancers detected in an early detection programme was 3.4% in the first year, but fell to 0.6% in year 2, to 0.7% in year 3 and was only 0.3% in the fourth year [6].

From this information, it is likely that an investment to establish mass screening will need to plan for an initial heavy workload for 1 to 2 years but that this is likely to diminish rapidly with time. Thereafter, the detection rate of early prostate cancer will approach baseline levels, for which a more modest investment will be adequate. This has been the experience of breast cancer screening in the UK.

Future considerations

It is not difficult to adopt a negative approach towards efforts to detect prostate cancer because of the frequent quote: 'more men die with it than from it'. The hard fact is that it is a major killer of men and as such is a major threat to health. Furthermore, while many men suffering from prostate cancer are registered to die from other causes, it is a fact that the quality of life of many of these people and their families is severely reduced by their illness. Surely, the core of scepticism towards screening for prostate cancer originates from the limitations of testing for the disease in its early stages and uncertainty about the best treatment, rather than the need to improve the care of a major malignancy. Nevertheless, while the consensus view at the present time is that there is insufficient evidence of potential benefit to recommend widespread population screening for prostate cancer, few will disagree that randomized trials of screening with control groups should be undertaken to test scientifically the effect of screening on mortality (see Chapter 19). This would give the opportunity to test the cost-effectiveness and cost-benefit of screening alongside clinical benefits. The investigators of the ACS-NPCDP undertook a cost analysis of prostate cancer screening, including dollar value of benefits accrued due to earlier detection and treatment. Calculations were made from future medical savings from treating earlier cancer, lost wages and reduced suffering from prevention of advanced disease and the authors arrived at a sum of $29 443 [7].

Conclusions

From these discussions it seems doubtful whether at the present time society will be able to afford to fund mass screening programmes to detect early prostate cancer unless a massive restructuring of national budgets occurs. The debate to date has centred around the clinical value of screening – will it reduce mortality? Randomized trials of screening and of treatment of screen-positive men should give the answer, but in 10 years or more. These trials must also address the economic aspect to give a value judgement of the affordability of screening – is it affordable even if it proves to be clinically justified?

In the meantime, however, a strong case could be made to establish without further delay screening facilities for men in high-risk groups such as those with family histories of prostate and/or breast cancer, and men of African descent. For lower-risk men in the general population, case-finding may prove to be the best value for money, for which many would be willing to pay a relatively modest fee. Whatever the conclusions of clinical trials to evaluate mass screening may be, it is unlikely that screening for prostate cancer will receive unqualified support until the costs for detection become equivalent to the costs of the mammogram and the costs of management of screen-positive men are within the budget of a district hospital. Nevertheless, economic arguments that appear at the present time to render screening for prostate cancer unrealistic and unaffordable should not prevent randomized screening trials from taking place because a proper scientific evaluation of the effectiveness of screening is needed anyway, and it is possible that future developments could discover more effective but less expensive tests and treatments for early prostate cancer, from which there could be both clinical and economic benefits. It is unlikely that public pressure for screening will go away.

References

1 Smith R. British government revamps screening policy. *Br Med J* 1994; **308**: 357–358.
2 Littrup PJ. Prostate cancer screening. Appropriate choices? *Cancer* 1994; **74**: 2016–2022.
3 Chodak GW & Schoenberg HW. Early detection of prostate cancer by routine screening *JAMA* 1984; **252**: 3261–3264.
* 4 Optenberg SA & Thompson IM. Economics of screening for carcinoma of the prostate. *Urol Clin North Am* 1990; **17**: 719–737.
5 Mettlin C. Early detection of prostate cancer following repeated examinations by multiple modalities: results of the American Cancer Society national prostate cancer detection project. *Clin Invest Med* 1993; **16**: 440–447.
6 Labrie F, Dupont A, Suburu R *et al.* Optimized strategy for detection of early stage curable prostate cancer: role of prescreening with prostate-specific antigen. *Clin Invest Med* 1993; **16**: 425–439.
* 7 Littrup PJ, Goodman AC, Mettlin CJ & Murphy GP. Cost analysis of prostate cancer screening. Frameworks for discussion. *J Urol* 1994; **152**: 1865.

* Reference of special interest.

Index

Index

Index